# THE DASH DIET
## Cookbook 2021

## 500 EASY AND DELICIOUS RECIPES TO NATURALLY LOWER BLOOD PRESSURE AND PROMOTE OVERALL HEALTH AND WELLNESS

*Gwenda Smith*

# TABLE OF CONTENTS

# INTRODUCTION

In the mid-1990s, dietary approaches to stop hypertension (DASH) was designed to lower blood pressure through a healthy diet, not a drug. Scientists have been studying the effect of diet on blood pressure for some time. The time has come to put this knowledge into practice. The researchers also observed that diets rich in calcium and potassium and, to a lesser extent, magnesium had helped lower blood pressure. Logically, it seemed that taking these dietary supplements would lower blood pressure.

Much research has been done, but unfortunately, most showed little or no benefit from calcium, potassium, or magnesium supplements, so the approach went back to the diet. As we have seen, it has been observed that, in general, vegetarians living in the United States had lower blood pressure and lower heart disease mortality rates than people who consumed a more traditional western diet. But few Americans would be willing to give up meat, even if it meant reducing the risk of a heart attack.

Frustrated by the inability of supplements to provide an easy solution for hypertension, the researchers decided to create a diet rich in foods that contain these nutrients. The menu was rich in plant foods such as fruits, vegetables, beans, nuts, seeds, mainly whole grains, and heart-healthy oils. Low-fat dairy products were an essential part of the diet, as were limited quantities of lean meat, poultry, and fish. It was based on the knowledge acquired in vegetarian diets. The first research on the DASH diet was published in 1997. It is a study that aimed to evaluate the effect of the dietary pattern on blood pressure, and it did it very effectively.

The DASH diet reduced blood pressure and first-line medications in just fourteen days. Surprisingly, the rise in blood pressure occurred even though researchers did not allow participants to lose weight. It contained many carbohydrates, mainly to prevent weight loss because if the participants had also lost weight, the researchers would not have known if weight loss or diet would have been helpful. As reported and stated by the New England Journal of

Medicine: "DASH is particularly effective in people with hypertension (variation of SBP and DBP: -10.7- and -4.7-mm Hg, respectively)." 8 In the late 1980s and 1990s, most heart specialists, recommended replacing saturated fat. (SFA) with so-called complex carbohydrates.

Another study (Omni-Heart) was conducted to evaluate whether the results of measuring blood pressure in the DASH diet would be better if, instead of replacing SFA with carbohydrates (particularly refined), SFAs were replaced with monounsaturated fats (MUFA) or protein. And actually, they have seen better results. 9, 10 both approaches reduced total cholesterol, but MUFA did not increase triglycerides (TG) or "good" cholesterol (HDL). Maintaining a higher HDL value and a lower TG is very beneficial for heart health. It is a vital sign that you are successfully managing or reducing the risk of metabolic syndrome. A particular advantage was that appetite seemed to be much easier to control. Instead of needing drugs with very unwanted side effects, participants can have very positive "side effects." Wouldn't you like to check your blood pressure with food instead of medications? Have you ever heard of the DASH diet before reading this book? Many people don't. So why isn't DASH adoption universal? Why didn't it explode?

Most educational material, including the National Heart, Lung, and Blood Institute (NHLBI), makes monitoring DASH difficult. Based on the complex information in this literature, many doctors believed that it would be tough for patients to follow them, so they did not. Don't even bother to recommend; what a pity! We thought this food model was too important to be a research curiosity. We made this cookbook about the Dash diet to show people how easy it is to take a life formula. And it worked. People have found that they can continue with this and that their health has improved significantly. So, let's follow the latest DASH improvements and include all the recipes here to make it the best plan in the world! And the best flavor!

# CHAPTER 1.
# THE DIETARY APPROACH TO STOP HYPERTENSION (DASH) BASICS

Unlike the regular diets out there, DASH is a tad bit different. It means Dietary Approaches to Stop Hypertension. Yes, you read that right. Finally, a diet that focuses on one of the greatest killers of the 21st century-hypertension. According to recent studies, one out of three adults suffers from hypertension or high blood pressure. It keeps increasing with age, with almost two-thirds of the population suffering from it from the age of 65. High blood pressure is not a single stroke disease- it brings heart trouble, kidney diseases, and even diabetes.

Our sedentary lifestyles, coupled with unhealthy eating habits, have fueled several hypertension-related diseases. Most can be corrected by following a healthy diet, which is what DASH aims at. This diet comprises foods and recipes that promote lower sodium levels and higher potassium, calcium, fiber, and magnesium levels in the body. It also helps lower the overall blood pressure to an optimum level without harming the body processes. When this happens, disorders related to hypertension disappear, such as osteoporosis, diabetes, and kidney failure.

The original diet plan aimed to lower blood pressure through natural foods and without medication aid. It was sponsored and endorsed by the US National Institute of Health. When the trials of the first DASH diet came out, it was found that lowering the blood pressure helped maintain the level even with some excess sodium in the blood. Not only this, but the diet was also found to be beneficial in keeping the extra pounds off and prevent many disorders related to hypertension.

## WHO SHOULD FOLLOW THIS DIET?

Is the diet for me? Or is it only for people with existing hypertension problems? According to the Dietary Guidelines for Americans, the DASH diet is a healthy eating model that anyone can follow. Of course, since the diet's primary objective is to lower blood pressure, people suffering from hypertension become the primary beneficiaries of the diet. But anyone who wishes to get healthy and scientifically lose weight can follow it, children included.

This diet works while other diets fail miserably because the body is kept full with the required nutrition. The fundamental nutrients, such as calcium, magnesium, and potassium, are elevated in the body through a wholesome diet plan, and sodium levels are also kept in control. And it is all done in a controlled, scientific, and disciplined manner without any crashes or spikes in the metabolism, ensuring a healthier you.

## THE IMPROVED DASH DIET PLAN

When research into diet plans for hypertension began, they did not focus too much on weight loss. They were more concerned with getting the blood pressure levels regulated. But soon, the researchers realized that healthy weight loss was the need of the hour, and therefore there were an additional need to create a systematic weight loss plan and reduced blood pressure levels. So, after a lot of deliberation, the DASH diet for weight loss was also formulated, including nuts, cereals, whole fruits and vegetables, and seeds.

Unlike other flyby diets, which are more word of mouth than scientific, the DASH diet is primarily based on scientific principles of good health. The research on DASH diets indicates that it is not merely a tool for reducing your blood pressure by eating a low sodium diet. The plan is designed for each person, keeping their specific needs in mind, and comprises wholesome foods, such as fruits, vegetables, grains, fresh produce, etc. which keeps the body in fighting fit condition. Top rung research institutes such as the American Heart Association, Dietary Guidelines for Americans, the National Heart, Lung, and Blood Institute- all endorse this diet plan.

Several more corroborating research reports after, the DASH diet was further improved to optimize health and reduce hypertension by increasing the protein intake and cutting down on empty carbs and bad fats. The DASH diet's primary hypothesis is based on sound scientific principles of attainable and sustainable weight loss. The meals and snacks prescribed in the diet plan comprise bulky, fibrous foods, which keep you filled for hours and do not let you snack mindlessly. They are designed to keep your blood sugar levels regulated, instead of the spike and crash cycles, as seen with other diets. By following this diet, you keep your blood sugar levels on an even keel, defeat other diseases like diabetes, reduce your triglycerides, melt your stubborn belly fat, lower your LDL, improve your HDL numbers, and generally feel healthier on average. Of course, a significant portion of the diet is protein-rich, so you build your muscle and lose body fat, and in the process, you avoid slowing your metabolism, which aids in sustaining your current weight.

Even if you're is not suffering from hypertension, you can adopt the DASH diet to keep your internal systems healthy and robust. In this part of your journey, you will learn how you can make this diet work for you.

Rome wasn't built in a day. Similarly, your body will not take too kindly to change if you do it suddenly. It will protest, and you will soon return to square one. To avoid that discomfort, take baby steps. Do not jump into the diet headlong. Try the meal plan for two days a week, then increase it to three times, and when you are comfortable with it, adopt it ultimately. You might already be eating some DASH diet foods and snacks and not be aware of it. Make a list and see which food items correspond to the diet's meal plan. And do not be under the impression that the DASH diet goes for a toss while dining out. There are plenty of options and strategies you can adopt while eating out. You need to be careful and select healthy choices.

## BEGINNING THE DASH DIET

Now that you are supplied with the necessary background information on the DASH diet let us see first what it entails. This meal plan is rich in vegetables, fruits, dairy products, whole grains, lean meats, poultry, fish, and legumes such as peas and beans. Additionally, it contains low fat from natural sources and high fiber from sweet potatoes, cabbage, and leafy vegetables. It adheres to the US guidelines about the sodium and potassium content. It is a flexible eating plan designed to meet the needs of a variety of people and keeps in mind their food preferences. There is a healthy alternative to almost any kind of food craving. It is what a typical DASH diet comprises:

# CHAPTER 2.
# BENEFITS OF DASH DIET

Although you're likely to go for the DASH diet because of a slimmer waist and better health, there are more reasons to consider the DASH diet. They include the following:

## WEIGHT LOSS

DASH advocates for much less fat than you'd find in a typical American diet. It means that it's lower in calories. This diet eliminates and reduces unhealthy fats, fast food, fried foods, as well as foods that are highly processed. Instead, it emphasizes healthy fats like saturated fats and healthy saturated fats like omega 3 fats that are good for your body and help weight loss. These are mostly present in foods with lower calories. The high fiber content in most of the foods recommended under the DASH diet is another great contributor to weight loss because fibers help you have a feeling of satiety while also aiding digestion so your body can eliminate wastes while slowing down the absorption of sugar and fat. It promotes efficient regulation and response to insulin, limiting the risk of and symptoms of metabolic syndrome.

The high absorption or consumption of fresh vegetables and fruits translates to high vitamin c and antioxidants levels. Vitamin C is instrumental in reducing the stress that reduces the amount of stress hormone, cortisol, produced. This hormone is also responsible for the storage of fat in the area around the abdomen. Therefore, what you eat will not be stored as fat in your abdomen. Additionally, vitamin C is a building block of L-carnitine that is instrumental in the transportation of fat. When your body receives a signal or cue that you no longer need the fat, it is turned to glucose for use as energy. The body needs sufficient amounts of vitamin C to make L-carnitine naturally. It means you need to consume vitamin C daily to contribute to weight loss because the primary role of vitamin C is fighting infection and rebuilding damaged cells.

The DASH diet also advocates for caloric intake that differs from one person to another, considering your weight loss goals, current weight, body shape, and activity level. This diet avoids consuming very few calories that eventually puts you at risk of losing lean muscle tissue instead of fat while ensuring you're getting enough nutrients to support your level of activity.

## HEART DISEASE

When you have a combination of high blood pressure, metabolic syndrome, and type 2 diabetes, you're likely to end up with heart disease. The fact that the DASH diet addresses all these conditions means that it can also eliminate your risk of heart disease. This diet is an excellent option even when you're not already experiencing any of these conditions. Heart disease records the most significant number of deaths among Americans. Health professionals recommend a diet low in unhealthy fats and high in healthy fats, and fiber will positively influence your heart health. The American Heart Association recommends DASH because it's a heart-healthy diet. Apart from improved heart health, this diet also reduces the risk of developing kidney stones and improving colon and digestive health.

## METABOLIC SYNDROME

The term metabolic syndrome is used for a group of symptoms associated with insulin and obesity. This syndrome is sometimes known as pre-diabetes because when not checked, it results in type 2 diabetes. Some of the typical metabolic syndrome markers include high blood sugar, large waist size, elevated HDL, and high triglycerides. The DASH diet can eliminate these unwanted symptoms. The DASH diet consists of reduced amounts of bad fats and an increase in the consumption of good fats and fiber, helping lower triglyceride levels and HDL cholesterol. The nutrients you obtain from the DASH diet with the fat loss you experience around the abdomen, account for a significant reduction in metabolic syndrome, helping you experience optimal health.

## TYPE 2 DIABETES

The DASH diet was rated as the best diet or battling Type 2 diabetes and for anyone facing the risk of developing diabetes by the U.S. News and World Report. It has been demonstrated that this diet is capable of lessening the symptoms and the severity of diabetes significantly. In some cases, the dietary change associated with this diet has helped in reversing the condition. The reason behind this is simple. The foods incorporated into the DASH diet help in improving the health of people who have diabetes. For instance, nuts help controlling glucose in people with diabetes. Simultaneously, the high fiber content will slow down the absorption of sugar, which helps prevent blood sugar levels. All the vegetables and fruits in the DASH diet are packed with antioxidants that help prevent and reduce or lower complications related to Type 2 diabetes. The DASH diet can also help reduce type 2 diabetes by promoting weight loss, especially abdominal fat, that triggers insulin insensitivity.

## CONTROLLED BLOOD PRESSURE

It is the main benefit of the DASH diet and the reason why nutritionists and physicians recommend it. Following DASH lets you keep your blood pressure in check. This diet is ideal for anyone who is taking medication to control blood pressure and those with prehypertension symptoms and are looking for better ways of managing these symptoms. DASH is specially designed to help tame blood pressure and has been scientifically proven to work.

## HEALTHY EATING

Let's face it. One of the grounds or reasons why most people experience high blood pressure is that being overweight or obese is associated with poor eating choices. Following the DASH diet helps you make a lifestyle change to healthy eating. Thus, you will be spending more time in the kitchen preparing fresh food instead of grabbing processed food on the go. You will also enjoy your mealtimes because your plate will be filled with more nutritious foods. DASH also stretches you a little to try out new vegetables and fruits and experiment with various seasonings that are salt-free to create meals that you will enjoy.

## REDUCED RISK OF OSTEOPOROSIS

The majority of dietary approaches to preventing and treating osteoporosis include increasing your intake of calcium and vitamin D that is found in abundance in foods recommended for the DASH diet. It, coupled with reduced sodium intake, is proof that the DASH diet is quite beneficial for bone health. Some studies found a notable decline in bone turnover for people who followed the DASH diet. When sustained over a more extended period, the DASH diet is instrumental in improving bone mineral status. Other nutrients in abundance in the DASH diet and are excellent at promoting bone health over time include vitamin C, antioxidants, magnesium, and polyphenols.

## HEALTHY CHOLESTEROL LEVELS

Since most of the fruits, beans, nuts, whole grains, and vegetables recommended under the DASH diet have high fiber content, you can eat them alongside fish and lean meat while limiting or regulating your intake of refined carbohydrates and sweets. It goes a long way in improving your cholesterol levels.

## HEALTHIER KIDNEYS

The DASH diet lowers the risk for kidney stones and kidney disease because of the abundance of magnesium, potassium, calcium, and fiber present in the foods encouraged. The focus on reducing sodium intake is also an advantage if you face developing kidney disease. Even then, the DASH diet should be restricted to patients who have chronic kidney disease and those undergoing dialysis without close guidance of qualified health care professionals.

## DECREASED RISK OF CERTAIN CANCERS

Researchers have studied the relationship between the DASH diet and certain types of cancers and found a positive association that relates to reducing salt intake and monitoring dietary fat consumption. The diet is also low in red meant that it is linked to cancer of the rectum, colon, esophagus, lung, stomach, kidney, and prostate. Eating plenty of fresh produce helps prevent various cancers while emphasizing dairy products that are low in fat contributes to a drop in the risk of colon cancer.

## BETTER MENTAL HEALTH

The DASH diet will boost your mood while decreasing symptoms of mental health disorders like anxiety or depression. It is associated with various lifestyle changes that include avoiding cigarettes, moderating alcohol consumption, and exercising regularly. Moreover, the inclusion of nutrient-rich foods in the diet also helps balance hormones and chemicals in the brain and body, thus contributing to improved mental health and overall well-being.

## ANTI-AGING PROPERTIES

Many people who follow the DASH diet have attested to the fact that this diet helps avoid some effects of aging so that they keep them feeling and looking younger. Increasing your consumption of fresh vegetables and fruits that are full of antioxidants will rejuvenate your hair and skin, revitalize and strengthen your joints, muscles, and bones, help you lose weight, and leave you feeling healthier.

## REDUCED RISK OF DEVELOPING HEART DISEASE

The DASH diet's ability to keep your blood pressure in check is instrumental in strengthening the body's resistance to heart disease. According to a 2010 study, DASH can substantially lower the risk of heart disease. It is particularly remarkable given the persistent and enormous burden of coronary heart disease. It is attributed to the fact that lowered blood pressure lets the heart function efficiently and effectively. Moreover, it can also be beneficial for those who are not struggling with hypertension but are keen on preventing the onset of heart disease.

# CHAPTER 3.
# BREAKFAST

# 1. BLUEBERRY WAFFLES

**COOKING: 15'**  **PREPARATION: 15'**  **SERVINGS: 8**

## INGREDIENTS

- » 2 cups whole wheat flour
- » 1 tablespoon baking powder
- » 1 teaspoon ground cinnamon
- » 2 tablespoons sugar
- » 2 large eggs
- » 3 tablespoons unsalted butter, melted
- » 3 tablespoons nonfat plain Greek yogurt
- » 1½ cups 1% milk
- » 2 teaspoons vanilla extract
- » 4 ounces blueberries
- » Nonstick cooking spray
- » ½ cup maple almond butter

## DIRECTIONS

1. Preheat waffle iron. Mix the flour, baking powder, cinnamon, plus sugar in a large bowl. Mix the eggs, melted butter, yogurt, milk, and vanilla in a small bowl. Combine well.

2. Put the wet fixing to the dry mix and whisk until well combined. Do not over whisk; it's okay if the mixture has some lumps. Fold in the blueberries.

3. Oiled the waffle iron with cooking spray, then cook 1/3 cup of the batter until the waffles are lightly browned and slightly crisp. Repeat with the rest of the batter.

4. Place 2 waffles in each of 4 storage containers. Store the almond butter in 4 condiment cups. To serve, top each warm waffle with 1 tablespoon of maple almond butter.

**NUTRITIONS:** Calories: 647, Fat: 37g, Carbohydrates: 67g, Protein: 22g, Sodium: 156mg

# 2. APPLE PANCAKES

**COOKING: 5'**  **PREPARATION: 15'**  **SERVINGS: 16**

## INGREDIENTS

- » ¼ cup extra-virgin olive oil, divided
- » 1 cup whole wheat flour
- » 2 teaspoons baking powder
- » 1 teaspoon baking soda
- » 1 teaspoon ground cinnamon
- » 1 cup 1% milk
- » 2 large eggs
- » 1 medium Gala apple, diced
- » 2 tablespoons maple syrup
- » ¼ cup chopped walnuts

## DIRECTIONS

1. Set aside 1 teaspoon of oil to use for greasing a griddle or skillet. In a large bowl, stir the flour, baking powder, baking soda, cinnamon, milk, eggs, apple, and the remaining oil.

2. Warm griddle or skillet on medium-high heat and coat with the reserved oil. Working in batches, pour in about ¼ cup of the batter for each pancake. Cook until browned on both sides.

3. Place 4 pancakes into each of 4 medium storage containers and the maple syrup in 4 small containers. Put each serving with 1 tablespoon of walnuts and drizzle with ½ tablespoon of maple syrup.

**NUTRITIONS:** Calories: 378, Fat: 22g, Carbohydrates: 39g, Protein: 10g, Sodium: 65mg

# 3. SUPER-SIMPLE GRANOLA

**COOKING: 25'**     **PREPARATION: 15'**     **SERVINGS: 8**

## INGREDIENTS

- » ¼ cup extra-virgin olive oil
- » ¼ cup honey
- » ½ teaspoon ground cinnamon
- » ½ teaspoon vanilla extract
- » ¼ teaspoon salt
- » 2 cups rolled oats
- » ½ cup chopped walnuts
- » ½ cup slivered almonds

## DIRECTIONS

1. Preheat the oven to 350°F. Mix the oil, honey, cinnamon, vanilla, and salt in a large bowl. Add the oats, walnuts, and almonds. Stir to coat. Put the batter out onto the prepared sheet pan. Bake for 20 minutes. Let cool.

**NUTRITIONS:** Calories: 254, Fat: 16g, Carbohydrates: 25g, Fiber: 3.5g, Protein: 5g, Potassium: 163mg, Sodium: 73mg

# 4. SAVORY YOGURT BOWLS

**COOKING: 0'**     **PREPARATION: 15'**     **SERVINGS: 4**

## INGREDIENTS

- » 1 medium cucumber, diced
- » ½ cup pitted Kalamata olives, halved
- » 2 tablespoons fresh lemon juice
- » 1 tablespoon extra-virgin olive oil
- » 1 teaspoon dried oregano
- » ¼ teaspoon freshly ground black pepper
- » 2 cups nonfat plain Greek yogurt
- » ½ cup slivered almonds

## DIRECTIONS

1. In a small bowl, mix the cucumber, olives, lemon juice, oil, oregano, and pepper. Divide the yogurt evenly among 4 storage containers. Top with the cucumber-olive mix and almonds.

**NUTRITIONS:** Calories: 240, Fat: 16g, Carbohydrates: 10g, Protein: 16g, Potassium: 353mg, Sodium: 350mg

# 5. ENERGY SUNRISE MUFFINS

**COOKING: 25'**        **PREPARATION: 15'**        **SERVINGS: 16**

## INGREDIENTS

» Nonstick cooking spray
» 2 cups whole wheat flour
» 2 teaspoons baking soda
» 2 teaspoons ground cinnamon
» 1 teaspoon ground ginger
» ¼ teaspoon salt
» 3 large eggs
» ½ cup packed brown sugar
» 1/3 cup unsweetened applesauce
» ¼ cup honey
» ¼ cup vegetable or canola oil
» 1 teaspoon grated orange zest
» Juice of 1 medium orange
» 2 teaspoons vanilla extract
» 2 cups shredded carrots
» 1 large apple, peeled and grated
» ½ cup golden raisins
» ½ cup chopped pecans
» ½ cup unsweetened coconut flakes

**NUTRITIONS:** Calories: 292, Fat: 14g,
Carbohydrates: 42g, Protein: 5g, Sodium: 84mg

## DIRECTIONS

1. If you can fit two 12-cup muffin tins side by side in your oven, then leave a rack in the middle, then preheat the oven to 350°F.

2. Coat 16 cups of the muffin tins with cooking spray or line with paper liners. Mix the flour, baking soda, cinnamon, ginger, and salt in a large bowl. Set aside.

3. Mix the eggs, brown sugar, applesauce, honey, oil, orange zest, orange juice, and vanilla until combined in a medium bowl. Add the carrots and apple and whisk again.

4. Mix the dry and wet ingredients with a spatula. Fold in the raisins, pecans, and coconut. Mix everything once again, just until well combined. Put the batter into the prepared muffin cups, filling them to the top.

5. Bake within 20 to 25 minutes, or until a wooden toothpick inserted into the middle of the center muffin comes out clean (switching racks halfway through if baking on 2 racks). Cool for 5 minutes in the tins, then transfers to a wire rack to cool for an additional 5 minutes. Cool completely before storing in containers.

# 6. SPINACH, EGG, AND CHEESE BREAKFAST QUESADILLAS

**COOKING: 15'**        **PREPARATION: 15'**        **SERVINGS: 4**

## INGREDIENTS

» 1½ tablespoons extra-virgin olive oil
» ½ medium onion, diced
» 1 medium red bell pepper, diced
» 4 large eggs
» 1/8 teaspoon salt
» 1/8 teaspoon freshly ground black pepper
» 4 cups baby spinach
» ½ cup crumbled feta cheese
» Nonstick cooking spray
» 4 (6-inch) whole-wheat tortillas, divided
» 1 cup shredded part-skim low-moisture mozzarella cheese, divided

**NUTRITIONS:** Calories: 453, Fat: 28g,
Carbohydrates: 28g, Fiber: 4.5g, Protein: 23g,
Potassium: 205mg, Sodium: 837mg

## DIRECTIONS

1. Warm-up oil over medium heat in a large skillet. Add the onion and bell pepper and sauté for about 5 minutes, or until soft.

2. Mix the eggs, salt, and black pepper in a medium bowl. Stir in the spinach and feta cheese. Put the egg batter in the skillet and scramble for about 2 minutes, or until the eggs are cooked. Remove from the heat.

3. Coat a clean skillet with cooking spray and add 2 tortillas. Place one-quarter of the spinach-egg mixture on one side of each tortilla. Sprinkle each with ¼ cup of mozzarella cheese. Fold the other halves of the tortillas down to close the quesadillas and brown for about 1 minute.

4. Turnover and cook again in a minute on the other side. Repeat with the remaining 2 tortillas and ½ cup of mozzarella cheese. Cut each quesadilla in half or wedges. Divide among 4 storage containers or reusable bags.

# 7. SIMPLE CHEESE AND BROCCOLI OMELETS

## COOKING: 10'       PREPARATION: 15'       SERVINGS: 4

## INGREDIENTS

- » 3 tablespoons extra-virgin olive oil, divided
- » 2 cups chopped broccoli
- » 8 large eggs
- » ¼ cup 1% milk
- » ½ teaspoon freshly ground black pepper
- » 8 tablespoons shredded reduced-fat Monterey Jack cheese, divided

## DIRECTIONS

1. In a nonstick skillet, heat 1 tablespoon of oil over medium-high heat. Add the broccoli and sauté, occasionally stirring, for 3 to 5 minutes, or until the broccoli turns bright green. Scrape into a bowl.

2. Mix the eggs, milk, plus pepper in a small bowl. Wipe out the skillet and heat ½ tablespoon of oil. Add one-quarter of the egg mixture and tilt the skillet to ensure an even layer. Cook for 2 minutes and then add 2 tablespoons of cheese and one-quarter of the broccoli. Use a spatula to fold into an omelet.

3. Repeat step 3 with the remaining 1½ tablespoons of oil, remaining egg mixture, 6 tablespoons of cheese, and remaining broccoli to make a total of 4 omelets. Divide into 4 storage containers.

**NUTRITIONS:** Calories: 292, Fat: 23g, Carbohydrates: 4g, Fiber: 1g, Protein: 18g, Potassium: 308mg, Sodium: 282mg

# 8. CREAMY AVOCADO AND EGG SALAD SANDWICHES

## COOKING: 0'       PREPARATION: 15'       SERVINGS: 4

## INGREDIENTS

- » 2 small avocados, halved and pitted
- » 2 tablespoons nonfat plain Greek yogurt
- » Juice of 1 large lemon
- » ¼ teaspoon salt
- » ½ teaspoon freshly ground black pepper
- » 8 large eggs, hardboiled, peeled, and chopped
- » 3 tablespoons finely chopped fresh dill
- » 3 tablespoons finely chopped fresh parsley
- » 8 whole wheat bread slices (or your choice)

## DIRECTIONS

1. Scoop the avocados into a large bowl and mash. Mix in the yogurt, lemon juice, salt, and pepper. Add the eggs, dill, and parsley and combine.

2. Store the bread and salad separately in 4 reusable storage bags and 4 containers and assemble the night before or serving. To serve, divide the mixture evenly among 4 of the bread slices and top with the other slices to make sandwiches.

**NUTRITIONS:** Calories: 488, Fat: 22g, Carbohydrates: 48g, Fiber: 8g, Protein: 23g, Potassium: 469mg, Sodium: 597mg

# 9. BREAKFAST HASH

**COOKING: 25'**     **PREPARATION: 15'**     **SERVINGS: 4**

## INGREDIENTS

» Nonstick cooking spray
» 2 large sweet potatoes, ½-inch cubes
» 1 scallion, finely chopped
» ¼ teaspoon salt
» ½ teaspoon freshly ground black pepper
» 8 ounces extra-lean ground beef (96% or leaner)
» 1 medium onion, diced
» 2 garlic cloves, minced
» 1 red bell pepper, diced
» ¼ teaspoon ground cumin
» ¼ teaspoon paprika
» 2 cups coarsely chopped kale leaves
» ¾ cup shredded reduced-fat Cheddar cheese
» 4 large eggs

## DIRECTIONS

1. Oiled a large skillet with cooking spray and heat over medium heat. Add the sweet potatoes, scallion, salt, and pepper. Sauté for 10 minutes, stirring often.

2. Add the beef, onion, garlic, bell pepper, cumin, and paprika. Sauté, frequently stirring, for about 4 minutes, or until the meat browns. Add the kale to the skillet and stir until wilted. Sprinkle with the Cheddar cheese.

3. Make four wells in the hash batter and crack an egg into each. Cover and let the eggs cook until the white is fully cooked and the yolk is to your liking. Divide into 4 storage containers.

**NUTRITIONS:** Calories: 323, Fat: 15g, Carbohydrates: 23g, Fiber: 4g, Protein: 25g, Potassium: 676mg, Sodium: 587mg

# 10. HEARTY BREAKFAST CASSEROLE

**COOKING: 30'**     **PREPARATION: 15'**     **SERVINGS: 4**

## INGREDIENTS

» ¼ cup extra-virgin olive oil, divided
» 1 cup whole wheat flour
» 2 teaspoons baking powder
» 1 teaspoon baking soda
» 1 teaspoon ground cinnamon
» 1 cup 1% milk
» 2 large eggs
» 1 medium Gala apple, diced
» 2 tablespoons maple syrup
» ¼ cup chopped walnuts

## DIRECTIONS

1. Preheat the oven to 350°F. Oiled at a 9-by-13-inch baking dish with cooking spray. Coat a large skillet with cooking spray and heat over medium heat. Add the bell pepper, mushrooms, onion, garlic, and sweet potato.

2. Sauté, frequently stirring, for 3 to 4 minutes, or until the onion is translucent. Add the spinach and continue to sauté while stirring, until the spinach has wilted. Remove, then set aside to cool slightly.

3. Mix the eggs, milk, mustard powder, paprika, black pepper, and salt in a large bowl. Add the sautéed vegetables. Put the batter into the prepared baking dish.

4. Bake for 30 minutes. Remove from the oven, sprinkle with the Colby-Jack cheese, return to the oven, and bake again within 5 minutes to melt the cheese. Divide into 4 storage containers.

**NUTRITIONS:** Calories: 378, Fat: 25g, Carbohydrates: 17g, Fiber: 3g, Protein: 26g, Potassium: 717mg, Sodium: 658mg

# 11. CREAMY APPLE-AVOCADO SMOOTHIE

**COOKING: 0'**      **PREPARATION: 15'**      **SERVINGS: 2**

## INGREDIENTS

- » ½ medium avocado, peeled and pitted
- » 1 medium apple, chopped
- » 1 cup baby spinach leaves
- » 1 cup nonfat vanilla Greek yogurt
- » ½ to 1 cup of water
- » 1 cup ice
- » Freshly squeezed lemon juice (optional)

## DIRECTIONS

1. Blend all of the fixing using a blender, and blend until smooth and creamy. Put a squeeze of lemon juice on top if desired, and serve immediately.

**NUTRITIONS:** Calories: 200, Fat: 7g, Sodium: 56mg, Potassium: 378mg, Carbohydrates: 27g, Fiber: 5g, Sugars: 20g, Protein: 10g

# 12. STRAWBERRY, ORANGE, AND BEET SMOOTHIE

**COOKING: 0'**      **PREPARATION: 5'**      **SERVINGS: 2**

## INGREDIENTS

- » 1 cup nonfat milk
- » 1 cup of frozen strawberries
- » 1 medium beet, cooked, peeled, and cubed
- » 1 orange, peeled and quartered
- » 1 frozen banana, peeled and chopped
- » 1 cup nonfat vanilla Greek yogurt
- » 1 cup ice

## DIRECTIONS

1. In a blender, combine all of the fixings, and blend until smooth. Serve immediately

**NUTRITIONS:** Calories: 266, Fat: 0g, Cholesterol: 7mg, Sodium: 104mg, Carbohydrates: 51g, Fiber: 6g, Sugars: 34g, Protein: 15g

# 13. BLUEBERRY-VANILLA YOGURT SMOOTHIE

**COOKING: 0'**     **PREPARATION: 5'**     **SERVINGS: 2**

## INGREDIENTS

» 1½ cups frozen blueberries
» 1 cup nonfat vanilla Greek yogurt
» 1 frozen banana, peeled and sliced
» ½ cup nonfat or low-fat milk
» 1 cup ice

## DIRECTIONS

1. In a blender, combine all of the fixing listed, and blend until smooth and creamy. Serve immediately.

**NUTRITIONS:** Calories: 228, Fat: 1g, Sodium: 63mg, Potassium: 470mg, Carbohydrates: 45g, Fiber: 5g, Sugars: 34g, Protein: 12g

# 14. GREEK YOGURT OAT PANCAKES

**COOKING: 10'**     **PREPARATION: 15'**     **SERVINGS: 2**

## INGREDIENTS

» 6 egg whites (or ¾ cup liquid egg whites)
» 1 cup rolled oats
» 1 cup plain nonfat Greek yogurt
» 1 medium banana, peeled and sliced
» 1 teaspoon ground cinnamon
» 1 teaspoon baking powder

## DIRECTIONS

1. Blend all of the listed fixing using a blender. Warm a griddle over medium heat. Spray the skillet with nonstick cooking spray.

2. Put 1/3 cup of the mixture or batter onto the griddle. Allow to cook and flip when bubbles on the top burst, about 5 minutes. Cook again within a minute until golden brown. Repeat with the remaining batter. Divide between two serving plates and enjoy.

**NUTRITIONS:** Calories: 318, Fat: 4g, Sodium: 467mg, Potassium: 634mg, Carbohydrates: 47g, Fiber: 6g, Sugars: 13g, Protein: 28g

# 15. SCRAMBLED EGG AND VEGGIE BREAKFAST QUESADILLAS

**COOKING: 15'**      **PREPARATION: 15'**      **SERVINGS: 2**

## INGREDIENTS

- » 2 eggs
- » 2 egg whites
- » 2 to 4 tablespoons nonfat or low-fat milk
- » ¼ teaspoon freshly ground black pepper
- » 1 large tomato, chopped
- » 2 tablespoons chopped cilantro
- » ½ cup canned black beans, rinsed and drained
- » 1½ tablespoons olive oil, divided
- » 4 corn tortillas
- » ½ avocado, peeled, pitted, and thinly sliced

## DIRECTIONS

1. Mix the eggs, egg whites, milk, and black pepper in a bowl. Using an electric mixer, beat until smooth. To the same bowl, add the tomato, cilantro, and black beans, and fold into the eggs with a spoon.

2. Warm-up half of the olive oil in a medium pan over medium heat. Add the scrambled egg mixture and cook for a few minutes, stirring, until cooked through. Remove from the pan.

3. Divide the scrambled-egg mixture between the tortillas, layering only on one half of the tortilla. Top with avocado slices and fold the tortillas in half.

4. Heat the remaining oil over medium heat, and add one of the folded tortillas to the pan. Cook within 1 to 2 minutes on each side or until browned. Repeat with remaining tortillas. Serve immediately.

**NUTRITIONS:** Calories: 445, Fat: 24g, Sodium: 228mg, Potassium: 614mg, Carbohydrates: 42g, Fiber: 11g, Sugars: 2g, Protein: 19g

# 16. STUFFED BREAKFAST PEPPERS

**COOKING: 45'**      **PREPARATION: 15'**      **SERVINGS: 4**

## INGREDIENTS

- » 4 bell peppers (any color)
- » 1 (16-ounce) bag frozen spinach
- » 4 eggs
- » ¼ cup shredded low-fat cheese (optional)
- » Freshly ground black pepper

## DIRECTIONS

1. Preheat the oven to 400°F. Line a baking dish with aluminum foil. Cut the tops off the pepper, then discard the seeds. Discard the tops and seeds. Put the peppers in the baking dish, and bake for about 15 minutes.

2. While the peppers bake, defrost the spinach and drain off the excess moisture. Remove the peppers, then stuff the bottoms evenly with the defrosted spinach.

3. Crack an egg over the spinach inside each pepper. Top each egg with a tablespoon of the cheese (if using) and season with black pepper to taste. Bake within 15 to 20 minutes, or until the egg whites are set and opaque.

**NUTRITIONS:** Calories: 136, Fat: 5g, Sodium: 131mg, Potassium: 576mg, Carbohydrates: 15g, Protein: 11g

# 17. SWEET POTATO TOAST THREE WAYS

**COOKING: 25'**     **PREPARATION: 15'**     **SERVINGS: 1**

## INGREDIENTS

- » 1 large sweet potato, unpeeled
- » Topping Choice #1:
- » 4 tablespoons peanut butter
- » 1 ripe banana, sliced
- » Dash ground cinnamon
- » Topping Choice #2:
- » ½ avocado, peeled, pitted, and mashed
- » 2 eggs (1 per slice)
- » Topping Choice #3:
- » 4 tablespoons nonfat or low-fat ricotta cheese
- » 1 tomato, sliced
- » Dash black pepper

## DIRECTIONS

1. Slice the sweet potato lengthwise into ¼-inch thick slices. Place the sweet potato slices in a toaster on high for about 5 minutes or until cooked through.

2. Repeat multiple times, if necessary, depending on your toaster settings. Top with your desired topping choices and enjoy.

**NUTRITIONS:** Calories: 137, Fat: 0g, Sodium: 17mg, Potassium: 265mg, Carbohydrates: 32g, Fiber: 4g, Sugars: 0g, Protein: 2g

# 18. APPLE-APRICOT BROWN RICE BREAKFAST PORRIDGE

**COOKING: 8'**     **PREPARATION: 15'**     **SERVINGS: 4**

## INGREDIENTS

- » 3 cups cooked brown rice
- » 1¾ cups nonfat or low-fat milk
- » 2 tablespoons lightly packed brown sugar
- » 4 dried apricots, chopped
- » 1 medium apple, cored and diced
- » ¾ teaspoon ground cinnamon
- » ¾ teaspoon vanilla extract

## DIRECTIONS

1. Combine the rice, milk, sugar, apricots, apple, and cinnamon in a medium saucepan. Boil it on medium heat, lower the heat down slightly and cook within 2 to 3 minutes. Turn it off, then stir in the vanilla extract. Serve warm.

**NUTRITIONS:** Calories: 260, Fat: 2g, Sodium: 50mg, Potassium: 421mg, Carbohydrates: 57g, Fiber: 4g, Sugars: 22g, Protein: 7g

# 19. CARROT CAKE OVERNIGHT OATS

**COOKING: 25'**     **PREPARATION: 15'**     **SERVINGS: 8**

## INGREDIENTS

- » ¼ cup extra-virgin olive oil
- » ¼ cup honey
- » ½ teaspoon ground cinnamon
- » ½ teaspoon vanilla extract
- » ¼ teaspoon salt
- » 2 cups rolled oats
- » ½ cup chopped walnuts
- » ½ cup slivered almonds

## DIRECTIONS

1. Preheat the oven to 350°F. Mix the oil, honey, cinnamon, vanilla, and salt in a large bowl. Add the oats, walnuts, and almonds. Stir to coat. Put the batter out onto the prepared sheet pan. Bake for 20 minutes. Let cool.

**NUTRITIONS:** Calories: 254, Fat: 16g, Carbohydrates: 25g, Fiber: 3.5g, Protein: 5g, Potassium: 163mg, Sodium: 73mg

# 20. STEEL-CUT OATMEAL WITH PLUMS AND PEAR

**COOKING: 25'** | **PREPARATION: 15'** | **SERVINGS: 4**

## INGREDIENTS

- » 2 cups of water
- » 1 cup nonfat or low-fat milk
- » 1 cup steel-cut oats
- » 1 cup dried plums, chopped
- » 1 medium pear, cored, and skin removed, diced
- » 4 tablespoons almonds, roughly chopped

## DIRECTIONS

1. Mix the water, milk, plus oats in a medium pot and bring to a boil over high heat. Reduce the heat and cover. Simmer for about 10 minutes, stirring occasionally.

2. Add the plums and pear, and cover. Simmer for another 10 minutes. Turn off the heat and let stand within 5 minutes until all of the liquid is absorbed. To serve, top each portion with a sprinkling of almonds.

**NUTRITIONS:** Calories: 307, Fat: 6g, Sodium: 132mg, Potassium: 640mg, Carbohydrates: 58g, Fiber: 9g, Sugars: 24g, Protein: 9g

# 21. FRENCH TOAST WITH APPLESAUCE

**COOKING: 5'** | **PREPARATION: 5'** | **SERVINGS: 6**

## INGREDIENTS

- » ¼ c. unsweetened applesauce
- » ½ c. skim milk
- » 2 packets Stevia
- » 2 eggs
- » 6 slices whole-wheat bread
- » 1 tsp. ground cinnamon

## DIRECTIONS

1. Mix well applesauce, sugar, cinnamon, milk, and eggs in a mixing bowl. Soak the bread into the applesauce mixture until wet. On medium fire, heat a large nonstick skillet.

2. Add soaked bread on one side and another on the other side. Cook in a single layer within 2-3 minutes per side on medium-low fire or until lightly browned. Serve and enjoy.

**NUTRITIONS:** Calories: 122.6, Fat:2.6 g, Carbs:18.3 g, Protein:6.5 g, Sugars:14.8 g, Sodium: 11mg

# 22. BANANA-PEANUT BUTTER AND GREENS SMOOTHIE

**COOKING: 0'**　　　　**PREPARATION: 5'**　　　　**SERVINGS: 1**

## INGREDIENTS

- » 1 c. chopped and packed Romaine lettuce
- » 1 frozen medium banana
- » 1 tbsp. all-natural peanut butter
- » 1 c. cold almond milk

## DIRECTIONS

1. In a heavy-duty blender, add all ingredients. Puree until smooth and creamy. Serve and enjoy.

**NUTRITIONS:** Calories: 349.3, Fat:9.7 g, Carbs:57.4 g, Protein:8.1 g, Sugars:4.3 g, Sodium:18 mg

# 23. BAKING POWDER BISCUITS

**COOKING: 5'**　　　　**PREPARATION: 5'**　　　　**SERVINGS: 1**

## INGREDIENTS

- » 1 egg white
- » 1 c. white whole-wheat flour
- » 4 tbsps. Non-hydrogenated vegetable shortening
- » 1 tbsp. sugar
- » 2/3 c. low-Fat milk
- » 1 c. unbleached all-purpose flour
- » 4 tsp.
- » Sodium-free baking powder

## DIRECTIONS

1. Warm oven to 450°F. Put the flour, sugar, plus baking powder into a mixing bowl and mix. Split the shortening into the batter using your fingers until it resembles coarse crumbs. Put the egg white plus milk and stir to combine.

2. Put the dough out onto a lightly floured surface and knead 1 minute. Roll dough to ¾ inch thickness and cut into 12 rounds. Place rounds on the baking sheet. Bake 10 minutes, then remove the baking sheet and place biscuits on a wire rack to cool.

**NUTRITIONS:** Calories: 118, Fat:4 g, Carbs:16 g, Protein:3 g, Sugars:0.2 g, Sodium: 6 mg

# 24. OATMEAL BANANA PANCAKES WITH WALNUTS

**COOKING: 5'**  **PREPARATION: 15'**  **SERVINGS: 8**

## INGREDIENTS

» 1 finely diced firm banana
» 1 c. whole wheat pancake mix
» 1/8 c. chopped walnuts
» ¼ c. old-fashioned oats

## DIRECTIONS

1. Make the pancake mix, as stated in the directions on the package. Add walnuts, oats, and chopped banana. Coat a griddle with cooking spray. Add about ¼ cup of the pancake batter onto the griddle when hot.

2. Turn pancake over when bubbles form on top. Cook until golden brown. Serve immediately.

**NUTRITIONS:** Calories: 155, Fat:4 g, Carbs:28 g, Protein:7 g, Sugars:2.2 g, Sodium:16 mg

# 25. CREAMY OATS, GREENS & BLUEBERRY SMOOTHIE

**COOKING: 0'**  **PREPARATION: 4'**  **SERVINGS: 1**

## INGREDIENTS

» 1 c. cold
» Fat-free milk
» 1 c. salad greens
» ½ c. fresh frozen blueberries
» ½ c. frozen cooked oatmeal
» 1 tbsp. sunflower seeds

## DIRECTIONS

1. Blend all ingredients using a powerful blender until smooth and creamy. Serve and enjoy.

**NUTRITIONS:** Calories: 280, Fat:6.8 g, Carbs:44.0 g, Protein:14.0 g, Sugars:32 g, Sodium:141 mg

# 26. BANANA & CINNAMON OATMEAL

**COOKING: 0'**      **PREPARATION: 5'**      **SERVINGS: 6**

## INGREDIENTS

» 2 c. quick-cooking oats
» 4 c. Fat-free milk
» 1 tsp. ground cinnamon
» 2 chopped large ripe banana
» 4 tsp. Brown sugar
» Extra ground cinnamon

## DIRECTIONS

1. Place milk in a skillet and bring to boil. Add oats and cook over medium heat until thickened, for two to four minutes.

2. Stir intermittently. Add cinnamon, brown sugar, and banana and stir to combine. If you want, serve with the extra cinnamon and milk.   Enjoy!

**NUTRITIONS:** Calories: 215, Fat:2 g, Carbs:42 g, Protein:10 g, Sugars:1 g, Sodium:40 mg

# 27. BAGELS MADE HEALTHY

**COOKING: 40'**      **PREPARATION: 5'**      **SERVINGS: 8**

## INGREDIENTS

» 1 ½ c. warm water
» 1 ¼ c. bread flour
» 2 tbsps. Honey
» 2 c. whole wheat flour
» 2 tsp. Yeast
» 1 ½ tbsps. Olive oil
» 1 tbsp. vinegar

## DIRECTIONS

1. In a bread machine, mix all ingredients, and then process on dough cycle. Once done, create 8 pieces shaped like a flattened ball. Create a donut shape using your thumb to make a hole at the center of each ball.

2. Place donut-shaped dough on a greased baking sheet then covers and let it rise about ½ hour.   Prepare about 2 inches of water to boil in a large pan.

3. In boiling water, drop one at a time the bagels and boil for 1 minute, then turn them once.   Remove them and return to the baking sheet and bake at 3500F for about 20 to 25 minutes until golden brown.

**NUTRITIONS:** Calories: 228, Fat:3.7 g, Carbs:41.8 g, Protein:6.9 g, Sugars:0 g, Sodium:15 mg

# 28. CEREAL WITH CRANBERRY-ORANGE TWIST

**COOKING: 0'**    **PREPARATION: 5'**    **SERVINGS: 1**

## INGREDIENTS

» ½ c. water
» ½ c. orange juice
» 1/3 c. oat bran
» ¼ c. dried cranberries
» Sugar
» Milk

## DIRECTIONS

1. In a bowl, combine all ingredients. For about 2 minutes, microwave the bowl, then serve with sugar and milk. Enjoy!

**NUTRITIONS:** Calories: 220, Fat:2.4 g, Carbs:43.5 g, Protein:6.2 g, Sugars:8 g, Sodium:1 mg

# 29. NO COOK OVERNIGHT OATS

**COOKING: 0'**    **PREPARATION: 5'**    **SERVINGS: 1**

## INGREDIENTS

» 1 ½ c. low-fat milk
» 5 whole almond pieces
» 1 tsp. chia seeds
» 2 tbsps. Oats
» 1 tsp. sunflower seeds
» 1 tbsp. Craisins

## DIRECTIONS

1. In a jar or mason bottle with a cap, mix all ingredients. Refrigerate overnight. Enjoy for breakfast.

**NUTRITIONS:** Calories: 271, Fat:9.8 g, Carbs:35.4 g, Protein:16.7 g, Sugars:9, Sodium:103 mg

# 30. AVOCADO CUP WITH EGG

**COOKING: 0'**     **PREPARATION: 5'**     **SERVINGS: 4**

## INGREDIENTS

- » 4 tsp. parmesan cheese
- » 1 chopped stalk scallion
- » 4 dashes pepper
- » 4 dashes paprika
- » 2 ripe avocados
- » 4 medium eggs

## DIRECTIONS

1. Preheat oven to 375 0F. Slice avocadoes in half and discard the seed. Slice the rounded portions of the avocado to make it level and sit well on a baking sheet.

2. Place avocadoes on a baking sheet and crack one egg in each hole of the avocado. Season each egg evenly with pepper and paprika. Bake within 25 minutes or until eggs is cooked to your liking. Serve with a sprinkle of parmesan.

**NUTRITIONS:** Calories: 206, Fat:15.4 g, Carbs:11.3 g, Protein:8.5 g, Sugars:0.4 g, Sodium:21 mg

# 31. MEDITERRANEAN TOAST

**COOKING: 0'**     **PREPARATION: 10'**     **SERVINGS: 2**

## INGREDIENTS

- » 1 ½ tsp. reduced-Fat crumbled feta
- » 3 sliced Greek olives
- » ¼ mashed avocado
- » 1 slice good whole wheat bread
- » 1 tbsp. roasted red pepper hummus
- » 3 sliced cherry tomatoes
- » 1 sliced hardboiled egg

## DIRECTIONS

1. First, toast the bread and top it with ¼ mashed avocado and 1 tablespoon hummus. Add the cherry tomatoes, olives, hardboiled egg, and feta. To taste, season with salt and pepper.

**NUTRITIONS:** Calories: 333.7, Fat:17 g, Carbs:33.3 g, Protein:16.3 g, Sugars:1 g, Sodium:19 mg

# 32. INSTANT BANANA OATMEAL

**COOKING: 2'**     **PREPARATION: 1'**     **SERVINGS: 1**

## INGREDIENTS

» 1 mashed ripe banana
» ½ c. water
» ½ c. quick oats

## DIRECTIONS

1. Measure the oats and water into a microwave-safe bowl and stir to combine. Place bowl in microwave and heat on high for 2 minutes. Remove the bowl, then stir in the mashed banana and serve.

**NUTRITIONS:** Calories: 243, Fat:3 g, Carbs:50 g, Protein:6 g, Sugars:20 g, Sodium:30 mg

# 33. ALMOND BUTTER-BANANA SMOOTHIE

**COOKING: 5'**     **PREPARATION: 0'**     **SERVINGS: 1**

## INGREDIENTS

» 1 tbsp. Almond butter
» ½ c. ice cubes
» ½ c. packed spinach
» 1 peeled and a frozen medium banana
» 1 c. Fat-free milk

## DIRECTIONS

1. Blend all the listed fixing above in a powerful blender until smooth and creamy. Serve and enjoy.

**NUTRITIONS:** Calories: 293, Fat:9.8 g, Carbs:42.5 g, Protein:13.5 g, Sugars:12 g, Sodium:40 mg

# 34. BROWN SUGAR CINNAMON OATMEAL

**COOKING: 3'**      **PREPARATION: 1'**      **SERVINGS: 4**

## INGREDIENTS

- » ½ tsp. ground cinnamon
- » 1 ½ tsp pure vanilla extract
- » ¼ c. light brown sugar
- » 2 c. low- Fat milk
- » 1 1/3 c. quick oats

## DIRECTIONS

1. Put the milk plus vanilla into a medium saucepan and boil over medium-high heat.

2. Lower the heat to medium once it boils. Mix in oats, brown sugar, plus cinnamon, and cook, stirring 2–3 minutes. Serve immediately.

**NUTRITIONS:** Calories: 208, Fat:3 g, Carbs:38 g, Protein:8 g, Sugars:15 g, Sodium:33 mg

# 35. BUCKWHEAT PANCAKES WITH VANILLA ALMOND MILK

**COOKING: 10'**      **PREPARATION: 10'**      **SERVINGS: 1**

## INGREDIENTS

- » ½ c. unsweetened vanilla almond milk
- » 2-4 packets natural sweetener
- » 1/8 tsp salt
- » ½ cup buckwheat flour
- » ½ tsp. double-acting baking powder

## DIRECTIONS

1. Prepare a nonstick pancake griddle and spray with the cooking spray, place over medium heat   Whisk the buckwheat flour, salt, baking powder, and stevia in a small bowl and stir in the almond milk after.

2. Onto the pan, scoop a large spoonful of batter, cook until bubbles no longer pop on the surface and the entire surface looks dry and (2-4 minutes). Flip and cook for another 2-4 minutes. Repeat with all the remaining batter.

**NUTRITIONS:** Calories: 240, Fat:4.5 g, Carbs:2 g, Protein:11 g, Sugars:17 g, Sodium:38 mg

# 36. SALMON AND EGG SCRAMBLE

**COOKING: 4'**    **PREPARATION: 15'**    **SERVINGS: 4**

## INGREDIENTS

- » 1 teaspoon of olive oil
- » 3 organic whole eggs
- » 3 tablespoons of water
- » 1 minced garlic
- » 6 Oz. Smoked salmon, sliced
- » 2 avocados, sliced
- » Black pepper to taste
- » 1 green onion, chopped

## DIRECTIONS

1. Warm-up olive oil in a large skillet and sauté onion in it. Take a medium bowl and whisk eggs in it, add water and make a scramble with the help of a fork. Add to the skillet the smoked salmon along with garlic and black pepper.

2. Stir for about 4 minutes until all ingredients get fluffy. At this stage, add the egg mixture. Once the eggs get firm, serve on a plate with a garnish of avocados.

**NUTRITIONS:** Calories: 120, Carbs: 3g, Fat: 4g, Protein: 19g, Sodium: 898 mg, Potassium: 129mg

# 37. PUMPKIN MUFFINS

**COOKING: 20'**    **PREPARATION: 15'**    **SERVINGS: 4**

## INGREDIENTS

- » 4 cups of almond flour
- » 2 cups of pumpkin, cooked and pureed
- » 2 large whole organic eggs
- » 3 teaspoons of baking powder
- » 2 teaspoons of ground cinnamon
- » 1/2 cup raw honey
- » 4 teaspoons almond butter

## DIRECTIONS

1. Preheat the oven at 400-degree F. Line the muffin paper on the muffin tray. Mix almond flour, pumpkin puree, eggs, baking powder, cinnamon, almond butter, and honey in a large bowl.

2. Put the prepared batter into a muffin tray and bake within 20 minutes. Once golden-brown, serve, and enjoy.

**NUTRITIONS:** Calories: 136, Carbs: 22g, Fat: 5g, Protein: 2g, Sodium: 11 mg, Potassium: 699 mg

# 38. SWEET BERRIES PANCAKE

**COOKING: 15'**     **PREPARATION: 15'**     **SERVINGS: 4**

## INGREDIENTS

- » 4 cups of almond flour
- » Pinch of sea salt
- » 2 organic eggs
- » 4 teaspoons of walnut oil
- » 1 cup of strawberries, mashed
- » 1 cup of blueberries, mashed
- » 1 teaspoon baking powder
- » Honey for topping, optional

## DIRECTIONS

1. Take a bowl and add almond flour, baking powder, and sea salt. Take another bowl and add eggs, walnut oil, strawberries, and blueberries mash. Combine ingredients of both bowls.

2. Heat a bit of walnut oil in a cooking pan and pour the spoonful mixture to make pancakes. Once the bubble comes on the top, flip the pancake to cook from the other side. Once done, serve with the glaze of honey on top.

**NUTRITIONS:** Calories: 161, Carbs: 23g, Fat: 6g, Protein: 3g, Cholesterol: 82 mg, Sodium: 91 mg, Potassium: 252mg

# 39. ZUCCHINI PANCAKES

**COOKING: 10'**     **PREPARATION: 15'**     **SERVINGS: 4**

## INGREDIENTS

- » 4 large zucchinis
- » 4 green onions, diced
- » 1/3 cup of milk
- » 1 organic egg
- » Sea Salt, just a pinch
- » Black pepper, grated
- » 2 tablespoons of olive oil

## DIRECTIONS

1. First, wash the zucchinis and grate it with a cheese grater. Mix the egg and add in the grated zucchinis and milk in a large bowl. Warm oil in a skillet and sauté onions in it.

2. Put the egg batter into the skillet and make pancakes. Once cooked from both sides. Serve by sprinkling salt and pepper on top.

**NUTRITIONS:** Calories: 70, Carbs: 8g, Fat: 3g, Protein: 2g, Cholesterol: 43 mg, Sodium: 60 mg, Potassium: 914mg

# 40. BREAKFAST BANANA SPLIT

**COOKING: 0'**       **PREPARATION: 15'**       **SERVINGS: 3**

## INGREDIENTS

- » 2 bananas, peeled
- » 1 cup oats, cooked
- » 1/2 cup low-fat strawberry yogurt
- » 1/3 teaspoon honey, optional
- » 1/2 cup pineapple, chunks

## DIRECTIONS

1. Peel the bananas and cut lengthwise. Place half of the banana in each separate bowl. Spoon strawberry yogurt on top and pour cooked oats with pineapple chunks on each banana. Serve immediately with a glaze of honey of liked.

**NUTRITIONS:** Calories: 145, Carbs: 18g, Fat: 7g, Protein: 3g, Sodium:2 mg, Potassium: 380 mg

# 41. EASY VEGGIE MUFFINS

**COOKING: 40'**       **PREPARATION: 10'**       **SERVINGS: 4**

## INGREDIENTS

- » ¾ cup cheddar cheese, shredded
- » 1 cup green onion, chopped
- » 1 cup tomatoes, chopped
- » 1 cup broccoli, chopped
- » 2 cups non-fat milk
- » 1 cup biscuit mix
- » 4 eggs
- » Cooking spray
- » 1 teaspoon Italian seasoning
- » A pinch of black pepper

## DIRECTIONS

1. Grease a muffin tray with cooking spray and divide broccoli, tomatoes, cheese, and onions in each muffin cup.

2. In a bowl, combine green onions with milk, biscuit mix, eggs, pepper, and Italian seasoning, whisk well and pour into the muffin tray as well.

3. Cook the muffins in the oven at 375 degrees F for 40 minutes, divide them between plates, and serve.

**NUTRITIONS:** Calories: 80, Carbs: 3g, Fat: 5g, Protein: 7g, Sodium: 25 mg

# 42. CARROT MUFFINS

**COOKING: 30'**     **PREPARATION: 10'**     **SERVINGS: 5**

## INGREDIENTS

- » 1 and ½ cups whole wheat flour
- » ½ cup stevia
- » 1 teaspoon baking powder
- » ½ teaspoon cinnamon powder
- » ½ teaspoon baking soda
- » ¼ cup natural apple juice
- » ¼ cup olive oil
- » 1 egg
- » 1 cup fresh cranberries
- » 2 carrots, grated
- » 2 teaspoons ginger, grated
- » ¼ cup pecans, chopped
- » Cooking spray

## DIRECTIONS

1. Mix the flour with the stevia, baking powder, cinnamon, and baking soda in a large bowl. Add apple juice, oil, egg, cranberries, carrots, ginger, and pecans and stir well.

2. Oiled a muffin tray with cooking spray, divide the muffin mix, put in the oven, and cook at 375 degrees F within 30 minutes. Divide the muffins between plates and serve for breakfast.

**NUTRITIONS:** Calories: 34, Carbs: 6g, Fat: 1g, Protein: 0g, Sodium: 52 mg

# 43. PINEAPPLE OATMEAL

**COOKING: 25'**     **PREPARATION: 10'**     **SERVINGS: 4**

## INGREDIENTS

- » 2 cups old-fashioned oats
- » 1 cup walnuts, chopped
- » 2 cups pineapple, cubed
- » 1 tablespoon ginger, grated
- » 2 cups non-fat milk
- » 2 eggs
- » 2 tablespoons stevia
- » 2 teaspoons vanilla extract

## DIRECTIONS

1. In a bowl, combine the oats with the pineapple, walnuts, and ginger, stir and divide into 4 ramekins. Mix the milk with the eggs, stevia, and vanilla in a bowl and pour over the oats mix. Bake at 400 degrees F within 25 minutes. 4. Serve for breakfast.

**NUTRITIONS:** Calories: 200, Carbs: 40g, Fat: 1g, Protein: 3g, Sodium: 275 mg

# 44. SPINACH MUFFINS

**COOKING: 30'**          **PREPARATION: 10'**          **SERVINGS: 6**

## INGREDIENTS

- » 6 eggs
- » ½ cup non-fat milk
- » 1 cup low-fat cheese, crumbled
- » 4 ounces spinach
- » ½ cup roasted red pepper, chopped
- » 2 ounces prosciutto, chopped
- » Cooking spray

## DIRECTIONS

1. Mix the eggs with the milk, cheese, spinach, red pepper, and prosciutto in a bowl. Grease a muffin tray with cooking spray, divide the muffin mix, introduce in the oven, and bake at 350 degrees F within 30 minutes. Divide between plates and serve for breakfast.

**NUTRITIONS:** Calories: 112, Carbs: 19g, Fat: 3g, Protein: 2g, Sodium: 274 mg

# 45. CHIA SEEDS BREAKFAST MIX

**COOKING: 0'**          **PREPARATION: 8 H**          **SERVINGS: 4**

## INGREDIENTS

- » 2 cups old-fashioned oats
- » 4 tablespoons chia seeds
- » 4 tablespoons coconut sugar
- » 3 cups of coconut milk
- » 1 teaspoon lemon zest, grated
- » 1 cup blueberries

## DIRECTIONS

1. In a bowl, combine the oats with chia seeds, sugar, milk, lemon zest, and blueberries, stir, divide into cups and keep in the fridge for 8 hours. 2. Serve for breakfast.

**NUTRITIONS:** Calories: 69, Carbs: 0g, Fat: 5g, Protein: 3g, Sodium: 0 mg

# 46. BREAKFAST FRUITS BOWLS

**COOKING: 0'**     **PREPARATION: 10'**     **SERVINGS: 2**

## INGREDIENTS

- » 1 cup mango, chopped
- » 1 banana, sliced
- » 1 cup pineapple, chopped
- » 1 cup almond milk

## DIRECTIONS

1. Mix the mango with the banana, pineapple, and almond milk in a bowl, stir, divide into smaller bowls, and serve.

**NUTRITIONS:** Calories: 10, Carbs: 0g, Fat: 1g, Protein: 0g, Sodium: 0mg

# 47. PUMPKIN COOKIES

**COOKING: 25'**     **PREPARATION: 10'**     **SERVINGS: 6**

## INGREDIENTS

- » 2 cups whole wheat flour
- » 1 cup old-fashioned oats
- » 1 teaspoon baking soda
- » 1 teaspoon pumpkin pie spice
- » 15 ounces pumpkin puree
- » 1 cup coconut oil, melted
- » 1 cup of coconut sugar
- » 1 egg
- » ½ cup pepitas, roasted
- » ½ cup cherries, dried

## DIRECTIONS

1. Mix the flour the oats, baking soda, pumpkin spice, pumpkin puree, oil, sugar, egg, pepitas, and cherries in a bowl, stir well, shape medium cookies out of this mix, arrange them all on a baking sheet, then bake within 25 minutes at 350 degrees F. Serve the cookies for breakfast.

**NUTRITIONS:** Calories: 150, Carbs: 24g, Fat: 8g, Protein: 1g, Sodium: 220 mg

# 48. VEGGIE SCRAMBLE

**COOKING: 2'**          **PREPARATION: 10'**          **SERVINGS: 1**

## INGREDIENTS

- » 1 egg
- » 1 tablespoon water
- » ¼ cup broccoli, chopped
- » ¼ cup mushrooms, chopped
- » A pinch of black pepper
- » 1 tablespoon low-fat mozzarella, shredded
- » 1 tablespoon walnuts, chopped
- » Cooking spray

## DIRECTIONS

1. Grease a ramekin with cooking spray, add the egg, water, pepper, mushrooms, and broccoli, and whisk well. Introduce in the microwave and cook for 2 minutes. Add mozzarella and walnuts on top and serve for breakfast.

**NUTRITIONS:** Calories: 128, Carbs: 24g, Fat: 0g, Protein: 9g, Sodium: 86 mg

# 49. MUSHROOMS AND TURKEY BREAKFAST

**COOKING: 1 H 5'**          **PREPARATION: 10'**          **SERVINGS: 12**

## INGREDIENTS

- » 8 ounces whole-wheat bread, cubed
- » 12 ounces turkey sausage, chopped
- » 2 cups fat-free milk
- » 5 ounces low-fat cheddar, shredded
- » 3 eggs
- » ½ cup green onions, chopped
- » 1 cup mushrooms, chopped
- » ½ teaspoon sweet paprika
- » A pinch of black pepper
- » 2 tablespoons low-fat parmesan, grated

## DIRECTIONS

1. Put the bread cubes on a prepared lined baking sheet, bake at 400 degrees F for 8 minutes. Meanwhile, heat a pan over medium-high heat, add turkey sausage, stir, and brown for 7 minutes.

2. In a bowl, combine the milk with the cheddar, eggs, parmesan, black pepper, and paprika and whisk well.

3. Add mushrooms, sausage, bread cubes, and green onions stir, pour into a baking dish, bake at 350 degrees F within 50 minutes. 5. Slice, divide between plates and serve for breakfast.

**NUTRITIONS:** Calories: 88, Carbs: 1g, Fat: 9g, Protein: 1g, Sodium: 74 mg

# 50. MUSHROOMS AND CHEESE OMELET

**COOKING: 15'**     **PREPARATION: 10'**     **SERVINGS: 4**

## INGREDIENTS

- » 2 tablespoons olive oil
- » A pinch of black pepper
- » 3 ounces mushrooms, sliced
- » 1 cup baby spinach, chopped
- » 3 eggs, whisked
- » 2 tablespoons low-fat cheese, grated
- » 1 small avocado, peeled, pitted, and cubed
- » 1 tablespoons parsley, chopped

## DIRECTIONS

1. Add mushrooms, stir, cook them for 5 minutes and transfer to a bowl on a heated pan with the oil over medium-high heat.

2. Heat-up the same pan over medium-high heat, add eggs and black pepper, spread into the pan, cook within 7 minutes, and transfer to a plate.

3. Spread mushrooms, spinach, avocado, and cheese on half of the omelet, fold the other half over this mix, sprinkle parsley on top, and serve.

**NUTRITIONS:** Calories: 136, Carbs: 5g, Fat: 5g, Protein: 16g, Sodium: 192 mg

# 51. EGG WHITE BREAKFAST MIX

**COOKING: 10'**     **PREPARATION: 10'**     **SERVINGS: 4**

## INGREDIENTS

- » 1 yellow onion, chopped
- » 3 plum tomatoes, chopped
- » 10 ounces spinach, chopped
- » A pinch of black pepper
- » 2 tablespoons water
- » 12 egg whites
- » Cooking spray

## DIRECTIONS

1. Mix the egg whites with water and pepper in a bowl. Grease a pan with cooking spray, heat up over medium heat, add ¼ of the egg whites, spread into the pan, and cook for 2 minutes.

2. Spoon ¼ of the spinach, tomatoes, and onion, fold, and add to a plate. 4. Serve for breakfast. Enjoy!

**NUTRITIONS:** Calories: 31, Carbs: 0g, Fat: 2g, Protein: 3g, Sodium: 55 mg

# 52. PESTO OMELET

**COOKING: 6'**     **PREPARATION: 10'**     **SERVINGS: 2**

## INGREDIENTS

- » 2 teaspoons olive oil
- » Handful cherry tomatoes, chopped
- » 3 tablespoons pistachio pesto
- » A pinch of black pepper
- » 4 eggs

## DIRECTIONS

1. In a bowl, combine the eggs with cherry tomatoes, black pepper, and pistachio pesto and whisk well. Add eggs mix, spread into the pan, cook for 3 minutes, flip, cook for 3 minutes more, divide between 2 plates, and serve on a heated pan with the oil over medium-high heat.

**NUTRITIONS:** Calories: 240, Carbs: 23g, Fat: 9g, Protein: 17g, Sodium: 292 mg

# 53. QUINOA BOWLS

**COOKING: 20'**     **PREPARATION: 10'**     **SERVINGS: 2**

## INGREDIENTS

- » 1 peach, sliced
- » 1/3 cup quinoa, rinsed
- » 2/3 cup low-fat milk
- » ½ teaspoon vanilla extract
- » 2 teaspoons brown sugar
- » 12 raspberries
- » 14 blueberries

## DIRECTIONS

1. Mix the quinoa with the milk, sugar, and vanilla in a small pan, simmer over medium heat, cover the pan, cook for 20 minutes and flip with a fork. Divide this mix into 2 bowls, top each with raspberries and blueberries and serve for breakfast.

**NUTRITIONS:** Calories: 170, Carbs: 31g, Fat: 3g, Protein: 6g, Sodium: 120 mg

# 54. STRAWBERRY SANDWICH

**COOKING: 0'**       **PREPARATION: 10'**       **SERVINGS: 4**

## INGREDIENTS

- » 8 ounces low-fat cream cheese, soft
- » 1 tablespoon stevia
- » 1 teaspoon lemon zest, grated
- » 4 whole-wheat English muffins, toasted
- » 2 cups strawberries, sliced

## DIRECTIONS

1. In your food processor, combine the cream cheese with the stevia and lemon zest and pulse well. Spread 1 tablespoon of this mix on 1 muffin half and top with some of the sliced strawberries. Repeat with the rest of the muffin halves and serve for breakfast. Enjoy!

**NUTRITIONS:** Calories: 150, Carbs: 23g, Fat: 7g, Protein: 2g, Sodium: 70 mg

# 55. APPLE QUINOA MUFFINS

**COOKING: 35'**       **PREPARATION: 10'**       **SERVINGS: 4**

## INGREDIENTS

- » ½ cup natural, unsweetened applesauce
- » 1 cup banana, peeled and mashed
- » 1 cup quinoa
- » 2 and ½ cups old-fashioned oats
- » ½ cup almond milk
- » 2 tablespoons stevia
- » 1 teaspoon vanilla extract
- » 1 cup of water
- » Cooking spray
- » 1 teaspoon cinnamon powder
- » 1 apple, cored, peeled, and chopped

## DIRECTIONS

1. Put the water in a small pan, bring to a simmer over medium heat, add quinoa, cook within 15 minutes, fluff with a fork, and transfer to a bowl.

2. Add all ingredients, stir, divide into a muffin pan greases with cooking spray, introduce in the oven, and bake within 20 minutes at 375 degrees F. Serve for breakfast.

**NUTRITIONS:** Calories: 241, Carbs: 31g, Fat: 11g, Protein: 5g, Sodium: 251 mg

# 56. VERY BERRY MUESLI

**COOKING: 0'**    **PREPARATION: 15'**    **SERVINGS: 2**

## INGREDIENTS

» 1 c. Oats
» 1 c. Fruit flavored Yogurt
» ½ c. Milk
» 1/8 tsp. Salt
» ½ c dried Raisins
» ½ c. Chopped Apple
» ½ c. Frozen Blueberries
» ¼ c. chopped Walnuts

## DIRECTIONS

1. Combine your yogurt, salt, and oats in a medium bowl, mix well, and then cover it tightly. Fridge for at least 6 hours. Add your raisins and apples the gently fold. Top with walnuts and serve. Enjoy!

**NUTRITIONS:** Calories: 195, Protein 6g, Carbs 31g, Fat 4g, Sodium 0mg

# 57. VEGGIE QUICHE MUFFINS

**COOKING: 40'**    **PREPARATION: 15'**    **SERVINGS: 12**

## INGREDIENTS

» ¾ c. shredded Cheddar
» 1 c. chopped Green Onion
» 1 c. chopped Broccoli
» 1 c. diced Tomatoes
» 2 c. Milk
» 4 Eggs
» 1 c. Pancake mix
» 1 tsp. Oregano
» ½ tsp. Salt
» ½ tsp. Pepper

## DIRECTIONS

1. Preheat your oven to 375 0F, and lightly grease a 12-cup muffin tin with oil. Sprinkle your tomatoes, broccoli, onions, and cheddar into your muffin cups.

2. Combine your remaining ingredients in a medium, whisk to combine, then pour evenly on top of your veggies.

3. Set to bake in your preheated oven for about 40 minutes or until golden brown. Allow to cool slightly (about 5 minutes), then serve. Enjoy!

**NUTRITIONS:** Calories: 58.5, Protein 5.1 g, Carbs 2.9 g, Fat 3.2 g, Sodium 340 mg

# 58. TURKEY SAUSAGE AND MUSHROOM STRATA

**COOKING: 8'**　　　　**PREPARATION: 15'**　　　　**SERVINGS: 12**

## INGREDIENTS

- » 8 oz. cubed Ciabatta bread
- » 12 oz. chopped turkey sausage
- » 2 c. Milk
- » 4 oz. shredded Cheddar
- » 3 large Eggs
- » 12 oz. Egg substitute
- » ½ c. chopped Green onion
- » 1 c. diced Mushroom
- » ½ tsp. Paprika
- » ½ tsp. Pepper
- » 2 tbsps. grated Parmesan cheese

## DIRECTIONS

1. Set oven to preheat to 400 0F. Lay your bread cubes flat on a baking tray and set it to toast for about 8 min. Meanwhile, add a skillet over medium heat with sausage and cook while stirring, until fully brown and crumbled.

2. Mix salt, pepper, paprika, parmesan cheese, egg substitute, eggs, cheddar cheese, and milk in a large bowl. Add in your remaining ingredients and toss well to incorporate.

3. Transfer mixture to a large baking dish (preferably a 9x13-inch), then tightly cover and allow to rest in the refrigerator overnight. Set your oven to preheat to 3500F, remove the cover from your casserole, and set to bake until golden brown and cooked through. Slice and serve.

**NUTRITIONS:** Calories: 288.2, Protein 24.3g, Carbs 18.2g, Fat. 12.4g, Sodium 355 mg

# 59. BACON BITS

**COOKING: 60'**　　　　**PREPARATION: 15'**　　　　**SERVINGS: 4**

## INGREDIENTS

- » 1 c. Millet
- » 5 c. Water
- » 1 c. diced Sweet potato
- » 1 tsp. ground Cinnamon
- » 2 tbsps. Brown sugar
- » 1 medium diced Apple
- » ¼ c. Honey

## DIRECTIONS

1. In a deep pot, add your sugar, sweet potato, cinnamon, water, and millet, then stir to combine, then boil on high heat. After that, simmer on low.

2. Cook like this for about an hour, until your water is fully absorbed and millet is cooked. Stir in your remaining ingredients and serve.

**NUTRITIONS:** Calories: 136, Protein 3.1g, Carbs 28.5g, Fat 1.0g, Sodium 120 mg

# 60. STEEL CUT OAT BLUEBERRY PANCAKES

**COOKING: 15'**     **PREPARATION: 15'**     **SERVINGS: 4**

## INGREDIENTS

- » 1½ c. Water
- » ½ c. steel-cut oats
- » 1/8 tsp. Salt
- » 1 c. Whole wheat Flour
- » ½ tsp. Baking powder
- » ½ tsp. Baking soda
- » 1 Egg
- » 1 c. Milk
- » ½ c. Greek yogurt
- » 1 c. Frozen Blueberries
- » ¾ c. Agave Nectar

## DIRECTIONS

1. Combine your oats, salt, and water in a medium saucepan, stir, and allow to come to a boil over high heat. Adjust the heat to low, and allow to simmer for about 10 min, or until oats get tender. Set aside.

2. Combine all your remaining ingredients, except agave nectar, in a medium bowl, then fold in oats. Preheat your skillet, and lightly grease it. Cook ¼ cup of milk batter at a time for about 3 minutes per side. Garnish with Agave Nectar.

**NUTRITIONS:** Calories: 257, Protein 14g, Carbs 46g, Fat 7g, Sodium 123 mg

# 61. SPINACH, MUSHROOM, AND FETA CHEESE SCRAMBLE

**COOKING: 4'**     **PREPARATION: 15'**     **SERVINGS: 1**

## INGREDIENTS

- » Olive oil cooking spray
- » ½ c. sliced Mushroom
- » 1 c. chopped Spinach
- » 3 Eggs
- » 2 tbsps. Feta cheese
- » Pepper

## DIRECTIONS

1. Set a lightly greased, medium skillet over medium heat. Add spinach and mushrooms, and cook until spinach wilts.

2. Combine egg whites, cheese, pepper, and whole egg in a medium bowl, whisk to combine. Pour into your skillet and cook, while stirring, until set (about 4 minutes). Serve.

**NUTRITIONS:** Calories: 236.5, Protein 22.2g, Carbs 12.9g, Fat 11.4g, Sodium 405 mg

# 62. RED VELVET PANCAKES WITH CREAM CHEESE TOPPING

**COOKING: 10'**                 **PREPARATION: 15'**                 **SERVINGS: 2**

## INGREDIENTS

**Cream Cheese Topping:**
» 2 oz. Cream cheese
» 3 tbsps. Yogurt
» 3 tbsps. Honey
» 1 tbsp. Milk

**Pancakes:**
» ½ c. Whole wheat Flour
» ½ c. all-purpose flour
» 2¼tsps. Baking powder
» ½ tsp. Unsweetened Cocoa powder
» ¼ tsp. Salt
» ¼ c. Sugar
» 1 large Egg
» 1 c. + 2 tbsps. Milk
» 1 tsp. Vanilla
» 1 tsp. Red paste food coloring

## DIRECTIONS

1. Combine all your topping ingredients in a medium bowl, and set aside. Add all your pancake ingredients in a large bowl and fold until combined. Set a greased skillet over medium heat to get hot.

2. Add ¼ cup of pancake batter onto the hot skillet and cook until bubbles begin to form on the top. Flip and cook until set. Repeat until your batter is done well. Add your toppings and serve.

**NUTRITIONS:** Calories: 231, Protein 7g, Carbs 43g, Fat 4g, Sodium 0mg

# 63. PEANUT BUTTER & BANANA BREAKFAST SMOOTHIE

**COOKING: 0'**                 **PREPARATION: 15'**                 **SERVINGS: 1**

## INGREDIENTS

» 1 c. Non-fat milk
» 1 tbsp. Peanut butter
» 1 Banana
» ½ tsp. Vanilla

## DIRECTIONS

1. Place non-fat milk, peanut butter, and banana in a blender. Blend until smooth.

**NUTRITIONS:** Calories: 295, Protein 133g, Carbs 42g, Fat 8.4g, Sodium 100 mg

# 64. NO-BAKE BREAKFAST GRANOLA BARS

**COOKING: 0'**          **PREPARATION: 15'**          **SERVINGS: 18**

## INGREDIENTS

- » 2 c. Old fashioned oatmeal
- » ½ c. Raisins
- » ½ c. Brown sugar
- » 2½ c. Corn rice cereal
- » ½ c. Syrup
- » ½ c. Peanut butter
- » ½ tsp. Vanilla

## DIRECTIONS

1. In a suitable size mixing bowl, mix using a wooden spoon, rice cereal, oatmeal, and raisins. In a saucepan, combine corn syrup and brown sugar. On a medium-high flame, continuously stir the mixture and bring to a boil.

2. On boiling, take away from heat. In a saucepan, stir vanilla and peanut into the sugar mixture. Stir until very smooth.

3. Spoon peanut butter mixture on the cereal and raisins into the mixing bowl and combine — shape mixture into a 9 x 13 baking tin. Allow to cool properly, then cut into bars (18 pcs).

**NUTRITIONS:** Calories: 152, Protein 4g, Carbs 26g, Fat 4.3g, Sodium 160 mg

# 65. MUSHROOM SHALLOT FRITTATA

**COOKING: 25'**          **PREPARATION: 15'**          **SERVINGS: 4**

## INGREDIENTS

- » 1 tsp. butter
- » 4 chopped shallots
- » ½ lb. chopped mushrooms
- » 2 tsp. chopped parsley
- » 1 tsp. dried thyme
- » Black pepper
- » 3 medium Eggs
- » 5 large Egg whites
- » 1 tbsp. Milk
- » ¼ c. grated parmesan cheese

## DIRECTIONS

1. Heat oven to 350 0F. In a suitable size oven-proof skillet, heat butter over medium flame. Add shallots and sauté for about 5 mins. or until golden brown. Add to pot, thyme, parsley, chopped mushroom, and black pepper to taste.

2. Whisk milk, egg whites, parmesan, and eggs into a bowl. Pour mixture into the skillet, ensuring the mushroom is covered completely. Transfer the skillet to the oven as soon as the edges begin to set.

3. Bake until frittata is cooked (15-20 mins). Should be served warm, cut into equal wedges (4 pcs).

**NUTRITIONS:** Calories: 346, Protein 19.1g, Carbs 48.3g, Fat 12g, Sodium 218 mg

# 66. JACK-O-LANTERN PANCAKES

**COOKING: 5'**          **PREPARATION: 15'**          **SERVINGS: 8**

## INGREDIENTS

- » 1 Egg
- » ½ c. Canned pumpkin
- » 1¾c. Low-fat milk
- » 2 tbsps. Vegetable oil
- » 2 c. Flour
- » 2 tbsps. Brown sugar
- » 1 tbsp. Baking powder
- » 1 tsp. Pumpkin pie spice
- » 1 tsp. Salt

## DIRECTIONS

1. In a mixing bowl, mix milk, pumpkin, eggs, and oil. Add dry ingredients to egg mixture. Stir gently. Coat skillet lightly with cooking spray and heat on medium.

2. When the skillet is hot, spoon (using a dessert spoon) batter onto the skillet. When bubbles start bursting, flip pancakes over and cook until it's a nice golden-brown color.

**NUTRITIONS:** Calories: 313, Protein 15g, Carbs 28g, Fat 16g, Sodium 1 mg

# 67. FRUIT PIZZA

**COOKING: 0'**          **PREPARATION: 15'**          **SERVINGS: 2**

## INGREDIENTS

- » 1 English muffin
- » 2 tbsps. Fat-free cream cheese
- » 2 tbsps. sliced strawberries
- » 2 tbsps. blueberries
- » 2 tbsps. crushed pineapple

## DIRECTIONS

1. Cut English muffin in half and toast halves until slightly browned. Coat both halves with cream cheese. Arrange fruits atop cream cheese on muffin halves. Serve soon after preparation. Any leftovers refrigerate within 2 hours.

**NUTRITIONS:** Calories: 119, Protein 6g, Carbs 23g, Fat 1g, Sodium 288 mg

# 68. FLAX BANANA YOGURT MUFFINS

**COOKING: 20'**  **PREPARATION: 15'**  **SERVINGS: 12**

## INGREDIENTS

- » 1 c. Whole wheat flour
- » 1 c. Old-fashioned rolled oats
- » 1 tsp. Baking soda
- » 2 tbsps. Ground flaxseed
- » 3 large ripe bananas
- » ½ c. Greek yogurt
- » ¼ c. Unsweetened applesauce
- » ¼ c. Brown sugar
- » 2 tsp. Vanilla extract

## DIRECTIONS

1. Set oven at 355 0F and preheat. Prepare muffin tin, or you can use cooking spray or cupcake liners. Combine dry ingredients in a mixing bowl.

2. In a separate bowl, mix yogurt, banana, sugar, vanilla, and applesauce. Combine both mixtures and mix. Do not over mix. The batter should not be smooth but lumpy. Bake for 20 mins, or when inserted, toothpick comes out clean.

**NUTRITIONS:** Calories: 136, Protein 4g, Carbs 30g, Fat 2g, Sodium 242 mg

# CHAPTER 4.
# LUNCH

# 69. CREAMY CHICKEN BREAST

**COOKING: 20'**  **PREPARATION: 10'**  **SERVINGS: 4**

## INGREDIENTS

»  1 tablespoon olive oil
»  A pinch of black pepper
»  2 pounds chicken breasts, skinless, boneless, and cubed
»  4 garlic cloves, minced
»  2 and ½ cups low-sodium chicken stock
»  2 cups coconut cream
»  ½ cup low-fat parmesan, grated
»  1 tablespoon basil, chopped

## DIRECTIONS

1.  Heat-up a pan with the oil over medium-high heat, add chicken cubes, and brown them for 3 minutes on each side. Add garlic, black pepper, stock, and cream, toss, cover the pan and cook everything for 10 minutes more. Add cheese and basil, toss, divide between plates and serve for lunch. Enjoy!

**NUTRITIONS:** Calories 221, Fat 6g, Fiber 9g, Carbs 14g, Protein 7g, Sodium 197 mg

# 70. INDIAN CHICKEN STEW

**COOKING: 20'**  **PREPARATION: 1 H**  **SERVINGS: 4**

## INGREDIENTS

»  1-pound chicken breasts, skinless, boneless, and cubed
»  1 tablespoon garam masala
»  1 cup fat-free yogurt
»  1 tablespoon lemon juice
»  A pinch of black pepper
»  ¼ teaspoon ginger, ground
»  15 ounces tomato sauce, no-salt-added
»  5 garlic cloves, minced
»  ½ teaspoon sweet paprika

## DIRECTIONS

1.  In a bowl, mix the chicken with garam masala, yogurt, lemon juice, black pepper, ginger, and fridge for 1 hour. Heat-up a pan over medium heat, add chicken mix, toss and cook for 5-6 minutes.

2.  Add tomato sauce, garlic and paprika, toss, cook for 15 minutes, divide between plates and serve for lunch. Enjoy!

**NUTRITIONS:** Calories 221, Fat 6g, Fiber 9g, Carbs 14g, Protein 16g, Sodium 4 mg

# 71. CHICKEN, BAMBOO, AND CHESTNUTS MIX

**COOKING: 20'**   **PREPARATION: 10'**   **SERVINGS: 4**

## INGREDIENTS

» 1-pound chicken thighs, boneless, skinless, and cut into medium chunks
» 1 cup low-sodium chicken stock
» 1 tablespoon olive oil
» 2 tablespoons coconut aminos
» 1-inch ginger, grated
» 1 carrot, sliced
» 2 garlic cloves, minced
» 8 ounces canned bamboo shoots, no-salt-added and drained
» 8 ounces water chestnuts

## DIRECTIONS

1. Heat-up a pan with the oil over medium-high heat, add chicken, stir, and brown for 4 minutes on each side. Add the stock, aminos, ginger, carrot, garlic, bamboo, and chestnuts, toss, cover the pan, and cook everything over medium heat for 12 minutes. Divide everything between plates and serve. Enjoy!

**NUTRITIONS:** Calories 281, Fat 7g, Fiber 9g, Carbs 14g, Protein 14g, Sodium 125mg

# 72. SALSA CHICKEN

**COOKING: 25'**   **PREPARATION:10'**   **SERVINGS: 4**

## INGREDIENTS

» 1 cup mild salsa, no-salt-added
» ½ teaspoon cumin, ground
» Black pepper to the taste
» 1 tablespoon chipotle paste
» 1-pound chicken thighs, skinless and boneless
» 2 cups corn
» Juice of 1 lime
» ½ tablespoon olive oil
» 2 tablespoons cilantro, chopped
» 1 cup cherry tomatoes, halved
» 1 small avocado, pitted, peeled, and cubed

## DIRECTIONS

1. In a pot, combine the salsa with the cumin, black pepper, chipotle paste, chicken thighs, and corn, toss, bring to a simmer and cook over medium heat for 25 minutes. Add lime juice, oil, cherry tomatoes, and avocado, toss, divide into bowls and serve for lunch. Enjoy!

**NUTRITIONS:** Calories 269, Fat 6g, Fiber 9g, Carbs 18g, Protein 7g, Sodium 500 mg

# 73. RICE WITH CHICKEN

**COOKING: 30'**      **PREPARATION: 10'**      **SERVINGS: 4**

## INGREDIENTS

- » ½ cup coconut aminos
- » 1/3 cup rice wine vinegar
- » 2 tablespoons olive oil
- » 1 chicken breast, skinless, boneless, and cubed
- » ½ cup red bell pepper, chopped
- » A pinch of black pepper
- » 2 garlic cloves, minced
- » ½ teaspoon ginger, grated
- » ½ cup carrots, grated
- » 1 cup white rice
- » 2 cups of water

## DIRECTIONS

1. Heat-up a pan with the oil over medium-high heat, add the chicken, stir and brown for 4 minutes on each side. Add aminos, vinegar, bell pepper, black pepper, garlic, ginger, carrots, rice and stock, stock, cover the pan and cook over medium heat for 20 minutes. Divide everything into bowls and serve for lunch. Enjoy!

**NUTRITIONS:** Calories: 70, Carbs: 13g, Fat: 2g, Protein: 2g, Sodium 5 mg

# 74. TOMATO SOUP

**COOKING: 20'**      **PREPARATION: 10'**      **SERVINGS: 4**

## INGREDIENTS

- » 3 garlic cloves, minced
- » 1 yellow onion, chopped
- » 3 carrots, chopped
- » 15 ounces tomato sauce, no-salt-added
- » 1 tablespoon olive oil
- » 15 ounces roasted tomatoes, no-salt-added
- » 1 cup low-sodium veggie stock
- » 1 tablespoon tomato paste, no-salt-added
- » 1 tablespoon basil, dried
- » ¼ teaspoon oregano, dried
- » 3 ounces coconut cream
- » A pinch of black pepper

## DIRECTIONS

1. Heat-up a pot with the oil over medium heat, add garlic and onion, stir and cook for 5 minutes. Add carrots, tomato sauce, tomatoes, stock, tomato paste, basil, oregano, and black pepper, stir, bring to a simmer, cook for 15 minutes, add cream, blend the soup using an immersion blender, divide into bowls and serve for lunch. Enjoy!

**NUTRITIONS:** Calories: 90, Carbs: 20g, Fat: 0g, Protein: 2g, Sodium 480 mg

# 75. COD SOUP

**COOKING: 25'**  **PREPARATION: 10'**  **SERVINGS: 4**

## INGREDIENTS

- » 1 yellow onion, chopped
- » 12 cups low-sodium fish stock
- » 1-pound carrots, sliced
- » 1 tablespoon olive oil
- » Black pepper to the taste
- » 2 tablespoons ginger, minced
- » 1 cup of water
- » 1-pound cod, skinless, boneless, and cut into medium chunks

## DIRECTIONS

1. Heat-up a pot with the oil over medium-high heat, add onion, stir and cook for 4 minutes. Add water, stock, ginger, and carrots, stir and cook for 10 minutes more.

2. Blend soup using an immersion blender, add the fish and pepper, stir, cook for 10 minutes more, ladle into bowls and serve. Enjoy!

**NUTRITIONS:** Calories: 344, Carbs: 35g, Fat: 4g, Protein: 46g, Sodium 334 mg

# 76. SWEET POTATO SOUP

**COOKING: 1H 40'**  **PREPARATION: 10'**  **SERVINGS: 6**

## INGREDIENTS

- » 4 big sweet potatoes
- » 28 ounces veggie stock
- » A pinch of black pepper
- » ¼ teaspoon nutmeg, ground
- » 1/3 cup low-sodium heavy cream

## DIRECTIONS

1. Put the sweet potatoes on a lined baking sheet, bake them at 350 degrees F for 1 hour and 30 minutes, cool them down, peel, roughly chop them, and put them in a pot.

2. Add stock, nutmeg, cream, and pepper pulse well using an immersion blender, heat the soup over medium heat, cook for 10 minutes, ladle into bowls and serve. Enjoy!

**NUTRITIONS:** Calories: 110, Carbs: 23g, Fat: 1g, Protein: 2g, Sodium 140 mg

# 77. SWEET POTATOES AND ZUCCHINI SOUP

**COOKING: 20'**      **PREPARATION: 10'**      **SERVINGS: 8**

## INGREDIENTS

- » 4 cups veggie stock
- » 2 tablespoons olive oil
- » 2 sweet potatoes, peeled and cubed
- » 8 zucchinis, chopped
- » 2 yellow onions, chopped
- » 1 cup of coconut milk
- » A pinch of black pepper
- » 1 tablespoon coconut aminos
- » 4 tablespoons dill, chopped
- » ½ teaspoon basil, chopped

## DIRECTIONS

1. Heat-up a pot with the oil over medium heat, add onion, stir and cook for 5 minutes. Add zucchinis, stock, basil, potato, and pepper, stir and cook for 15 minutes more. Add milk, aminos, and dill, pulse using an immersion blender, ladle into bowls and serve for lunch.

**NUTRITIONS:** Calories: 270, Carbs: 50g, Fat: 4g, Protein: 11g, Sodium 416 mg

# 78. LEMONGRASS AND CHICKEN SOUP

**COOKING: 25'**      **PREPARATION: 10'**      **SERVINGS: 4**

## INGREDIENTS

- » 4 lime leaves, torn
- » 4 cups veggie stock, low-sodium
- » 1 lemongrass stalk, chopped
- » 1 tablespoon ginger, grated
- » 1-pound chicken breast, skinless, boneless, and cubed
- » 8 ounces mushrooms, chopped
- » 4 Thai chilies, chopped
- » 13 ounces of coconut milk
- » ¼ cup lime juice
- » ¼ cup cilantro, chopped
- » A pinch of black pepper

## DIRECTIONS

1. Put the stock into a pot, bring to a simmer over medium heat, add lemongrass, ginger, and lime leaves, stir, cook for 10 minutes, strain into another pot, and heat up over medium heat again.

2. Add chicken, mushrooms, milk, cilantro, black pepper, chilies, and lime juice, stir, simmer for 15 minutes, ladle into bowls and serve.

**NUTRITIONS:** Calories: 105, Carbs: 1g, Fat: 2g, Protein: 15g, Sodium 200 mg

# 79. EASY LUNCH SALMON STEAKS

**COOKING: 20'**     **PREPARATION: 10'**     **SERVINGS: 4**

## INGREDIENTS

- » 1 big salmon fillet, cut into 4 steaks
- » 3 garlic cloves, minced
- » 1 yellow onion, chopped
- » Black pepper to the taste
- » 2 tablespoons olive oil
- » ¼ cup parsley, chopped
- » Juice of 1 lemon
- » 1 tablespoon thyme, chopped
- » 4 cups of water

## DIRECTIONS

1. Heat a pan with the oil on medium-high heat, cook onion and garlic within 3 minutes.

2. Add black pepper, parsley, thyme, water, and lemon juice, stir, bring to a gentle boil, add salmon steaks, cook them for 15 minutes, drain, divide between plates and serve with a side salad for lunch.

**NUTRITIONS:** Calories: 110, Carbs: 3g, Fat: 4g, Protein: 15g, Sodium 330 mg

# 80. LIGHT BALSAMIC SALAD

**COOKING: 0'**     **PREPARATION: 10'**     **SERVINGS: 3**

## INGREDIENTS

- » 1 orange, cut into segments
- » 2 green onions, chopped
- » 1 romaine lettuce head, torn
- » 1 avocado, pitted, peeled, and cubed
- » ¼ cup almonds, sliced
- » For the salad dressing:
- » 1 teaspoon mustard
- » ¼ cup olive oil
- » 2 tablespoons balsamic vinegar
- » Juice of ½ orange
- » Salt and black pepper

## DIRECTIONS

1. In a salad bowl, mix oranges with avocado, lettuce, almonds, and green onions. In another bowl, mix olive oil with vinegar, mustard, orange juice, salt, and pepper, whisk well, add this to your salad, toss and serve.

**NUTRITIONS:** Calories: 35, Carbs: 5g, Fat: 2g, Protein: 0g, Sodium 400 mg

# 81. PURPLE POTATO SOUP

**COOKING: 1H 15'**    **PREPARATION: 10'**    **SERVINGS: 6**

## INGREDIENTS

- » 6 purple potatoes, chopped
- » 1 cauliflower head, florets separated
- » Black pepper to the taste
- » 4 garlic cloves, minced
- » 1 yellow onion, chopped
- » 3 tablespoons olive oil
- » 1 tablespoon thyme, chopped
- » 1 leek, chopped
- » 2 shallots, chopped
- » 4 cups chicken stock, low-sodium

## DIRECTIONS

1. In a baking dish, mix potatoes with onion, cauliflower, garlic, pepper, thyme, and half of the oil, toss to coat, introduce in the oven and bake for 45 minutes at 400 degrees F.

2. Heat a pot with the rest of the oil over medium-high heat, add leeks and shallots, stir and cook for 10 minutes.

3. Add roasted veggies and stock, stir, bring to a boil, cook for 20 minutes, transfer soup to your food processor, blend well, divide into bowls, and serve.

**NUTRITIONS:** Calories: 70, Carbs: 15g, Fat: 0g, Protein: 2g, Sodium 6 mg

# 82. LEEKS SOUP

**COOKING: 1 H 15'**    **PREPARATION: 10'**    **SERVINGS: 6**

## INGREDIENTS

- » 2 gold potatoes, chopped
- » 1 cup cauliflower florets
- » Black pepper to the taste
- » 5 leeks, chopped
- » 4 garlic cloves, minced
- » 1 yellow onion, chopped
- » 3 tablespoons olive oil
- » Handful parsley, chopped
- » 4 cups low-sodium chicken stock

## DIRECTIONS

1. Heat-up a pot with the oil over medium-high heat, add onion and garlic, stir and cook for 5 minutes.

2. Add potatoes, cauliflower, black pepper, leeks, and stock, stir, bring to a simmer, cook over medium heat for 30 minutes, blend using an immersion blender, add parsley, stir, ladle into bowls and serve.

**NUTRITIONS:** Calories: 125, Carbs: 29g, Fat: 1g, Protein: 4g, Sodium 52 mg

# 83. CAULIFLOWER LUNCH SALAD

**COOKING: 10'**          **PREPARATION: 2 H**          **SERVINGS: 4**

## INGREDIENTS

- » 1/3 cup low-sodium veggie stock
- » 2 tablespoons olive oil
- » 6 cups cauliflower florets, grated
- » Black pepper to the taste
- » ¼ cup red onion, chopped
- » 1 red bell pepper, chopped
- » Juice of ½ lemon
- » ½ cup kalamata olives halved
- » 1 teaspoon mint, chopped
- » 1 tablespoon cilantro, chopped

## DIRECTIONS

1. Heat-up a pan with the oil over medium-high heat, add cauliflower, pepper and stock, stir, cook within 10 minutes, transfer to a bowl, and keep in the fridge for 2 hours. Mix cauliflower with olives, onion, bell pepper, black pepper, mint, cilantro, and lemon juice, toss to coat, and serve.

**NUTRITIONS:** Calories: 102, Carbs: 3g, Fat: 10g, Protein: 0g, Sodium 97 mg

# CHAPTER 5.
# DINNER

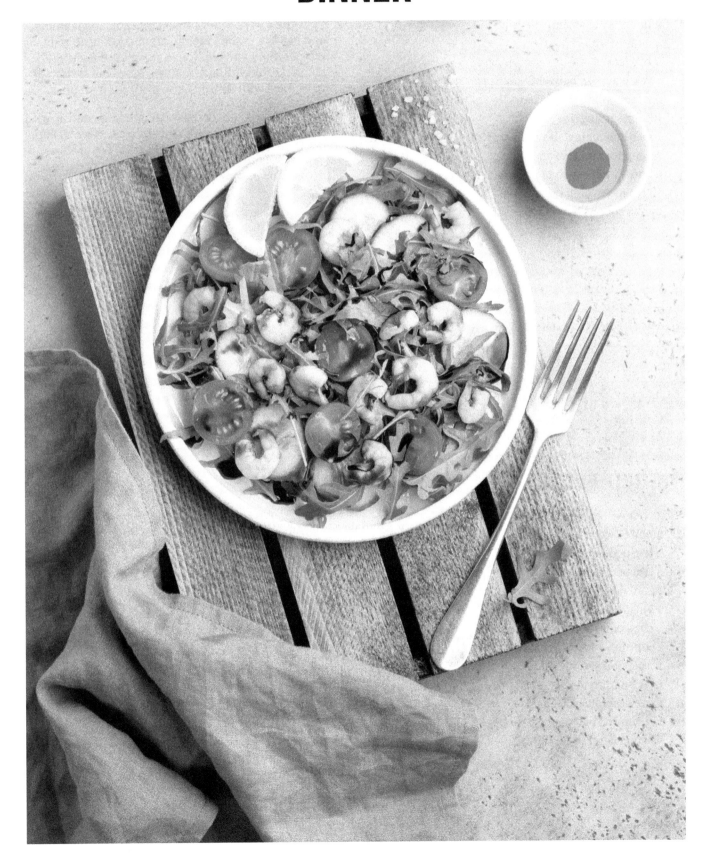

# 84. SHRIMP COCKTAIL

**COOKING: 5'**　　　　**PREPARATION: 10'**　　　　**SERVINGS: 8**

## INGREDIENTS

- » 2 pounds big shrimp, deveined
- » 4 cups of water
- » 2 bay leaves
- » 1 small lemon, halved
- » Ice for cooling the shrimp
- » Ice for serving
- » 1 medium lemon sliced for serving
- » ¾ cup tomato passata
- » 2 and ½ tablespoons horseradish, prepared
- » ¼ teaspoon chili powder
- » 2 tablespoons lemon juice

## DIRECTIONS

1. Pour the 4 cups water into a large pot, add lemon and bay leaves. Boil over medium-high heat, reduce temperature, and boil for 10 minutes. Put shrimp, stir and cook within 2 minutes. Move the shrimp to a bowl filled with ice and leave aside for 5 minutes.

2. In a bowl, mix tomato passata with horseradish, chili powder, and lemon juice and stir well. Place shrimp in a serving bowl filled with ice, with lemon slices, and serve with the cocktail sauce you've prepared.

**NUTRITIONS:** Calories: 276, Carbs: 0g, Fat: 8g, Protein: 25g, Sodium: 182 mg

# 85. QUINOA AND SCALLOPS SALAD

**COOKING: 35'**　　　　**PREPARATION: 10'**　　　　**SERVINGS: 6**

## INGREDIENTS

- » 12 ounces dry sea scallops
- » 4 tablespoons canola oil
- » 2 teaspoons canola oil
- » 4 teaspoons low sodium soy sauce
- » 1 and ½ cup quinoa, rinsed
- » 2 teaspoons garlic, minced
- » 3 cups of water
- » 1 cup snow peas, sliced diagonally
- » 1 teaspoon sesame oil
- » 1/3 cup rice vinegar
- » 1 cup scallions, sliced
- » 1/3 cup red bell pepper, chopped
- » ¼ cup cilantro, chopped

## DIRECTIONS

1. In a bowl, mix scallops with 2 teaspoons soy sauce, stir gently, and leave aside for now. Heat a pan with 1 tablespoon canola oil over medium-high heat, add the quinoa, stir and cook for 8 minutes. Put garlic, stir and cook within 1 more minute.

2. Put the water, boil over medium heat, stir, cover, and cook for 15 minutes. Remove from heat and leave aside covered for 5 minutes. Add snow peas, cover again and leave for 5 more minutes.

3. Meanwhile, in a bowl, mix 3 tablespoons canola oil with 2 teaspoons soy sauce, vinegar, and sesame oil and stir well. Add quinoa and snow peas to this mixture and stir again. Add scallions, bell pepper, and stir again.

4. Pat dry the scallops and discard marinade. Heat another pan with 2 teaspoons canola oil over high heat, add scallops, and cook for 1 minute on each side. Add them to the quinoa salad, stir gently, and serve with chopped cilantro.

**NUTRITIONS:** Calories: 181, Carbs: 12g, Fat: 6g, Protein: 13g, Sodium: 153 mg

# 86. SQUID AND SHRIMP SALAD

**COOKING: 15'**     **PREPARATION: 10'**     **SERVINGS: 4**

## INGREDIENTS

- » 8 ounces squid, cut into medium pieces
- » 8 ounces shrimp, peeled and deveined
- » 1 red onion, sliced
- » 1 cucumber, chopped
- » 2 tomatoes, cut into medium wedges
- » 2 tablespoons cilantro, chopped
- » 1 hot jalapeno pepper, cut in rounds
- » 3 tablespoons rice vinegar
- » 3 tablespoons dark sesame oil
- » Black pepper to the taste

## DIRECTIONS

1. In a bowl, mix the onion with cucumber, tomatoes, pepper, cilantro, shrimp, and squid and stir well. Cut a big parchment paper in half, fold it in half heart shape and open. Place the seafood mixture in this parchment piece, fold over, seal edges, place on a baking sheet, and introduce in the oven at 400 degrees F for 15 minutes.

2. Meanwhile, in a small bowl, mix sesame oil with rice vinegar and black pepper and stir very well. Take the salad out of the oven, leave to cool down for a few minutes, and transfer to a serving plate. Put the dressing over the salad and serve right away.

**NUTRITIONS:** Calories: 235, Carbs: 9g, Fat: 8g, Protein: 30g, Sodium: 165 mg

# 87. PARSLEY SEAFOOD COCKTAIL

**COOKING: 1H 30'**     **PREPARATION: 2H 10'**     **SERVINGS: 4**

## INGREDIENTS

- » 1 big octopus, cleaned
- » 1-pound mussels
- » 2 pounds clams
- » 1 big squid cut in rings
- » 3 garlic cloves, chopped
- » 1 celery rib, cut crosswise into thirds
- » ½ cup celery rib, sliced
- » 1 carrot, cut crosswise into 3 pieces
- » 1 small white onion, chopped
- » 1 bay leaf
- » ¾ cup white wine
- » 2 cups radicchio, sliced
- » 1 red onion, sliced
- » 1 cup parsley, chopped
- » 1 cup olive oil
- » 1 cup red wine vinegar
- » Black pepper to the taste

## DIRECTIONS

1. Put the octopus in a pot with celery rib cut in thirds, garlic, carrot, bay leaf, white onion, and white wine. Add water to cover the octopus, cover with a lid, bring to a boil over high heat, reduce to low, and simmer within 1 and ½ hours.

2. Drain octopus, reserve boiling liquid, and leave aside to cool down. Put ¼ cup octopus cooking liquid in another pot, add mussels, heat up over medium-high heat, cook until they open, transfer to a bowl, and leave aside.

3. Add clams to the pan, cover, cook over medium-high heat until they open, transfer to the bowl with mussels, and leave aside. Add squid to the pan, cover and cook over medium-high heat for 3 minutes, transfer to the bowl with mussels and clams.

4. Meanwhile, slice octopus into small pieces and mix with the rest of the seafood. Add sliced celery, radicchio, red onion, vinegar, olive oil, parsley, salt, and pepper, stir gently, and leave aside in the fridge within 2 hours before serving.

**NUTRITIONS:** Calories: 102, Carbs: 7g, Fat: 1g, Protein: 16g, Sodium: 0mg

# 88. SHRIMP AND ONION GINGER DRESSING

**COOKING: 5'**       **PREPARATION: 10'**       **SERVINGS: 2**

## INGREDIENTS

- » 8 medium shrimp, peeled and deveined
- » 12 ounces package mixed salad leaves
- » 10 cherry tomatoes, halved
- » 2 green onions, sliced
- » 2 medium mushrooms, sliced
- » 1/3 cup rice vinegar
- » ¼ cup sesame seeds, toasted
- » 1 tablespoon low-sodium soy sauce
- » 2 teaspoons ginger, grated
- » 2 teaspoons garlic, minced
- » 2/3 cup canola oil
- » 1/3 cup sesame oil

## DIRECTIONS

1. In a bowl, mix rice vinegar with sesame seeds, soy sauce, garlic, ginger, and stir well. Pour this into your kitchen blender, add canola oil and sesame oil, pulse very well, and leave aside. Brush shrimp with 3 tablespoons of the ginger dressing you've prepared.

2. Heat your kitchen grill over high heat, add shrimp and cook for 3 minutes, flipping once. In a salad bowl, mix salad leaves with grilled shrimp, mushrooms, green onions, and tomatoes. Drizzle ginger dressing on top and serve right away!

**NUTRITIONS:** Calories: 360, Carbs: 14g, Fat: 11g, Protein: 49g, Sodium: 469 mg

# 89. FRUIT SHRIMP SOUP

**COOKING: 25'**       **PREPARATION: 10'**       **SERVINGS: 6**

## INGREDIENTS

- » 8 ounces shrimp, peeled and deveined
- » 1 stalk lemongrass, smashed
- » 2 small ginger pieces, grated
- » 6 cup chicken stock
- » 2 jalapenos, chopped
- » 4 lime leaves
- » 1 and ½ cups pineapple, chopped
- » 1 cup shiitake mushroom caps, chopped
- » 1 tomato, chopped
- » ½ bell pepper, cubed
- » 2 tablespoons fish sauce
- » 1 teaspoon sugar
- » ¼ cup lime juice
- » 1/3 cup cilantro, chopped
- » 2 scallions, sliced

## DIRECTIONS

1. In a pot, mix ginger with lemongrass, stock, jalapenos, and lime leaves, stir, boil over medium heat, cook within 15 minutes. Strain liquid in a bowl and discard solids.

2. Return soup to the pot again, add pineapple, tomato, mushrooms, bell pepper, sugar, and fish sauce, stir, boil over medium heat, cook for 5 minutes, add shrimp and cook for 3 more minutes. Remove from heat, add lime juice, cilantro, and scallions, stir, ladle into soup bowls and serve.

**NUTRITIONS:** Calories: 290, Carbs: 39g, Fat: 12g, Protein: 7g, Sodium: 21 mg

# 90. MUSSELS AND CHICKPEA SOUP

**COOKING: 10'**     **PREPARATION: 10'**     **SERVINGS: 6**

## INGREDIENTS

» 3 garlic cloves, minced
» 2 tablespoons olive oil
» A pinch of chili flakes
» 1 and ½ tablespoons fresh mussels, scrubbed
» 1 cup white wine
» 1 cup chickpeas, rinsed
» 1 small fennel bulb, sliced
» Black pepper to the taste
» Juice of 1 lemon
» 3 tablespoons parsley, chopped

## DIRECTIONS

1. Heat a big saucepan with the olive oil over medium-high heat, add garlic and chili flakes, stir and cook within a couple of minutes. Add white wine and mussels, stir, cover, and cook for 3-4 minutes until mussels open.

2. Transfer mussels to a baking dish, add some of the cooking liquid over them, and fridge until they are cold enough. Take mussels out of the fridge and discard shells.

3. Heat another pan over medium-high heat, add mussels, reserved cooking liquid, chickpeas, and fennel, stir well, and heat them. Add black pepper to the taste, lemon juice, and parsley, stir again, divide between plates and serve.

**NUTRITIONS:** Calories: 286, Carbs: 49g, Fat: 4g, Protein: 14g, Sodium: 145mg

# 91. FISH STEW

**COOKING: 30'**     **PREPARATION: 10'**     **SERVINGS: 4**

## INGREDIENTS

» 1 red onion, sliced
» 2 tablespoons olive oil
» 1-pound white fish fillets, boneless, skinless, and cubed
» 1 avocado, pitted and chopped
» 1 tablespoon oregano, chopped
» 1 cup chicken stock
» 2 tomatoes, cubed
» 1 teaspoon sweet paprika
» A pinch of salt and black pepper
» 1 tablespoon parsley, chopped
» Juice of 1 lime

## DIRECTIONS

1. Warm-up oil in a pot over medium heat, add the onion, and sauté within 5 minutes. Add the fish, the avocado, and the other ingredients, toss, cook over medium heat for 25 minutes more, divide into bowls and serve for lunch.

**NUTRITIONS:** Calories: 78, Carbs: 8g, Fat: 1g, Protein: 11g, Sodium: 151 mg

# 92. SHRIMP AND BROCCOLI SOUP

**COOKING: 25'**　　　**PREPARATION: 5'**　　　**SERVINGS: 4**

## INGREDIENTS

- » 2 tablespoons olive oil
- » 1 yellow onion, chopped
- » 4 cups chicken stock
- » Juice of 1 lime
- » 1-pound shrimp, peeled and deveined
- » ½ cup coconut cream
- » ½ pound broccoli florets
- » 1 tablespoon parsley, chopped

## DIRECTIONS

1. Heat a pot with the oil over medium heat, add the onion and sauté for 5 minutes. Add the shrimp and the other ingredients, simmer over medium heat for 20 minutes more. Ladle the soup into bowls and serve.

**NUTRITIONS:** Calories: 220, Carbs: 12g, Fat: 7g, Protein: 26g, Sodium: 577 mg

# 93. COCONUT TURKEY MIX

**COOKING: 30'**　　　**PREPARATION: 10'**　　　**SERVINGS: 4**

## INGREDIENTS

- » 1 yellow onion, chopped
- » 1-pound turkey breast, skinless, boneless, and cubed
- » 2 tablespoons olive oil
- » 2 garlic cloves, minced
- » 1 zucchini, sliced
- » 1 cup coconut cream
- » A pinch of sea salt
- » black pepper

## DIRECTIONS

1. Bring the pan to medium heat, add the onion and the garlic and sauté for 5 minutes. Put the meat and brown within 5 minutes more. Add the rest of the ingredients, toss, bring to a simmer and cook over medium heat for 20 minutes more. Serve for lunch.

**NUTRITIONS:** Calories 200, Fat 4g, Fiber 2g, Carbs 14g, Protein 7g, Sodium 111mg

# 94. LIME SHRIMP AND KALE

**COOKING: 20'**          **PREPARATION: 10'**          **SERVINGS: 4**

## INGREDIENTS

- » 1-pound shrimp, peeled and deveined
- » 4 scallions, chopped
- » 1 teaspoon sweet paprika
- » 1 tablespoon olive oil
- » Juice of 1 lime
- » Zest of 1 lime, grated
- » A pinch of salt and black pepper
- » 2 tablespoons parsley, chopped

## DIRECTIONS

1. Bring the pan to medium heat, add the scallions and sauté for 5 minutes. Add the shrimp and the other ingredients, toss, cook over medium heat for 15 minutes more, divide into bowls and serve.

**NUTRITIONS:** Calories: 149, Carbs: 12g, Fat: 4g, Protein: 21g, Sodium: 250 mg

# 95. PARSLEY COD MIX

**COOKING: 20'**          **PREPARATION: 10'**          **SERVINGS: 4**

## INGREDIENTS

- » 1 tablespoon olive oil
- » 2 shallots, chopped
- » 4 cod fillets, boneless and skinless
- » 2 garlic cloves, minced
- » 2 tablespoons lemon juice
- » 1 cup chicken stock
- » A pinch of salt and black pepper

## DIRECTIONS

1. Bring the pan to medium heat -high heat, add the shallots and the garlic and sauté for 5 minutes. Add the cod and the other ingredients, cook everything for 15 minutes more, divide between plates and serve for lunch.

**NUTRITIONS:** Calories: 216, Carbs: 7g, Fat: 5g, Protein: 34g, Sodium: 380 mg

# 96. SALMON AND CABBAGE MIX

**COOKING: 25'**      **PREPARATION: 5'**      **SERVINGS: 4**

## INGREDIENTS

» 4 salmon fillets, boneless
» 1 yellow onion, chopped
» 2 tablespoons olive oil
» 1 cup red cabbage, shredded
» 1 red bell pepper, chopped
» 1 tablespoon rosemary, chopped
» 1 tablespoon coriander, ground
» 1 cup tomato sauce
» A pinch of sea salt
» black pepper

## DIRECTIONS

1. Bring the pan to medium heat, add the onion and sauté for 5 minutes. Put the fish and sear it within 2 minutes on each side. Add the cabbage and the remaining ingredients, toss, cook over medium heat for 20 minutes more, divide between plates and serve.

**NUTRITIONS:** Calories: 130, Carbs: 8g, Fat: 6g, Protein: 12g, Sodium: 345 mg

# CHAPTER 6.
# MAINS

# 97. TOFU & GREEN BEAN STIR-FRY

**COOKING: 20'**        **PREPARATION: 15'**        **SERVINGS: 4**

## INGREDIENTS

**For the guacamole:**
- » 2 ripe avocados, peeled and pitted
- » ½ jalapeño, seeded and finely minced
- » ¼ red onion, peeled and finely diced
- » ¼ cup fresh cilantro leaves, chopped
- » Zest and juice of 1 lime
- » ¼ teaspoon kosher or sea salt

**For the cakes:**
- » 3 sweet potatoes, cooked and peeled
- » ½ cup cooked black beans
- » 1 large egg
- » ½ cup panko bread crumbs
- » 1 teaspoon ground cumin
- » 1 teaspoon chili powder
- » ½ teaspoon kosher or sea salt
- » ¼ teaspoon ground black pepper
- » 2 tablespoons canola oil

**NUTRITIONS:** Calories: 369, Fat: 22g, Sodium: 521mg, Carbohydrate: 38g, Protein: 8g

## DIRECTIONS

1. Mash the avocado, then stir in the jalapeño, red onion, cilantro, lime zest and juice, and salt in a bowl. Taste and adjust the seasoning, if necessary.

2. Put the cooked sweet potatoes plus black beans in a bowl and mash until a paste form. Stir in the egg, bread crumbs, cumin, chili powder, salt, and black pepper until combined.

3. Warm-up canola oil in a large skillet at medium heat. Form the sweet potato mixture into 4 patties, place them in the hot skillet, and cook within 3 to 4 minutes per side, until browned and crispy. Serve the sweet potato cakes with guacamole on top.

# 98. PEANUT VEGETABLE PAD THAI

**COOKING: 20'**        **PREPARATION: 15'**        **SERVINGS: 6**

## INGREDIENTS

- » 8 ounces brown rice noodles
- » 1/3 cup natural peanut butter
- » 3 tablespoons unsalted vegetable broth
- » 1 tablespoon low-sodium soy sauce
- » 2 tablespoons of rice wine vinegar
- » 1 tablespoon honey
- » 2 teaspoons sesame oil
- » 1 teaspoon sriracha (optional)
- » 1 tablespoon canola oil
- » 1 red bell pepper, thinly sliced
- » 1 zucchini, cut into matchsticks
- » 2 large carrots, cut into matchsticks
- » 3 large eggs, beaten
- » ¾ teaspoon kosher or sea salt
- » ½ cup unsalted peanuts, chopped
- » ½ cup cilantro leaves, chopped

**NUTRITIONS:** Calories: 393, Fat: 19g, Sodium: 561mg, Carbohydrate: 45g, Protein: 13g

## DIRECTIONS

1. Boil a large pot of water. Cook the rice noodles as stated in package directions. Mix the peanut butter, vegetable broth, soy sauce, rice wine vinegar, honey, sesame oil, and sriracha in a bowl. Set aside.

2. Warm-up canola oil over medium heat in a large nonstick skillet. Add the red bell pepper, zucchini, and carrots, and sauté for 2 to 3 minutes, until slightly soft. Stir in the eggs and fold with a spatula until scrambled. Add the cooked rice noodles, sauce, and salt. Toss to combine. Spoon into bowls and evenly top with the peanuts and cilantro.

# 99. SPICY TOFU BURRITO BOWLS WITH CILANTRO AVOCADO SAUCE

**COOKING: 15'**     **PREPARATION: 15'**     **SERVINGS: 4**

## INGREDIENTS

**For the sauce:**
- » ¼ cup plain nonfat Greek yogurt
- » ½ cup fresh cilantro leaves
- » ½ ripe avocado, peeled
- » Zest and juice of 1 lime
- » 2 garlic cloves, peeled
- » ¼ teaspoon kosher or sea salt
- » 2 tablespoons water

**For the burrito bowls:**
- » 1 (14-ounce) package extra-firm tofu
- » 1 tablespoon canola oil
- » 1 yellow or orange bell pepper, diced
- » 2 tablespoons Taco Seasoning
- » ¼ teaspoon kosher or sea salt
- » 2 cups Fluffy Brown Rice
- » 1 (15-ounce) can black beans, drained

## DIRECTIONS

1. Place all the sauce ingredients in the bowl of a food processor or blender and purée until smooth. Taste and adjust the seasoning, if necessary. Refrigerate until ready for use.

2. Put the tofu on your plate lined with a kitchen towel. Put another kitchen towel over the tofu and place a heavy pot on top, changing towels if they become soaked. Let it stand within 15 minutes to remove the moisture. Cut the tofu into 1-inch cubes.

3. Warm-up canola oil in a large skillet over medium heat. Add the tofu and bell pepper and sauté, breaking up the tofu into smaller pieces for 4 to 5 minutes. Stir in the taco seasoning, salt, and ¼ cup of water. Evenly divide the rice and black beans among 4 bowls. Top with the tofu/bell pepper mixture and top with the cilantro avocado sauce.

**NUTRITIONS:** Calories: 383, Fat: 13g, Sodium: 438mg, Carbohydrate: 48g, Protein: 21g

# 100. SWEET POTATO CAKES WITH CLASSIC GUACAMOLE

**COOKING: 20'**     **PREPARATION: 15'**     **SERVINGS: 4**

## INGREDIENTS

**For the guacamole:**
- » 2 ripe avocados, peeled and pitted
- » ½ jalapeño, seeded and finely minced
- » ¼ red onion, peeled and finely diced
- » ¼ cup fresh cilantro leaves, chopped
- » Zest and juice of 1 lime
- » ¼ teaspoon kosher or sea salt

**For the cakes:**
- » 3 sweet potatoes, cooked and peeled
- » ½ cup cooked black beans
- » 1 large egg
- » ½ cup panko bread crumbs
- » 1 teaspoon ground cumin
- » 1 teaspoon chili powder
- » ½ teaspoon kosher or sea salt
- » ¼ teaspoon ground black pepper
- » 2 tablespoons canola oil

## DIRECTIONS

1. Mash the avocado, then stir in the jalapeño, red onion, cilantro, lime zest and juice, and salt in a bowl. Taste and adjust the seasoning, if necessary.

2. Put the cooked sweet potatoes plus black beans in a bowl and mash until a paste form. Stir in the egg, bread crumbs, cumin, chili powder, salt, and black pepper until combined.

3. Warm-up canola oil in a large skillet at medium heat. Form the sweet potato mixture into 4 patties, place them in the hot skillet, and cook within 3 to 4 minutes per side, until browned and crispy. Serve the sweet potato cakes with guacamole on top.

**NUTRITIONS:** Calories: 369, Fat: 22g, Sodium: 521mg, Carbohydrate: 38g, Protein: 8g

# 101. CHICKPEA CAULIFLOWER TIKKA MASALA

**COOKING: 40'**　　　　**PREPARATION: 15'**　　　　**SERVINGS: 6**

## INGREDIENTS

- » 2 tablespoons olive oil
- » 1 yellow onion, peeled and diced
- » 4 garlic cloves, peeled and minced
- » 1-inch piece fresh ginger, peeled and minced
- » 2 tablespoons Garam Masala
- » 1 teaspoon kosher or sea salt
- » ½ teaspoon ground black pepper
- » ¼ teaspoon ground cayenne pepper
- » ½ small head cauliflower, small florets
- » 2 (15-ounce) cans no-salt-added chickpeas, rinsed and drained
- » 1 (15-ounce) can no-salt-added petite diced tomatoes, drained
- » 1½ cups unsalted vegetable broth
- » ½ (15-ounce) can coconut milk
- » Zest and juice of 1 lime
- » ½ cup fresh cilantro leaves, chopped, divided
- » 1½ cups cooked Fluffy Brown Rice, divided

## DIRECTIONS

1. Warm-up olive oil over medium heat, then put the onion and sauté within 4 to 5 minutes in a large Dutch oven or stockpot. Stir in the garlic, ginger, garam masala, salt, black pepper, and cayenne pepper and toast for 30 to 60 seconds, until fragrant.

2. Stir in the cauliflower florets, chickpeas, diced tomatoes, and vegetable broth and increase to medium-high. Simmer within 15 minutes, until the cauliflower is fork-tender.

3. Remove, then stir in the coconut milk, lime juice, lime zest, and half of the cilantro. Taste and adjust the seasoning, if necessary. Serve over the rice and the remaining chopped cilantro.

**NUTRITIONS:** Calories: 323, Fat: 12g, Sodium: 444mg, Carbohydrate: 44g, Protein: 11g

# 102. EGGPLANT PARMESAN STACKS

**COOKING: 20'**　　　　**PREPARATION: 15'**　　　　**SERVINGS: 4**

## INGREDIENTS

- » 1 large eggplant, cut into thick slices
- » 2 tablespoons olive oil, divided
- » ¼ teaspoon kosher or sea salt
- » ¼ teaspoon ground black pepper
- » 1 cup panko bread crumbs
- » ¼ cup freshly grated Parmesan cheese
- » 5 to 6 garlic cloves, minced
- » ½ pound fresh mozzarella, sliced
- » 1½ cups lower-sodium marinara
- » ½ cup fresh basil leaves, torn

## DIRECTIONS

1. Preheat the oven to 425°F. Coat the eggplant slices in 1 tablespoon olive oil and sprinkle with the salt and black pepper. Put on a large baking sheet, then roast for 10 to 12 minutes, until soft with crispy edges. Remove the eggplant and set the oven to a low broil.

2. In a bowl, stir the remaining tablespoon of olive oil, bread crumbs, Parmesan cheese, and garlic. Remove the cooled eggplant from the baking sheet and clean it.

3. Create layers on the same baking sheet by stacking a roasted eggplant slice with a slice of mozzarella, a tablespoon of marinara, and a tablespoon of the bread crumb mixture, repeating with 2 layers of each ingredient. Cook under the broiler within 3 to 4 minutes until the cheese is melted and bubbly.

**NUTRITIONS:** Calories: 377, Fat: 22g, Sodium: 509mg, Carbohydrate: 29g, Protein: 16g

# 103. ROASTED VEGETABLE ENCHILADAS

**COOKING: 45'**  **PREPARATION: 15'**  **SERVINGS: 8**

## INGREDIENTS

- » 2 zucchinis, diced
- » 1 red bell pepper, seeded and sliced
- » 1 red onion, peeled and sliced
- » 2 ears corn
- » 2 tablespoons canola oil
- » 1 can no-salt-added black beans, drained
- » 1½ tablespoons chili powder
- » 2 teaspoon ground cumin
- » 1/8 teaspoon kosher or sea salt
- » ½ teaspoon ground black pepper
- » 8 (8-inch) whole-wheat tortillas
- » 1 cup Enchilada Sauce or store-bought enchilada sauce
- » ½ cup shredded Mexican-style cheese
- » ½ cup plain nonfat Greek yogurt
- » ½ cup cilantro leaves, chopped

**NUTRITIONS:** Calories: 10, Carbs: 0g, Fat: 1g, Protein: 0g, Sodium: 0mg

## DIRECTIONS

1. Preheat oven to 400°F. Place the zucchini, red bell pepper, and red onion on a baking sheet. Place the ears of corn separately on the same baking sheet. Drizzle all with the canola oil and toss to coat. Roast for 10 to 12 minutes, until the vegetables are tender. Remove and reduce the temperature to 375°F.

2. Cut the corn from the cob. Transfer the corn kernels, zucchini, red bell pepper, and onion to a bowl and stir in the black beans, chili powder, cumin, salt, and black pepper until combined.

3. Oiled a 9-by-13-inch baking dish with cooking spray. Line up the tortillas in the greased baking dish. Evenly distribute the vegetable bean filling into each tortilla. Pour half of the enchilada sauce and sprinkle half of the shredded cheese on top of the filling.

4. Roll each tortilla into enchilada shape and place them seam-side down. Pour the remaining enchilada sauce and sprinkle the remaining cheese over the enchiladas. Bake for 25 minutes until the cheese is melted and bubbly. Serve the enchiladas with Greek yogurt and chopped cilantro.

# 104. LENTIL AVOCADO TACOS

**COOKING: 35'**  **PREPARATION: 15'**  **SERVINGS: 6**

## INGREDIENTS

- » 1 tablespoon canola oil
- » ½ yellow onion, peeled and diced
- » 2-3 garlic cloves, minced
- » 1½ cups dried lentils
- » ½ teaspoon kosher or sea salt
- » 3 to 3½ cups unsalted vegetable or chicken stock
- » 2½ tablespoons Taco Seasoning or store-bought low-sodium taco seasoning
- » 16 (6-inch) corn tortillas, toasted
- » 2 ripe avocados, peeled and sliced

## DIRECTIONS

1. Heat-up the canola oil in a large skillet or Dutch oven over medium heat. Cook the onion within 4 to 5 minutes, until soft. Mix in the garlic and cook within 30 seconds until fragrant. Then add the lentils, salt, and stock. Bring to a simmer for 25 to 35 minutes, adding additional stock if needed.

2. When there's only a small amount of liquid left in the pan, and the lentils are al dente, stir in the taco seasoning and let simmer for 1 to 2 minutes. Taste and adjust the seasoning, if necessary. Spoon the lentil mixture into tortillas and serve with the avocado slices.

**NUTRITIONS:** Calories: 400, Fat: 14g, Sodium: 336mg, Carbohydrate: 64g, Fiber: 15g, Protein: 16g

# 105. TOMATO & OLIVE ORECCHIETTE WITH BASIL PESTO

**COOKING: 25'**  **PREPARATION: 15'**  **SERVINGS: 6**

## INGREDIENTS

- » 12 ounces orecchiette pasta
- » 2 tablespoons olive oil
- » 1-pint cherry tomatoes, quartered
- » ½ cup Basil Pesto or store-bought pesto
- » ¼ cup kalamata olives, sliced
- » 1 tablespoon dried oregano leaves
- » ¼ teaspoon kosher or sea salt
- » ½ teaspoon freshly cracked black pepper
- » ¼ teaspoon crushed red pepper flakes
- » 2 tablespoons freshly grated Parmesan cheese

## DIRECTIONS

1. Boil a large pot of water. Cook the orecchiette, drain and transfer the pasta to a large nonstick skillet.

2. Put the skillet over medium-low heat, then heat the olive oil. Stir in the cherry tomatoes, pesto, olives, oregano, salt, black pepper, and crushed red pepper flakes. Cook within 8 to 10 minutes, until heated throughout. Serve the pasta with the freshly grated Parmesan cheese.

**NUTRITIONS:** Calories: 332, Fat: 13g, Sodium: 389mg, Carbohydrate: 44g, Protein: 9g

# 106. ITALIAN STUFFED PORTOBELLO MUSHROOM BURGERS

**COOKING: 25'**  **PREPARATION: 15'**  **SERVINGS: 4**

## INGREDIENTS

- » 1 tablespoon olive oil
- » 4 large portobello mushrooms, washed and dried
- » ½ yellow onion, peeled and diced
- » 4 garlic cloves, peeled and minced
- » 1 can cannellini beans, drained
- » ½ cup fresh basil leaves, torn
- » ½ cup panko bread crumbs
- » 1/8 teaspoon kosher or sea salt
- » ¼ teaspoon ground black pepper
- » 1 cup lower-sodium marinara, divided
- » ½ cup shredded mozzarella cheese
- » 4 whole-wheat buns, toasted
- » 1 cup fresh arugula

## DIRECTIONS

1. Heat-up the olive oil in a large skillet to medium-high heat. Sear the mushrooms for 4 to 5 minutes per side, until slightly soft. Place on a baking sheet. Preheat the oven to a low broil.

2. Put the onion in the skillet and cook for 4 to 5 minutes, until slightly soft. Mix in the garlic then cooks within 30 to 60 seconds. Move the onions plus garlic to a bowl. Add the cannellini beans and smash with the back of a fork to form a chunky paste. Stir in the basil, bread crumbs, salt, and black pepper and half of the marinara. Cook for 5 minutes.

3. Remove the bean mixture from the stove and divide among the mushroom caps. Spoon the remaining marinara over the stuffed mushrooms and top each with the mozzarella cheese. Broil within 3 to 4 minutes, until the cheese is melted and bubbly. Transfer the burgers to the toasted whole-wheat buns and top with the arugula.

**NUTRITIONS:** Calories: 407, Fat: 9g, Sodium: 575mg, Carbohydrate: 63g, Protein: 25g

# 107. GNOCCHI WITH TOMATO BASIL SAUCE

**COOKING: 25'**  **PREPARATION: 15'**  **SERVINGS: 6**

## INGREDIENTS

- » 2 tablespoons olive oil
- » ½ yellow onion, peeled and diced
- » 3 cloves garlic, peeled and minced
- » 1 (32-ounce) can no-salt-added crushed San Marzano tomatoes
- » ¼ cup fresh basil leaves
- » 2 teaspoons Italian seasoning
- » ½ teaspoon kosher or sea salt
- » 1 teaspoon granulated sugar
- » ½ teaspoon ground black pepper
- » 1/8 teaspoon crushed red pepper flakes
- » 1 tablespoon heavy cream (optional)
- » 12 ounces gnocchi
- » ¼ cup freshly grated Parmesan cheese

## DIRECTIONS

1. Heat-up the olive oil in a Dutch oven or stockpot over medium heat. Add the onion and sauté for 5 to 6 minutes, until soft. Stir in the garlic and stir until fragrant, 30 to 60 seconds. Then stir in the tomatoes, basil, Italian seasoning, salt, sugar, black pepper, and crushed red pepper flakes.

2. Bring to a simmer for 15 minutes. Stir in the heavy cream, if desired. For a smooth, puréed sauce, use an immersion blender or transfer sauce to a blender and purée until smooth. Taste and adjust the seasoning, if necessary.

3. While the sauce simmers, cook the gnocchi according to the package instructions, remove with a slotted spoon, and transfer to 6 bowls. Pour the sauce over the gnocchi and top with the Parmesan cheese.

**NUTRITIONS:** Calories: 287, Fat: 7g, Sodium: 527mg, Carbohydrate: 41g, Protein: 10g

# 108. CREAMY PUMPKIN PASTA

**COOKING: 30'**  **PREPARATION: 15'**  **SERVINGS: 6**

## INGREDIENTS

- » 1-pound whole-grain linguine
- » 1 tablespoon olive oil
- » 3 garlic cloves, peeled and minced
- » 2 tablespoons chopped fresh sage
- » 1½ cups pumpkin purée
- » 1 cup unsalted vegetable stock
- » ½ cup low-fat evaporated milk
- » ¾ teaspoon kosher or sea salt
- » ½ teaspoon ground black pepper
- » ½ teaspoon ground nutmeg
- » ¼ teaspoon ground cayenne pepper
- » ½ cup freshly grated Parmesan cheese, divided

## DIRECTIONS

1. Cook the whole-grain linguine in a large pot of boiled water. Reserve ½ cup of pasta water and drain the rest. Set the pasta aside.

2. Warm-up olive oil over medium heat in a large skillet. Add the garlic and sage and sauté for 1 to 2 minutes, until soft and fragrant. Whisk in the pumpkin purée, stock, milk, and reserved pasta water and simmer for 4 to 5 minutes, until thickened.

3. Whisk in the salt, black pepper, nutmeg, and cayenne pepper and half of the Parmesan cheese. Stir in the cooked whole-grain linguine. Evenly divide the pasta among 6 bowls and top with the remaining Parmesan cheese.

**NUTRITIONS:** Calories: 381, Fat: 8g, Sodium: 175mg, Carbohydrate: 63g, Protein: 15g

# 109. MEXICAN-STYLE POTATO CASSEROLE

**COOKING: 60'**          **PREPARATION: 15'**          **SERVINGS: 8**

## INGREDIENTS

- » Cooking spray
- » 2 tablespoons canola oil
- » ½ yellow onion, peeled and diced
- » 4 garlic cloves, peeled and minced
- » 2 tablespoons all-purpose flour
- » 1¼ cups milk
- » 1 tablespoon chili powder
- » ½ tablespoon ground cumin
- » 1 teaspoon kosher salt or sea salt
- » ½ teaspoon ground black pepper
- » ¼ teaspoon ground cayenne pepper
- » 1½ cups shredded Mexican-style cheese, divided
- » 1 (4-ounce) can green chilis, drained
- » 1½ pounds baby Yukon Gold or red potatoes, thinly sliced
- » 1 red bell pepper, thinly sliced

## DIRECTIONS

1. Preheat the oven to 400°F. Oiled a 9-by-13-inch baking dish with cooking spray. In a large saucepan, warm canola oil on medium heat. Add the onion and sauté for 4 to 5 minutes, until soft. Mix in the garlic, then cook until fragrant, 30 to 60 seconds.

2. Mix in the flour, then put in the milk while whisking. Slow simmer for about 5 minutes, until thickened. Whisk in the chili powder, cumin, salt, black pepper, and cayenne pepper.

3. Remove from the heat and whisk in half of the shredded cheese and the green chilis. Taste and adjust the seasoning, if necessary. Line up one-third of the sliced potatoes and sliced bell pepper in the baking dish and top with a quarter of the remaining shredded cheese.

4. Repeat with 2 more layers. Pour the cheese sauce over the top and sprinkle with the remaining shredded cheese. Cover it with aluminum foil and bake within 45 to 50 minutes, until the potatoes are tender.

5. Remove the foil and bake again within 5 to 10 minutes, until the topping is slightly browned. Let cool within 20 minutes before slicing into 8 pieces. Serve.

**NUTRITIONS:** Calories: 195, Fat: 10g, Sodium: 487mg, Carbohydrate: 19g, Protein: 8g

# 110. BLACK BEAN STEW WITH CORNBREAD

## COOKING: 55'　　　PREPARATION: 15'　　　SERVINGS: 6

## INGREDIENTS

**For the black bean stew:**

» 2 tablespoons canola oil
» 1 yellow onion, peeled and diced
» 4 garlic cloves, peeled and minced
» 1 tablespoon chili powder
» 1 tablespoon ground cumin
» ¼ teaspoon kosher or sea salt
» ½ teaspoon ground black pepper
» 2 cans no-salt-added black beans, drained
» 1 (10-ounce) can fire-roasted diced tomatoes
» ½ cup fresh cilantro leaves, chopped

**For the cornbread topping:**

» 1¼ cups cornmeal
» ½ cup all-purpose flour
» ½ teaspoon baking powder
» ¼ teaspoon baking soda
» 1/8 teaspoon kosher or sea salt
» 1 cup low-fat buttermilk
» 2 tablespoons honey
» 1 large egg

## DIRECTIONS

1. Warm-up canola oil over medium heat in a large Dutch oven or stockpot. Add the onion and sauté for 4 to 6 minutes, until the onion is soft. Stir in the garlic, chili powder, cumin, salt, and black pepper.

2. Cook within 1 to 2 minutes, until fragrant. Add the black beans and diced tomatoes. Bring to a simmer and cook for 15 minutes. Remove, then stir in the fresh cilantro. Taste and adjust the seasoning, if necessary.

3. Preheat the oven to 375°F. While the stew simmers, prepare the cornbread topping. Mix the cornmeal, baking soda, flour, baking powder, plus salt in a bowl. In a measuring cup, whisk the buttermilk, honey, and egg until combined. Put the batter into the dry fixing until just combined.

4. In oven-safe bowls or dishes, spoon out the black bean soup. Distribute dollops of the cornbread batter on top and then spread it out evenly with a spatula. Bake within 30 minutes, until the cornbread is just set.

**NUTRITIONS:** Calories: 359, Fat: 7g, Sodium: 409mg, Carbohydrate: 61g, Protein: 14g

# 111. MUSHROOM FLORENTINE

**COOKING: 20'**         **PREPARATION: 15'**         **SERVINGS: 4**

## INGREDIENTS

- » 5 oz whole-grain pasta
- » ¼ cup low-sodium vegetable broth
- » 1 cup mushrooms, sliced
- » ¼ cup of soy milk
- » 1 teaspoon olive oil
- » ½ teaspoon Italian seasonings

## DIRECTIONS

1. Cook the pasta according to the direction of the manufacturer. Then pour olive oil into the saucepan and heat it. Add mushrooms and Italian seasonings. Stir the mushrooms well and cook for 10 minutes.

2. Then add soy milk and vegetable broth. Add cooked pasta and mix up the mixture well. Cook it for 5 minutes on low heat.

**NUTRITIONS:** Calories 287, Protein 12.4g, Carbohydrates 50.4g, Fat 4.2g, Sodium 26mg

# 112. HASSELBACK EGGPLANT

**COOKING: 25'**         **PREPARATION: 15'**         **SERVINGS: 2**

## INGREDIENTS

- » 2 eggplants, trimmed
- » 2 tomatoes, sliced
- » 1 tablespoon low-fat yogurt
- » 1 teaspoon curry powder
- » 1 teaspoon olive oil

## DIRECTIONS

1. Make the cuts in the eggplants in the shape of the Hasselback. Then rub the vegetables with curry powder and fill with sliced tomatoes. Sprinkle the eggplants with olive oil and yogurt and wrap in the foil (each Hasselback eggplant wrap separately). Bake the vegetables at 375F for 25 minutes.

**NUTRITIONS:** Calories 188, Protein 7g, Carbohydrates 38.1g, Fat 3g, Sodium 23mg

# 113. VEGETARIAN KEBABS

**COOKING: 6'**  **PREPARATION: 15'**  **SERVINGS: 4**

## INGREDIENTS

» 2 tablespoons balsamic vinegar
» 1 tablespoon olive oil
» 1 teaspoon dried parsley
» 2 tablespoons water
» 2 sweet peppers
» 2 red onions, peeled
» 2 zucchinis, trimmed

## DIRECTIONS

1. Cut the sweet peppers and onions into medium size squares. Then slice the zucchini. String all vegetables into the skewers. After this, in the shallow bowl, mix up olive oil, dried parsley, water, and balsamic vinegar.

2. Sprinkle the vegetable skewers with olive oil mixture and transfer in the preheated to 390F grill. Cook the kebabs within 3 minutes per side or until the vegetables are light brown.

**NUTRITIONS:** Calories 88, Protein 2.4g, Carbohydrates 13g, Fat 3.9g, Sodium 14mg

# 114. WHITE BEANS STEW

**COOKING: 55'**  **PREPARATION: 15'**  **SERVINGS: 4**

## INGREDIENTS

» 1 cup white beans, soaked
» 1 cup low-sodium vegetable broth
» 1 cup zucchini, chopped
» 1 teaspoon tomato paste
» 1 tablespoon avocado oil
» 4 cups of water
» ½ teaspoon peppercorns
» ½ teaspoon ground black pepper
» ¼ teaspoon ground nutmeg

## DIRECTIONS

1. Heat avocado oil in the saucepan, add zucchinis, and roast them for 5 minutes. After this, add white beans, vegetable broth, tomato paste, water, peppercorns, ground black pepper, and ground nutmeg. Simmer the stew within 50 minutes on low heat.

**NUTRITIONS:** Calories 184, Protein 12.3g, Carbohydrates 32.6g, Fat 1g, Sodium 55mg

# 115. VEGETARIAN LASAGNA

**COOKING: 30'**      **PREPARATION: 15'**      **SERVINGS: 6**

## INGREDIENTS

- » 1 cup carrot, diced
- » ½ cup bell pepper, diced
- » 1 cup spinach, chopped
- » 1 tablespoon olive oil
- » 1 teaspoon chili powder
- » 1 cup tomatoes, chopped
- » 4 oz low-fat cottage cheese
- » 1 eggplant, sliced
- » 1 cup low-sodium vegetable broth

## DIRECTIONS

1. Put carrot, bell pepper, and spinach in the saucepan. Add olive oil and chili powder and stir the vegetables well. Cook them for 5 minutes.

2. Make the sliced eggplant layer in the casserole mold and top it with vegetable mixture. Add tomatoes, vegetable stock, and cottage cheese. Bake the lasagna for 30 minutes at 375F.

**NUTRITIONS:** Calories 77, Protein 4.1g, Carbohydrates 9.7g, Fat 3g, Sodium 124mg

# 116. CARROT CAKES

**COOKING: 10'**      **PREPARATION: 15'**      **SERVINGS: 4**

## INGREDIENTS

- » 1 cup carrot, grated
- » 1 tablespoon semolina
- » 1 egg, beaten
- » 1 teaspoon Italian seasonings
- » 1 tablespoon sesame oil

## DIRECTIONS

1. In the mixing bowl, mix up grated carrot, semolina, egg, and Italian seasonings. Heat sesame oil in the skillet. Make the carrot cakes with the help of 2 spoons and put in the skillet. Roast the cakes for 4 minutes per side.

**NUTRITIONS:** Calories 70, Protein 1.9g, Carbohydrates 4.8g, Fat 4.9g, Sodium 35mg

# 117. VEGAN CHILI

**COOKING: 25'**     **PREPARATION: 15'**     **SERVINGS: 4**

## INGREDIENTS

- » ½ cup bulgur
- » 1 cup tomatoes, chopped
- » 1 chili pepper, chopped
- » 1 cup red kidney beans, cooked
- » 2 cups low-sodium vegetable broth
- » 1 teaspoon tomato paste
- » ½ cup celery stalk, chopped

## DIRECTIONS

1. Put all ingredients in the big saucepan and stir well. Close the lid and simmer the chili for 25 minutes over medium-low heat.

**NUTRITIONS:** Calories 234, Protein 13.1g, Carbohydrates 44.9g, Fat 0.9g, Sodium 92mg

# 118. AROMATIC WHOLE GRAIN SPAGHETTI

**COOKING: 10'**     **PREPARATION: 15'**     **SERVINGS: 2**

## INGREDIENTS

- » 1 teaspoon dried basil
- » ¼ cup of soy milk
- » 6 oz whole-grain spaghetti
- » 2 cups of water
- » 1 teaspoon ground nutmeg

## DIRECTIONS

1. Bring the water to boil, add spaghetti, and cook them for 8-10 minutes. Meanwhile, bring the soy milk to boil. Drain the cooked spaghetti and mix them up with soy milk, ground nutmeg, and dried basil. Stir the meal well.

**NUTRITIONS:** Calories 128, Protein 5.6g, Carbohydrates 25g, Fat 1.4g, Sodium 25mg

# 119. CHUNKY TOMATOES

**COOKING: 15'**　　　**PREPARATION: 15'**　　　**SERVINGS: 3**

## INGREDIENTS

- » 2 cups plum tomatoes, roughly chopped
- » ½ cup onion, diced
- » ½ teaspoon garlic, diced
- » 1 teaspoon Italian seasonings
- » 1 teaspoon canola oil
- » 1 chili pepper, chopped

## DIRECTIONS

1. Heat canola oil in the saucepan. Add chili pepper and onion. Cook the vegetables for 5 minutes. Stir them from time to time. After this, add tomatoes, garlic, and Italian seasonings. Close the lid and sauté the dish for 10 minutes.

**NUTRITIONS:** Calories 550, Protein 1.7g, Carbohydrates 8.4g, Fat 2.3g, Sodium 17mg

# 120. BAKED FALAFEL

**COOKING: 25'**　　　**PREPARATION: 15'**　　　**SERVINGS: 6**

## INGREDIENTS

- » 2 cups chickpeas, cooked
- » 1 yellow onion, diced
- » 3 tablespoons olive oil
- » 1 cup fresh parsley, chopped
- » 1 teaspoon ground cumin
- » ½ teaspoon coriander
- » 2 garlic cloves, diced

## DIRECTIONS

1. Blend all fixing in the food processor. Preheat the oven to 375F. Then line the baking tray with the baking paper. Make the balls from the chickpeas mixture and press them gently in the shape of the falafel. Put the falafel in the tray and bake in the oven for 25 minutes.

**NUTRITIONS:** Calories 316, Protein 13.5g, Carbohydrates 43.3g, Fat 11.2g, Fiber 12.4g, Sodium 23mg

# 121. PAELLA

**COOKING: 25'**　　　**PREPARATION: 15'**　　　**SERVINGS:6**

## INGREDIENTS

» 1 teaspoon dried saffron
» 1 cup short-grain rice
» 1 tablespoon olive oil
» 2 cups of water
» 1 teaspoon chili flakes
» 6 oz artichoke hearts, chopped
» ½ cup green peas
» 1 onion, sliced
» 1 cup bell pepper, sliced

## DIRECTIONS

1. Pour water into the saucepan. Add rice and cook it for 15 minutes. Meanwhile, heat olive oil in the skillet. Add dried saffron, chili flakes, onion, and bell pepper. Roast the vegetables for 5 minutes.

2. Add them to the cooked rice. Then add artichoke hearts and green peas. Stir the paella well and cook it for 10 minutes over low heat.

**NUTRITIONS:** Calories 170, Protein 4.2g, Carbohydrates 32.7g, Fat 2.7g, Sodium 33mg

# 122. MUSHROOM CAKES

**COOKING: 10'**　　　**PREPARATION: 15'**　　　**SERVINGS: 4**

## INGREDIENTS

» 2 cups mushrooms, chopped
» 3 garlic cloves, chopped
» 1 tablespoon dried dill
» 1 egg, beaten
» ¼ cup of rice, cooked
» 1 tablespoon sesame oil
» 1 teaspoon chili powder

## DIRECTIONS

1. Grind the mushrooms in the food processor. Add garlic, dill, egg, rice, and chili powder. Blend the mixture for 10 seconds. After this, heat sesame oil for 1 minute.

2. Make the medium size mushroom cakes and put in the hot sesame oil. Cook the mushroom cakes for 5 minutes per side on medium heat.

**NUTRITIONS:** Calories 103, Protein 3.7g, Carbohydrates 12g, Fat 4.8g, Sodium 27mg

# 123. GLAZED EGGPLANT RINGS

**COOKING: 10'**          **PREPARATION: 15'**          **SERVINGS: 4**

## INGREDIENTS

- » 3 eggplants, sliced
- » 1 tablespoon liquid honey
- » 1 teaspoon minced ginger
- » 2 tablespoons lemon juice
- » 3 tablespoons avocado oil
- » ½ teaspoon ground coriander
- » 3 tablespoons water

## DIRECTIONS

1. Rub the eggplants with ground coriander. Then heat the avocado oil in the skillet for 1 minute. When the oil is hot, add the sliced eggplant and arrange it in one layer.

2. Cook the vegetables for 1 minute per side. Transfer the eggplant to the bowl. Then add minced ginger, liquid honey, lemon juice, and water in the skillet. Bring it to boil and add cooked eggplants. Coat the vegetables in the sweet liquid well and cook for 2 minutes more.

**NUTRITIONS:** Calories 136, Protein 4.3g, Carbohydrates 29.6g, Fat 2.2g, Sodium 11mg

# 124. SWEET POTATO BALLS

**COOKING: 10'**          **PREPARATION: 15'**          **SERVINGS: 4**

## INGREDIENTS

- » 1 cup sweet potato, mashed, cooked
- » 1 tablespoon fresh cilantro, chopped
- » 1 egg, beaten
- » 3 tablespoons ground oatmeal
- » 1 teaspoon ground paprika
- » ½ teaspoon ground turmeric
- » 2 tablespoons coconut oil

## DIRECTIONS

1. Mix mashed sweet potato, fresh cilantro, egg, ground oatmeal, paprika, and turmeric in a bowl. Stir the mixture until smooth and make the small balls. Heat the coconut oil in the saucepan. Put the sweet potato balls, then cook them until golden brown.

**NUTRITIONS:** Calories 133, Protein 2.8g, Carbohydrates 13.1g, Fat 8.2g, Sodium 44mg

# 125. CHICKPEA CURRY

**COOKING: 10'**  **PREPARATION: 15'**  **SERVINGS: 4**

## INGREDIENTS

- » 1 ½ cup chickpeas, boiled
- » 1 teaspoon curry powder
- » ½ teaspoon garam masala
- » 1 cup spinach, chopped
- » 1 teaspoon coconut oil
- » ¼ cup of soy milk
- » 1 tablespoon tomato paste
- » ½ cup of water

## DIRECTIONS

1. Heat coconut oil in the saucepan. Add curry powder, garam masala, tomato paste, and soy milk. Whisk the mixture until smooth and bring it to boil.

2. Add water, spinach, and chickpeas. Stir the meal and close the lid. Cook it within 5 minutes over medium heat.

**NUTRITIONS:** Calories 298, Protein 15.4g, Carbohydrates 47.8g, Fat 6.1g, Sodium 37mg

# 126. PAN-FRIED SALMON WITH SALAD

**COOKING: 20'**  **PREPARATION: 15'**  **SERVINGS: 4**

## INGREDIENTS

- » Pinch of salt and pepper
- » 1 tablespoon extra-virgin olive oil
- » 2 tablespoon unsalted butter
- » ½ teaspoon fresh dill
- » 1 tablespoon fresh lemon juice
- » 100g salad leaves, or bag of mixed leaves
- » Salad Dressing:
- » 3 tablespoons olive oil
- » 2 tablespoons balsamic vinaigrette
- » 1/2 teaspoon maple syrup (honey)

## DIRECTIONS

1. Pat-dry the salmon fillets with a paper towel and season with a pinch of salt and pepper. In a skillet, warm-up oil over medium-high heat and add fillets. Cook each side within 5 to 7 minutes until golden brown.

2. Dissolve butter, dill, and lemon juice in a small saucepan. Put the butter mixture onto the cooked salmon. Lastly, combine all the salad dressing ingredients and drizzle to mixed salad leaves in a large bowl. Toss to coat. Serve with fresh salads on the side. Enjoy!

**NUTRITIONS:** Calories 307, Fat 22g, Protein 34.6g, Sodium 80mg, Carbohydrate 1.7g

# 127. VEGGIE VARIETY

**COOKING: 15'**     **PREPARATION: 15'**     **SERVINGS: 2**

## INGREDIENTS

- » ½ onion, diced
- » 1 teaspoon vegetable oil (corn or sunflower oil)
- » 200 g Tofu/ bean curd
- » 4 cherry tomatoes, halved
- » 30ml vegetable milk (soy or oat milk)
- » ½ tsp curry powder
- » 0.25 tsp paprika
- » Pinch of Salt & Pepper
- » 2 slices of Vegan protein bread/ Whole grain bread
- » Chives for garnish

## DIRECTIONS

1. Dice the onion and fry in a frying pan with the oil. Break the tofu by hand into small pieces and put them in the pan. Sauté 7-8 min. Season with curry, paprika, salt, and pepper. The cherry tomatoes and milk and cook it all over roast a few minutes. Serve with bread as desired and sprinkle with chopped chives.

**NUTRITIONS:** Calories 216, Fat 8.4g, Protein 14.1g, Sodium 140mg, Carbohydrate 24.8g

# 128. VEGETABLE PASTA

**COOKING: 15'**     **PREPARATION: 15'**     **SERVINGS: 4**

## INGREDIENTS

- » 1 kg of thin zucchini
- » 20 g of fresh ginger
- » 350g smoked tofu
- » 1 lime
- » 2 cloves of garlic
- » 2 tbsp sunflower oil
- » 2 tablespoons of sesame seeds
- » Pinch of salt and pepper
- » 4 tablespoons fried onions

## DIRECTIONS

1. Wash and clean the zucchini and, using a julienne cutter, cut the pulp around the kernel into long thin strips (noodles). Ginger peel and finely chop. Crumble tofu. Halve lime, squeeze juice. Peel and chop garlic.

2. Warm-up 1 tbsp of oil in a large pan and fry the tofu for about 5 minutes. After about 3 minutes, add ginger, garlic, and sesame. Season with soy sauce. Remove from the pan and keep warm.

3. Wipe out the pan, then warm 2 tablespoons of oil in it. Stir fry zucchini strips for about 4 minutes while turning. Season with salt, pepper, and lime juice. Arrange pasta and tofu. Sprinkle with fried onions.

**NUTRITIONS:** Calories 262, Fat 17.7g, Protein 15.4g, Sodium 62mg, Carbohydrate 17.1g

# 129. VEGETABLE NOODLES WITH BOLOGNESE

**COOKING: 15'**          **PREPARATION: 15'**          **SERVINGS: 4**

## INGREDIENTS

- » 1.5 kg of small zucchini (e.g., green and yellow)
- » 600g of carrots
- » 1 onion
- » 1 tbsp olive oil
- » 250g of beef steak
- » Pinch of Salt and pepper
- » 2 tablespoons tomato paste
- » 1 tbsp flour
- » 1 teaspoon vegetable broth (instant)
- » 40g pecorino or parmesan
- » 1 small potty of basil

## DIRECTIONS

1. Clean and peel zucchini and carrots and wash. Using a sharp, long knife, cut first into thin slices, then into long, fine strips. Clean or peel the soup greens, wash and cut into tiny cubes. Peel the onion and chop finely. Heat the Bolognese oil in a large pan. Fry hack in it crumbly. Season with salt and pepper.

2. Briefly sauté the prepared vegetable and onion cubes. Stir in tomato paste. Dust the flour, sweat briefly. Pour in 400 ml of water and stir in the vegetable stock. Boil everything, simmer for 7-8 minutes.

3. Meanwhile, cook the vegetable strips in plenty of salted water for 3-5 minutes. Drain, collecting some cooking water. Add the vegetable strips to the pan and mix well. If the sauce is not liquid enough, stir in some vegetable cooking water and season everything again.

4. Slicing cheese into fine shavings. Wash the basil, shake dry, peel off the leaves, and cut roughly. Arrange vegetable noodles, sprinkle with parmesan and basil

**NUTRITIONS:** Calories 269, Fat 9.7g, Protein 25.6g, Sodium 253mg, Carbohydrate 21.7g

# 130. HARISSA BOLOGNESE WITH VEGETABLE NOODLES

**COOKING: 30'**          **PREPARATION: 15'**          **SERVINGS: 4**

## INGREDIENTS

- » 2 onions
- » 1 clove of garlic
- » 3-4 tbsp oil
- » 400g ground beef
- » Pinch salt, pepper, cinnamon
- » 1 tsp Harissa (Arabic seasoning paste, tube)
- » 1 tablespoon tomato paste
- » 2 sweet potatoes
- » 2 medium Zucchini
- » 3 stems/basil
- » 100g of feta

## DIRECTIONS

1. Peel onions and garlic, finely dice. Warm-up 1 tbsp of oil in a wide saucepan. Fry hack in it crumbly. Fry onions and garlic for a short time. Season with salt, pepper, and ½ teaspoon cinnamon. Stir in harissa and tomato paste.

2. Add tomatoes and 200 ml of water, bring to the boil and simmer for about 15 minutes with occasional stirring. Peel sweet potatoes and zucchini or clean and wash. Cut vegetables into spaghetti with a spiral cutter.

3. Warm-up 2-3 tablespoons of oil in a large pan. Braise sweet potato spaghetti in it for about 3 minutes. Add the zucchini spaghetti and continue to simmer for 3-4 minutes while turning.

4. Season with salt and pepper. Wash the basil, shake dry and peel off the leaves. Garnish vegetable spaghetti and Bolognese on plates. Feta crumbles over. Sprinkle with basil.

**NUTRITIONS:** Calories 452, Fat 22.3g, Protein 37.1g, Sodium 253mg, Carbohydrate 27.6g

# 131. CURRY VEGETABLE NOODLES WITH CHICKEN

**COOKING: 15'**    **PREPARATION: 15'**    **SERVINGS: 2**

## INGREDIENTS

- » 600g of zucchini
- » 500g chicken fillet
- » Pinch of salt and pepper
- » 2 tbsp oil
- » 150 g of red and yellow cherry tomatoes
- » 1 teaspoon curry powder
- » 150g fat-free cheese
- » 200 ml vegetable broth
- » 4 stalk (s) of fresh basil

## DIRECTIONS

1. Wash the zucchini, clean, and cut into long thin strips with a spiral cutter. Wash meat, pat dry, and season with salt. Heat 1 tbsp oil in a pan. Roast chicken in it for about 10 minutes until golden brown.

2. Wash cherry tomatoes and cut in half. Approximately 3 minutes before the end of the cooking time to the chicken in the pan. Heat 1 tbsp oil in another pan. Sweat curry powder into it then stirs in cream cheese and broth. Flavor the sauce with salt plus pepper and simmer for about 4 minutes.

3. Wash the basil, shake it dry and pluck the leaves from the stems. Cut small leaves of 3 stems. Remove meat from the pan and cut it into strips. Add tomatoes, basil, and zucchini to the sauce and heat for 2-3 minutes. Serve vegetable noodles and meat on plates and garnish with basil.

**NUTRITIONS:** Calories 376, Fat 17.2g, Protein 44.9g, Sodium 352mg, Carbohydrate 9.5, Cholesterol 53mg

# 132. SWEET AND SOUR VEGETABLE NOODLES

**COOKING: 30'**    **PREPARATION: 15'**    **SERVINGS: 4**

## INGREDIENTS

- » 4 chicken fillets (75 g each)
- » 300g of whole-wheat spaghetti
- » 750g carrots
- » ½ liter clear chicken broth (instant)
- » 1 tablespoon sugar
- » 1 tbsp of green peppercorns
- » 2-3 tbsp balsamic vinegar
- » Capuchin flowers
- » Pinch of salt

## DIRECTIONS

1. Cook spaghetti in boiling water for about 8 minutes. Then drain. In the meantime, peel and wash carrots. Cut into long strips (best with a special grater). Blanch within 2 minutes in boiling salted water, drain. Wash chicken fillets. Add to the boiling chicken soup and cook for about 15 minutes.

2. Melt the sugar until golden brown. Measure 1/4 liter of chicken stock and deglaze the sugar with it. Add peppercorns, cook for 2 minutes. Season with salt and vinegar. Add the fillets, then cut into thin slices. Then turn the pasta and carrots in the sauce and serve garnished with capuchin blossoms. Serve and enjoy.

**NUTRITIONS:** Calories 374, Fat 21g, Protein 44g, Sodium 295mg, Carbohydrate 23.1

# 133. TUNA SANDWICH

**COOKING: 0'**  **PREPARATION: 15'**  **SERVINGS: 1**

## INGREDIENTS

- » 2 slices whole-grain bread
- » 1 6-oz. can low sodium tuna in water, in its juice
- » 2 tsp Yogurt (1.5% fat) or low-fat mayonnaise
- » 1 medium tomato, diced
- » ½ small sweet onion, finely diced
- » Lettuce leaves

## DIRECTIONS

1. Toast whole grain bread slices. Mix tuna, yogurt, or mayonnaise, diced tomato, and onion. Cover a toasted bread with lettuce leaves and spread the tuna mixture on the sandwich. Spread tuna mixed on toasted bread with lettuce leaves. Place another disc as a cover on top. Enjoy the sandwich.

**NUTRITIONS:** Calories 235, Fat 3g, Protein 27.8g, Sodium 350mg, Carbohydrate 25.9

# 134. FRUITED QUINOA SALAD

**COOKING: 0'**  **PREPARATION: 15'**  **SERVINGS: 2**

## INGREDIENTS

- » 2 cups cooked quinoa
- » 1 mango, sliced and peeled
- » 1 cup strawberry, quartered
- » ½ cup blueberries
- » 2 tablespoon pine nuts
- » Chopped mint leave for garnish
- » Lemon vinaigrette:
- » ¼ cup olive oil
- » ¼ cup apple cider vinegar
- » Zest of lemon
- » 3 tablespoon lemon juice
- » 1 teaspoon sugar

## DIRECTIONS

1. For the Lemon Vinaigrette, whisk olive oil, apple cider vinegar, lemon zest and juice, and sugar to a bowl; set aside. Combine quinoa, mango strawberries, blueberries, and pine nuts in a large bowl. Stir the lemon vinaigrette and garnish with mint. Serve and enjoy!

**NUTRITIONS:** Calories 425, Carbohydrates 76.1g, Proteins 11.3g, Fat 10.9, Sodium 16mg

# 135. TURKEY WRAP

**COOKING: 0'**       **PREPARATION: 15'**       **SERVINGS: 2**

## INGREDIENTS

- » 2 slices of low-fat Turkey breast (deli-style)
- » 4 tablespoon non-fat cream cheese
- » ½ cup lettuce leaves
- » ½ cup carrots, slice into a stick
- » 2 Homemade wraps or store-bought whole-wheat tortilla wrap

## DIRECTIONS

1. Prepare all the ingredients. Spread 2 tablespoons of non-fat cream cheese on each wrap. Arrange lettuce leaves, then add a slice of turkey breast; a slice of carrots stick on top. Roll and cut into half. Serve and enjoy!

**NUTRITIONS:** Calories 224, Carbohydrates 35g, Protein 10.3g, Fat 3.8g, Sodium 293mg

# 136. CHICKEN WRAP

**COOKING: 15'**       **PREPARATION: 15'**       **SERVINGS: 2**

## INGREDIENTS

- » 1 tablespoon extra- virgin olive oil
- » Lemon juice, divided into 3 parts
- » 2 cloves garlic, minced
- » 1 lb. boneless skinless chicken breasts
- » ½ cup non- fat plain Greek yogurt
- » ½ teaspoon paprika
- » Pinch of salt and pepper
- » Hot sauce to taste
- » Pita bread
- » Tomato slice

## DIRECTIONS

1. For the marinade, whisk 1 tablespoon olive oil, juice of 2 lemons, garlic, salt, and pepper in a bowl. Add chicken breasts to the marinade and place it into a large Ziploc. Let marinate for 30 mins. to 4 hours.

2. For the yogurt sauce, mix yogurt, hot sauce, and the remaining lemon juice season with paprika and a pinch of salt and pepper.

3. Warm skillet over medium heat and coat it with oil. Add chicken breast and cook until golden brown and cook about 8 minutes per side. Remove from pan and rest for few minutes, then slice.

4. To a piece of pita bread, add lettuce, tomato, and chicken slices. Drizzle with the prepared spicy yogurt sauce. Serve and enjoy!

**NUTRITIONS:** Calories 348, Carbohydrates 8.7g, Proteins 56g, Fat 10.2g, Sodium 198mg

# 137. VEGGIE WRAP

**COOKING: 0'**      **PREPARATION: 15'**      **SERVINGS: 2**

## INGREDIENTS

» 2 Homemade wraps or any flour tortillas
» ½ cup spinach
» 1/2 cup alfalfa sprouts
» ½ cup avocado, sliced thinly
» 1 medium tomato, sliced thinly
» ½ cup cucumber, sliced thinly
» Pinch of salt and pepper

## DIRECTIONS

1. Put 2 tablespoons of cream cheese on each tortilla. Layer each veggie according to your liking. Pinch of salt and pepper. Roll and cut into half. Serve and Enjoy!

**NUTRITIONS:** Calories 249, Carbohydrates 12.3g, Protein 5.7g, Fat 21.5g, Sodium 169mg

# 138. SALMON WRAP

**COOKING: 0'**      **PREPARATION: 15'**      **SERVINGS: 1**

## INGREDIENTS

» 2 oz. Smoke Salmon
» 2 teaspoon low-fat cream cheese
» ½ medium-size red onion, finely sliced
» ½ teaspoon fresh basil or dried basil
» Pinch of pepper
» Arugula leaves
» 1 Homemade wrap or any whole-meal tortilla

## DIRECTIONS

1. Warm wraps or tortilla into a heated pan or oven. Combine cream cheese, basil, pepper, and spread into the tortilla. Top with salmon, arugula, and sliced onion. Roll up and slice. Serve and Enjoy!

**NUTRITIONS:** Calories 151, Carbohydrates 19.2g, Protein 10.4g, Fat 3.4g, Sodium 316mg

# 139. DILL CHICKEN SALAD

**COOKING: 15'**       **PREPARATION: 15'**       **SERVINGS: 3**

## INGREDIENTS

- » 1 tablespoon unsalted butter
- » 1 small onion, diced
- » 2 cloves garlic, minced
- » 500g boneless skinless chicken breasts

**Salad:**
- » 2/3 cup Fat-free yogurt
- » ¼ cup mayonnaise light
- » 2 large shallots, minced
- » ½ cup fresh dill, finely chopped

## DIRECTIONS

1. Dissolve the butter over medium heat in a wide pan. Sauté onion and garlic in the butter and chicken breasts. Put water to cover the chicken breasts by 1 inch. Bring to boil. Cover and reduce the heat to a bare simmer.

2. Cook within 8 to 10 minutes or until the chicken is cooked through. Cool thoroughly. The shred chicken finely using 2 forks. Set aside. Whisk yogurt and mayonnaise. Then toss with the chicken. Add shallots and dill. Mix again all. Serve and Enjoy!

**NUTRITIONS:** Calories 253, Carbohydrates 9g, Protein 33.1g, Fat 9.5g, Sodium 236mg

# CHAPTER 7.
## SIDE DISHES

# 140. TURMERIC ENDIVES

**COOKING: 20'**     **PREPARATION: 10'**     **SERVINGS: 4**

## INGREDIENTS

- » 2 endives, halved lengthwise
- » 2 tablespoons olive oil
- » 1 teaspoon rosemary, dried
- » ½ teaspoon turmeric powder
- » A pinch of black pepper

## DIRECTIONS

1. Mix the endives with the oil and the other ingredients in a baking pan, toss gently, bake at 400 degrees F within 20 minutes. Serve as a side dish.

**NUTRITIONS:** Calories 64, Protein 0.2g, Carbohydrates 0.8g, Fat 7.1g, Fiber 0.6g, Sodium 3mg, Potassium 50mg

# 141. PARMESAN ENDIVES

**COOKING: 20'**     **PREPARATION: 10'**     **SERVINGS: 4**

## INGREDIENTS

- » 4 endives, halved lengthwise
- » 1 tablespoon lemon juice
- » 1 tablespoon lemon zest, grated
- » 2 tablespoons fat-free parmesan, grated
- » 2 tablespoons olive oil
- » A pinch of black pepper

## DIRECTIONS

1. In a baking dish, combine the endives with the lemon juice and the other ingredients except for the parmesan and toss. Sprinkle the parmesan on top, bake the endives at 400 degrees F for 20 minutes, and serve.

**NUTRITIONS:** Calories 71, Protein 0.9g, Carbohydrates 2.2g, Fat 7.1g, Fiber 0.9g, Sodium 71mg, Potassium 88mg

# 142. LEMON ASPARAGUS

**COOKING: 20'**       **PREPARATION: 10'**       **SERVINGS: 4**

## INGREDIENTS

» 1-pound asparagus, trimmed
» 2 tablespoons basil pesto
» 1 tablespoon lemon juice
» A pinch of black pepper
» 3 tablespoons olive oil
» 2 tablespoons cilantro, chopped
»

## DIRECTIONS

1. Arrange the asparagus n a lined baking sheet, add the pesto and the other ingredients, toss, bake at 400 degrees F within 20 minutes. Serve as a side dish.

**NUTRITIONS:** Calories 114, Protein 2.6g, Carbohydrates 4.5g, Fat 10.7g, Fiber 2.4g, Sodium 3mg, Potassium 240mg

# 143. LIME CARROTS

**COOKING: 30'**       **PREPARATION: 10'**       **SERVINGS: 4**

## INGREDIENTS

» 1 pound baby carrots, trimmed
» 1 tablespoon sweet paprika
» 1 teaspoon lime juice
» 3 tablespoons olive oil
» A pinch of black pepper
» 1 teaspoon sesame seeds

## DIRECTIONS

1. Arrange the carrots on a lined baking sheet, add the paprika and the other ingredients except for the sesame seeds, toss, bake at 400 degrees F within 30 minutes. Divide the carrots between plates, sprinkle sesame seeds on top and serve as a side dish.

**NUTRITIONS:** Calories 139, Protein 1.1g, Carbohydrates 10.5g, Fat 11.2g, 4g fiber, Sodium 89mg, Potassium 313mg

# 144. GARLIC POTATO PAN

**COOKING: 1H**     **PREPARATION: 10'**     **SERVINGS: 8**

## INGREDIENTS

- » 1-pound gold potatoes, peeled and cut into wedges
- » 2 tablespoons olive oil
- » 1 red onion, chopped
- » 2 garlic cloves, minced
- » 2 cups coconut cream
- » 1 tablespoon thyme, chopped
- » ¼ teaspoon nutmeg, ground
- » ½ cup low-fat parmesan, grated

## DIRECTIONS

1. Warm-up a pan with the oil over medium heat, put the onion plus the garlic, and sauté for 5 minutes. Add the potatoes and brown them for 5 minutes more.

2. Add the cream and the rest of the ingredients, toss gently, bring to a simmer and cook over medium heat within 40 minutes more. Divide the mix between plates and serve as a side dish.

**NUTRITIONS:** Calories 230, Protein 3.6g, Carbohydrates 14.3g, Fat 19.1g, Fiber 3.3g, Cholesterol 6mg, Sodium 105mg, Potassium 426mg

# 145. BALSAMIC CABBAGE

**COOKING: 20'**     **PREPARATION: 10'**     **SERVINGS: 4**

## INGREDIENTS

- » 1-pound green cabbage, roughly shredded
- » 2 tablespoons olive oil
- » A pinch of black pepper
- » 1 shallot, chopped
- » 2 garlic cloves, minced
- » 2 tablespoons balsamic vinegar
- » 2 teaspoons hot paprika
- » 1 teaspoon sesame seeds

## DIRECTIONS

1. Heat-up a pan with the oil over medium heat, add the shallot and the garlic, and sauté for 5 minutes. Add the cabbage and the other ingredients, toss, cook over medium heat for 15 minutes, divide between plates and serve.

**NUTRITIONS:** Calories 100, Protein 1.8g, Carbohydrates 8.2g, Fat 7.5g, Fiber 3g, Sodium 22mg, Potassium 225mg

# 146. CHILI BROCCOLI

**COOKING: 30'**          **PREPARATION: 10'**          **SERVINGS: 4**

## INGREDIENTS

- » 2 tablespoons olive oil
- » 1-pound broccoli florets
- » 2 garlic cloves, minced
- » 2 tablespoons chili sauce
- » 1 tablespoon lemon juice
- » A pinch of black pepper
- » 2 tablespoons cilantro, chopped

## DIRECTIONS

1. In a baking pan, combine the broccoli with the oil, garlic, and the other, toss a bit, and bake at 400 degrees F for 30 minutes. Divide the mix between plates and serve as a side dish.

**NUTRITIONS:** Calories 103, Protein 3.4g, Carbohydrates 8.3gz, 7.4g fat, 3g fiber, Sodium 229mg, Potassium 383mg

# 147. HOT BRUSSELS SPROUTS

**COOKING: 25'**          **PREPARATION: 10'**          **SERVINGS: 4**

## INGREDIENTS

- » 1 tablespoon olive oil
- » 1-pound Brussels sprouts, trimmed and halved
- » 2 garlic cloves, minced
- » ½ cup low-fat mozzarella, shredded
- » A pinch of pepper flakes, crushed

## DIRECTIONS

1. In a baking dish, combine the sprouts with the oil and the other ingredients except for the cheese and toss. Sprinkle the cheese on top, introduce in the oven and bake at 400 degrees F for 25 minutes. Divide between plates and serve as a side dish.

**NUTRITIONS:** Calories 111, Protein 10g, Carbohydrates 11.6g, Fat 3.9g, Fiber 5g, Cholesterol 4mg, Sodium 209mg, Potassium 447mg

# 148. PAPRIKA BRUSSELS SPROUTS

**COOKING: 25'**     **PREPARATION: 10'**     **SERVINGS: 4**

## INGREDIENTS

» 2 tablespoons olive oil
» 1-pound Brussels sprouts, trimmed and halved
» 3 green onions, chopped
» 2 garlic cloves, minced
» 1 tablespoon balsamic vinegar
» 1 tablespoon sweet paprika
» A pinch of black pepper

## DIRECTIONS

1. In a baking pan, combine the Brussels sprouts with the oil and the other ingredients, toss and bake at 400 degrees F within 25 minutes. Divide the mix between plates and serve.

**NUTRITIONS:** Calories 121, Protein 4.4g, Carbohydrates 12.6g, Fat 7.6g, Fiber 5.2g, Sodium 31mg, Potassium 521mg

# 149. CREAMY CAULIFLOWER MASH

**COOKING: 25'**     **PREPARATION: 10'**     **SERVINGS: 4**

## INGREDIENTS

» 2 pounds cauliflower florets
» ½ cup of coconut milk
» A pinch of black pepper
» ½ cup low-fat sour cream
» 1 tablespoon cilantro, chopped
» 1 tablespoon chives, chopped

## DIRECTIONS

1. Put the cauliflower in a pot, add water to cover, bring to a boil over medium heat, cook for 25 minutes and drain. Mash the cauliflower, add the milk, black pepper, and the cream, whisk well, divide between plates, sprinkle the rest of the ingredients on top, and serve.

**NUTRITIONS:** Calories 188, Protein 6.1g, Carbohydrates 15g, Fat 13.4g, Fiber 6.4g, Cholesterol 13mg, Sodium 88mg, Potassium 811mg

# 150. AVOCADO, TOMATO, AND OLIVES SALAD

**COOKING: 0'**          **PREPARATION: 5'**          **SERVINGS: 4**

## INGREDIENTS

- » 2 tablespoons olive oil
- » 2 avocados, cut into wedges
- » 1 cup kalamata olives, pitted and halved
- » 1 cup tomatoes, cubed
- » 1 tablespoon ginger, grated
- » A pinch of black pepper
- » 2 cups baby arugula
- » 1 tablespoon balsamic vinegar

## DIRECTIONS

1. In a bowl, combine the avocados with the kalamata and the other ingredients, toss and serve as a side dish.

**NUTRITIONS:** Calories 320, Protein 3g, Carbohydrates 13.9g, Fat 30.4g, Fiber 8.7g, Sodium 305mg, Potassium 655mg

# 151. RADISH AND OLIVES SALAD

**COOKING: 0'**          **PREPARATION: 5'**          **SERVINGS: 4**

## INGREDIENTS

- » 2 green onions, sliced
- » 1-pound radishes, cubed
- » 2 tablespoons balsamic vinegar
- » 2 tablespoon olive oil
- » 1 teaspoon chili powder
- » 1 cup black olives, pitted and halved
- » A pinch of black pepper

## DIRECTIONS

1. Mix radishes with the onions and the other ingredients in a large salad bowl, toss, and serve as a side dish.

**NUTRITIONS:** Calories 123, Protein 1.3g, Carbohydrates 6.9g, Fat 10.8g, Fiber 3.3g, Sodium 345mg, Potassium 306mg

# 152. SPINACH AND ENDIVES SALAD

**COOKING: 0'**     **PREPARATION: 5'**     **SERVINGS: 4**

## INGREDIENTS

- » 2 endives, roughly shredded
- » 1 tablespoon dill, chopped
- » ¼ cup lemon juice
- » ¼ cup olive oil
- » 2 cups baby spinach
- » 2 tomatoes, cubed
- » 1 cucumber, sliced
- » ½ cups walnuts, chopped

## DIRECTIONS

1. In a large bowl, combine the endives with the spinach and the other ingredients, toss and serve as a side dish.

**NUTRITIONS:** Calories 238, Protein 5.7g, Carbohydrates 8.4g, Fat 22.3g, Fiber 3.1g, Sodium 24mg, Potassium 506mg

# 153. BASIL OLIVES MIX

**COOKING: 0'**     **PREPARATION: 5'**     **SERVINGS: 4**

## INGREDIENTS

- » 2 tablespoons olive oil
- » 1 tablespoon balsamic vinegar
- » A pinch of black pepper
- » 4 cups corn
- » 2 cups black olives, pitted and halved
- » 1 red onion, chopped
- » ½ cup cherry tomatoes halved
- » 1 tablespoon basil, chopped
- » 1 tablespoon jalapeno, chopped
- » 2 cups romaine lettuce, shredded

## DIRECTIONS

1. Mix the corn with the olives, lettuce, and the other ingredients in a large bowl, toss well, divide between plates and serve as a side dish.

**NUTRITIONS:** Calories 290, Protein 6.2g, Carbohydrates 37.6g, Fat 16.1g, Fiber 7.4g, Sodium 613mg, Potassium 562mg

# 154. ARUGULA SALAD

**COOKING: 0'**     **PREPARATION: 5'**     **SERVINGS: 4**

## INGREDIENTS

- ¼ cup pomegranate seeds
- 5 cups baby arugula
- 6 tablespoons green onions, chopped
- 1 tablespoon balsamic vinegar
- 2 tablespoons olive oil
- 3 tablespoons pine nuts
- ½ shallot, chopped

## DIRECTIONS

1. In a salad bowl, combine the arugula with the pomegranate and the other ingredients, toss and serve.

**NUTRITIONS:** Calories 120, Protein 1.8g, Carbohydrates 4.2g, Fat 11.6g, Fiber 0.9g, Sodium 9mg, Potassium 163mg

# 155. SPANISH RICE

**COOKING: 1H 35'**     **PREPARATION: 15'**     **SERVINGS: 8**

## INGREDIENTS

- Brown rice – 2 cups
- Extra virgin olive oil – .25 cup
- Garlic, minced – 2 cloves
- Onion, diced – 1
- Tomatoes, diced – 2
- Jalapeno, seeded and diced – 1
- Tomato paste – 1 tablespoon
- Cilantro, chopped - .5 cup
- Chicken broth, low-sodium – 2.5 cups

## DIRECTIONS

1. Warm the oven to Fahrenheit 375 degrees. Puree the tomatoes, onion, plus garlic using a blender or food processor. Measure out two cups of this vegetable puree to use and discard the excess.

2. Into a large oven-safe Dutch pan, heat the extra virgin olive oil over medium heat until hot and shimmering. Add in the jalapeno and rice to toast, cooking while occasionally stirring for two to three minutes.

3. Slowly stir the chicken broth into the rice, followed by the vegetable puree and tomato paste. Stir until combine and increase the heat to medium-high until the broth reaches a boil.

4. Cover the Dutch pan with an oven-safe lid, transfer the pot to the preheated oven, and bake within 1 hour and 15 minutes. Remove and stir the cilantro into the rice. Serve.

**NUTRITIONS:** Calories: 265, Sodium: 32mg, Potassium: 322mg, Carbs: 40g, Fat: 3g, Protein: 5g

# 156. SWEET POTATOES AND APPLES

**COOKING: 40'**       **PREPARATION: 15'**       **SERVINGS: 4**

## INGREDIENTS

- » Sweet potatoes, sliced into 1" cubes – 2
- » Apples, cut into 1" cubes – 2
- » Extra virgin olive oil, divided – 3 tablespoons
- » Black pepper, ground - .25 teaspoon
- » Cinnamon, ground – 1 teaspoon
- » Maple syrup – 2 tablespoons

## DIRECTIONS

1. Warm the oven to Fahrenheit 425 degrees and grease a large baking sheet with non-stick cooking spray. Toss the cubed sweet potatoes with two tablespoons of the olive oil and black pepper until coated. Roast the potatoes within twenty minutes, stirring them once halfway through the process.

2. Meanwhile, toss the apples with the remaining tablespoon of olive oil, cinnamon, and maple syrup until evenly coated. After the sweet potatoes have cooked for twenty minutes, add the apples to the baking sheet and toss the sweet potatoes and apples.

3. Return to the oven, then roast it for twenty more minutes, once again giving it a good stir halfway through. Once the potatoes and apples are caramelized from the maple syrup, remove them from the oven and serve hot.

**NUTRITIONS:** Calories: 100, Carbs: 22g, Fat: 0g, Protein: 2g, Sodium: 38mg, Potassium: 341mg

# 157. ROASTED TURNIPS

**COOKING: 30'**       **PREPARATION: 15'**       **SERVINGS: 4**

## INGREDIENTS

- » Turnips, peels, and cut into ½" cubes – 2 cups
- » Black pepper, ground - .25 teaspoon
- » Garlic powder - .5 teaspoon
- » Onion powder - .5 teaspoon
- » Extra virgin olive oil – 1 tablespoon

## DIRECTIONS

1. Warm the oven to Fahrenheit 400 degrees and prepare a large baking sheet, setting it aside. Begin by trimming the top and bottom edges off of the turnips and peeling them if you wish. Slice them into 1/2-inch cubes.

2. Toss the turnips with the extra virgin olive oil and seasonings and then spread them out on the prepared baking sheet. Roast the turnips until tender, stirring them halfway through, about thirty minutes in total.

**NUTRITIONS:** Calories: 50, Carbs: 5g, Fat: 4g, Protein: 1g, Sodium: 44mg, Potassium: 134mg

# 158. NO-MAYO POTATO SALAD

**COOKING: 20'**          **PREPARATION: 15'**          **SERVINGS: 8**

## INGREDIENTS

- Red potatoes – 3 pounds
- Extra virgin olive oil - .5 cup
- White wine vinegar, divided – 5 tablespoons
- Dijon mustard – 2 teaspoons
- Red onion, sliced – 1 cup
- Black pepper, ground - .5 teaspoon
- Basil, fresh, chopped – 2 tablespoons
- Dill weed, fresh, chopped – 2 tablespoons
- Parsley, fresh, chopped – 2 tablespoons

**NUTRITIONS:** Calories: 144, Carbs: 19g, Fat: 7g, Protein: 2g, Sodium: 46mg, Potassium: 814mg

## DIRECTIONS

1. Add the red potatoes to a large pot and cover them with water until the water level is two inches above the potatoes. Put the pot on high heat, then boil potatoes until they are tender when poked with a fork, about fifteen to twenty minutes. Drain off the water.

2. Let the potatoes to cool until they can easily be handled but are still warm, then cut it in half and put them in a large bowl. Stir in three tablespoons of the white wine vinegar, giving the potatoes a good stir so that they can evenly absorb the vinegar.

3. Mix the rest of two tablespoons of vinegar, extra virgin olive oil, Dijon mustard, and black pepper in a small bowl. Add this mixture to the potatoes and give them a good toss to thoroughly coat the potatoes.

4. Toss in the red onion and minced herbs. Serve at room temperature or chilled. Serve immediately or store in the fridge for up to four days.

# 159. ZUCCHINI TOMATO BAKE

**COOKING: 30'**          **PREPARATION: 15'**          **SERVINGS: 4**

## INGREDIENTS

- Grape tomatoes, cut in half – 10 ounces
- Zucchini – 2
- Garlic, minced – 5 cloves
- Italian herb seasoning – 1 teaspoon
- Black pepper, ground - .25 teaspoon
- Parsley, fresh, chopped - .33 cup
- Parmesan cheese, low-sodium, grated - .5 cup

## DIRECTIONS

1. Warm the oven to Fahrenheit 350 degrees and coat a large baking sheet with non stick cooking spray. Mix the tomatoes, zucchini, garlic, Italian herb seasoning, Black pepper, and Parmesan cheese in a bowl.

2. Put the mixture out on the baking sheet and roast until the zucchini for thirty minutes. Remove, and garnish with parsley over the top before serving.

**NUTRITIONS:** Calories: 35, Carbs: 4g, Fat: 2g, Protein: 2g, Sodium: 30mg, Potassium: 649mg

# 160. CREAMY BROCCOLI CHEDDAR RICE

**COOKING: 40'**　　　**PREPARATION: 15'**　　　**SERVINGS: 6**

## INGREDIENTS

- » Brown rice – 1 cup
- » Chicken broth, low-sodium – 2 cups
- » Onion, minced – 1
- » Extra virgin olive oil, divided – 3 tablespoons
- » Garlic, minced – 2 cloves
- » Skim milk - .5 cup
- » Black pepper, ground - .25 teaspoon
- » Broccoli, chopped – 1.5 cups
- » Cheddar cheese, low-sodium, shredded – 1 cup

## DIRECTIONS

1. Put one tablespoon of the extra virgin olive oil in a large pot and sauté the onion plus garlic over medium heat within two minutes.

2. Put the chicken broth in a pot and wait for it to come to a boil before adding in the rice. Simmer the rice over low heat for twenty-five minutes.

3. Stir the skim milk, black pepper, and remaining two tablespoons of olive oil into the rice. Simmer again within five more minutes. Stir in the broccoli and cook the rice for five more minutes, until the broccoli is tender. Stir in the rice and serve while warm.

**NUTRITIONS:** Calories: 200, Carbs: 33g, Fat: 3g, Protein: 10g, Sodium: 50mg, Potassium: 344mg

# 161. SMASHED BRUSSELS SPROUTS

**COOKING: 40'**　　　**PREPARATION: 15'**　　　**SERVINGS: 6**

## INGREDIENTS

- » Brussels sprouts – 2 pounds
- » Garlic, minced – 3 cloves
- » Balsamic vinegar – 3 tablespoons
- » Extra virgin olive oil - .5 cup
- » Black pepper, ground - .5 teaspoon
- » Leek washed and thinly sliced – 1
- » Parmesan cheese, low-sodium, grated - .5 cup

## DIRECTIONS

1. Warm the oven to Fahrenheit 450 degrees and prepare two large baking sheets. Trim the yellow leaves and stems off of the Brussels sprouts and then steam them until tender, about twenty to twenty-five minutes.

2. Mix the garlic, black pepper, balsamic vinegar, and extra virgin olive oil in a large bowl. Add the steamed Brussels sprouts and leeks to the bowl and toss until evenly coated.

3. Spread the Brussels sprouts and leaks divided onto the prepared baking sheets.

4. Use a fork or a glass and press down on each of the Brussels sprouts to create flat patties. Put the Parmesan cheese on top and place the smashed sprouts in the oven for fifteen minutes until crispy. Enjoy hot and fresh from the oven.

**NUTRITIONS:** Calories: 116, Carbs: 11g, Fat: 5g, Protein: 10g, Sodium: 49mg, Potassium: 642mg

# 162. CILANTRO LIME RICE

**COOKING: 40'**     **PREPARATION: 15'**     **SERVINGS: 6**

## INGREDIENTS

- » Brown rice – 1.5 cups
- » Lime juice – 2 tablespoons
- » Lemon juice – 1.5 teaspoons
- » Lime zest - .5 teaspoon
- » Cilantro, chopped - .25 cup
- » Bay leaf – 1
- » Extra virgin olive oil – 1 tablespoon
- » Water

## DIRECTIONS

1. Cook rice and bay leaf in a pot with boiling water. Mix the mixture and allow it to boil for thirty minutes, reducing the heat slightly if need be.

2. Once the rice is tender, drain off the water and return the rice to the pot. Let it sit off of the heat within ten minutes. Remove the bay leaf and use a fork to fluff the rice. Stir the rest of the fixing into the rice and then serve immediately.

**NUTRITIONS:** Calories: 94, Carbs: 15g, Fat: 3g, Protein: 2g, Sodium: 184mg, Potassium: 245mg

# 163. CORN SALAD WITH LIME VINAIGRETTE

**COOKING: 7'**     **PREPARATION: 15'**     **SERVINGS: 6**

## INGREDIENTS

- » Corn kernels, fresh – 4.5 cups
- » Lemon juice – 1 tablespoon
- » Red bell pepper, diced – 1
- » Grape tomatoes halved – 1 cup
- » Cilantro, chopped - .25 cup
- » Green onion, chopped - .25 cup
- » Jalapeno, diced – 1
- » Red onion, thinly sliced - .25
- » Feta cheese - .5 cup
- » Truvia baking blend – 2 tablespoons
- » Extra virgin olive oil – 2 tablespoons
- » Honey - .5 tablespoon
- » Lime juice – 3 tablespoons
- » Black pepper, ground - .125 teaspoon
- » Cayenne pepper, ground - .125 teaspoon
- » Garlic powder - .125 teaspoon
- » Onion powder - .125 teaspoon

## DIRECTIONS

1. To create your lime vinaigrette, add the lime juice, onion powder, garlic powder, black pepper, cayenne pepper, and honey to a bowl. Mix, then slowly add in the extra virgin olive oil while whisking vigorously.

2. Boil a pot of water and add in the lemon juice, Baking Truvia, and corn kernels. Allow the corn to boil for seven minutes until tender. Strain the boiling water and add the corn kernels to a bowl of ice water to stop the cooking process and cool the kernels. Drain off the ice water and reserve the corn.

3. Add the tomatoes, red pepper, jalapeno, green onion, red onion, cilantro, and cooked corn to a large bowl and toss it until the vegetables are well distributed. Add the feta cheese and vinaigrette to the vegetables and then toss until well combined and evenly coated. Serve immediately.

**NUTRITIONS:** Calories: 88, Carbs: 23g, Fat: 0g, Protein: 3g, Sodium: 124mg, Potassium: 508mg

# 164. MEDITERRANEAN CHICKPEA SALAD

**COOKING: 0'**    **PREPARATION: 15'**    **SERVINGS: 6**

## INGREDIENTS

- » Chickpeas, cooked – 4 cups
- » Bell pepper, diced – 2 cups
- » Cucumber, chopped – 1 cup
- » Tomato, chopped – 1 cup
- » Avocado, diced – 1
- » Red wine vinegar – 2.5 tablespoons
- » Lemon juice – 1 tablespoon
- » Extra virgin olive oil – 3 tablespoons
- » Parsley, fresh, chopped – 1 teaspoon
- » Oregano, dried - .5 teaspoon
- » Garlic, minced – 1 teaspoon
- » Dill weed, dried - .25 teaspoon
- » Black pepper, ground - .25 teaspoon

## DIRECTIONS

1. Add the diced vegetables except for the avocado and the chickpeas to a large bowl and toss them. In a separate bowl, whisk the seasonings, lemon juice, red wine vinegar, and extra virgin olive oil to create a vinaigrette. Once combined, pour the mixture over the salad and toss to combine.

2. Place the salad in the fridge and allow it to marinate for at least a couple of hours before serving or up to two days. Immediately before serving the salad, dice the avocado and toss it in.

**NUTRITIONS:** Calories: 120, Carbs: 14g, Fat: 5g, Protein: 4g, Sodium: 15mg, Potassium: 696mg

# 165. ITALIAN ROASTED CABBAGE

**COOKING: 15'**    **PREPARATION: 15'**    **SERVINGS: 8**

## INGREDIENTS

- » Cabbage, sliced into 8 wedges – 1
- » Black pepper, ground – 1.5 teaspoons
- » Extra virgin olive oil - .66 cup
- » Italian herb seasoning – 2 teaspoons
- » Parmesan cheese, low-sodium, grated - .66 cup

## DIRECTIONS

1. Warm the oven to Fahrenheit 425 degrees. Prepare a large lined baking sheet with aluminum foil and then spray it with non-stick cooking spray.

2. Slice your cabbage in half, remove the stem, and then cut each half into four wedges so that you are left with eight wedges in total.

3. Arrange the cabbage wedges on the baking sheet and then drizzle half of the extra virgin olive oil over them. Sprinkle half of the seasonings and Parmesan cheese over the top.

4. Place the baking sheet in the hot oven, allow the cabbage to roast for fifteen minutes, and then flip the wedges. Put the rest of the olive oil over the top and then sprinkle the remaining seasonings and cheese over the top as well.

5. Return the cabbage to the oven and allow it to roast for fifteen more minutes, until tender. Serve fresh and hot.

**NUTRITIONS:** Calories: 17, Carbs: 4g, Fat: 0g, Protein: 1g, Sodium: 27mg, Potassium: 213mg

# 166. TEX-MEX COLE SLAW

**COOKING: 0'**     **PREPARATION: 15'**     **SERVINGS: 12**

## INGREDIENTS

- » Black beans, cooked – 2 cups
- » Grape tomatoes, sliced in half – 1.5 cups
- » Grilled corn kernels – 1.5 cups
- » Jalapeno, seeded and minced – 1
- » Cilantro, chopped – .5 cup
- » Bell pepper, diced – 1
- » Coleslaw cabbage mix – 16 ounces
- » Lime juice – 3 tablespoons
- » Light sour cream - .66 cup
- » Olive oil mayonnaise, reduced-fat – 1 cup
- » Chili powder – 1 tablespoon
- » Cumin, ground – 1 teaspoon
- » Onion powder – 1 teaspoon
- » Garlic powder – 1 teaspoon

## DIRECTIONS

1. Mix the sour cream, mayonnaise, lime juice, garlic powder, onion powder, cumin, and chili powder in a bowl to create the dressing.

2. In a large bowl, toss the vegetables and then add in the prepared dressing and toss again until evenly coated. Chill the mixture in the fridge for thirty minutes to twelve hours before serving.

**NUTRITIONS:** Calories: 50, Carbs: 10g, Fat: 1g, Protein: 3g, Sodium: 194mg, Potassium: 345mg

# 167. ROASTED OKRA

**COOKING: 20'**     **PREPARATION: 15'**     **SERVINGS: 4**

## INGREDIENTS

- » Okra, fresh – 1 pound
- » Extra virgin olive oil – 2 tablespoons
- » Cayenne pepper, ground - .125 teaspoon
- » Paprika – 1 teaspoon
- » Garlic powder - .25 teaspoon

## DIRECTIONS

1. Warm the oven to Fahrenheit 450 degrees and prepare a large baking sheet. Cut the okra into pieces appropriate 1/2-inch in size.

2. Place the okra on the baking pan and top it with the olive oil and seasonings, giving it a good toss until evenly coated. Roast the okra in the heated oven until it is tender and lightly browned and seared. Serve immediately while hot.

**NUTRITIONS:** Calories: 65, Carbs: 6g, Fat: 5g, Protein: 2g, Sodium: 9mg, Potassium: 356mg

# 168. BROWN SUGAR GLAZED CARROTS

**COOKING: 25'**      **PREPARATION: 15'**      **SERVINGS: 6**

## INGREDIENTS

- » Carrots, sliced into 1-inch pieces – 2 pounds
- » Light olive oil - .33 cup
- » Truvia Brown Sugar Blend - .25 cup
- » Black pepper, ground - .25 teaspoon

## DIRECTIONS

1. Warm the oven to Fahrenheit 400 degrees and prepare a large baking sheet. Toss the carrots with the oil, Truvia, and black pepper until evenly coated and then spread them out on the prepared baking sheet.

2. Place the carrots in the oven and allow them to roast until tender, about twenty to twenty-five minutes. Halfway through the cooking time, give the carrots a good serve. Remove the carrots from the oven and serve them alone or topped with fresh parsley.

**NUTRITIONS:** Calories: 110, Carbs: 16g, Fat: 4g, Protein: 1g, Sodium: 105mg, Potassium: 486mg

# 169. OVEN-ROASTED BEETS WITH HONEY RICOTTA

**COOKING: 40'**      **PREPARATION: 15'**      **SERVINGS: 6**

## INGREDIENTS

- » Purple beets – 1 pound
- » Golden beets – 1 pound
- » Ricotta cheese, low-fat - .5 cup
- » Extra virgin olive oil – 3 tablespoons
- » Honey – 1 tablespoon
- » Rosemary, fresh, chopped – 1 teaspoon
- » Black pepper, ground - .25 teaspoon

## DIRECTIONS

1. Warm the oven to Fahrenheit 375 degrees and prepare a large baking sheet by lining it with kitchen parchment. Slice the beets into 1/2-inch cubes before tossing them with the extra virgin olive oil and black pepper.

2. Put the beets on the prepared baking sheet and allow them to roast until tender, about thirty-five to forty minutes. Halfway through the cooking process, flip the beets over.

3. Meanwhile, in a small bowl, whisk the ricotta with the rosemary and honey. Fridge until ready to serve. Once the beets are done cooking, serve them topped with the ricotta mixture, and enjoy.

**NUTRITIONS:** Calories: 195, Carbs: 24g, Fat: 8g, Protein: 8g, Sodium: 139mg, Potassium: 521mg

# 170. EASY CARROTS MIX

**COOKING: 40'**        **PREPARATION: 10'**        **SERVINGS: 6**

## INGREDIENTS

- » 15 carrots, halved lengthwise
- » 2 tablespoons coconut sugar
- » ¼ cup olive oil
- » ½ teaspoon rosemary, dried
- » ½ teaspoon garlic powder
- » A pinch of black pepper

## DIRECTIONS

1. In a bowl, combine the carrots with the sugar, oil, rosemary, garlic powder, and black pepper, toss well, spread on a lined baking sheet, introduce in the oven and bake at 400 degrees F for 40 minutes. Serve.

**NUTRITIONS:** Calories: 60, Carbs: 9g, Fat: 0g, Protein: 2g, Sodium: 0 mg

# 171. TASTY GRILLED ASPARAGUS

**COOKING: 6'**        **PREPARATION: 10'**        **SERVINGS: 4**

## INGREDIENTS

- » 2 pounds asparagus, trimmed
- » 2 tablespoons olive oil
- » A pinch of salt and black pepper

## DIRECTIONS

1. In a bowl, combine the asparagus with salt, pepper, and oil and toss well. Place the asparagus on a preheated grill over medium-high heat, cook for 3 minutes on each side, then serve.

**NUTRITIONS:** Calories: 50, Carbs: 8g, Fat: 1g, Protein: 5g, Sodium: 420 mg

# 172. ROASTED CARROTS

**COOKING: 30'**          **PREPARATION: 10'**          **SERVINGS: 4**

## INGREDIENTS

- » 2 pounds carrots, quartered
- » A pinch of black pepper
- » 3 tablespoons olive oil
- » 2 tablespoons parsley, chopped

## DIRECTIONS

1. Arrange the carrots on a lined baking sheet, add black pepper and oil, toss, introduce in the oven, and cook within 30 minutes at 400 degrees F. Add parsley, toss, divide between plates and serve as a side dish.

**NUTRITIONS:** Calories: 89, Carbs: 10g, Fat: 6g, Protein: 1g, Sodium: 0 mg

# 173. OVEN ROASTED ASPARAGUS

**COOKING: 25'**          **PREPARATION: 10'**          **SERVINGS: 4**

## INGREDIENTS

- » 2 pounds asparagus spears, trimmed
- » 3 tablespoons olive oil
- » A pinch of black pepper
- » 2 teaspoons sweet paprika
- » 1 teaspoon sesame seeds

## DIRECTIONS

1. Arrange the asparagus on a lined baking sheet, add oil, black pepper, and paprika, toss, introduce in the oven and bake within 25 minutes at 400 degrees F. Divide the asparagus between plates, sprinkle sesame seeds on top, and serve as a side dish.

**NUTRITIONS:** Calories: 45, Carbs: 5g, Fat: 2g, Protein: 2g, Sodium: 0 mg

# 174. BAKED POTATO WITH THYME

**COOKING: 1H 15'**    **PREPARATION: 10'**    **SERVINGS: 8**

## INGREDIENTS

- » 6 potatoes, peeled and sliced
- » 2 garlic cloves, minced
- » 2 tablespoons olive oil
- » 1 and ½ cups of coconut cream
- » ¼ cup of coconut milk
- » 1 tablespoon thyme, chopped
- » ¼ teaspoon nutmeg, ground
- » A pinch of red pepper flakes
- » 1 and ½ cups low-fat cheddar, shredded
- » ½ cup low-fat parmesan, grated

## DIRECTIONS

1. Heat-up a pan with the oil over medium heat, add garlic, stir and cook for 1 minute. Add coconut cream, coconut milk, thyme, nutmeg, and pepper flakes, stir, bring to a simmer, adjust to low and cook within 10 minutes.

2. Put one-third of the potatoes in a baking dish, add 1/3 of the cream, repeat the process with the remaining potatoes and the cream, sprinkle the cheddar on top, cover with tin foil, introduce in the oven and cook at 375 degrees F for 45 minutes. Uncover the dish, sprinkle the parmesan, bake everything for 20 minutes, divide between plates, and serve as a side dish.

**NUTRITIONS:** Calories: 132, Carbs: 21g, Fat: 4g, Protein: 2g, Sodium: 56 mg

# 175. SPICY BRUSSELS SPROUTS

**COOKING: 20'**    **PREPARATION: 10'**    **SERVINGS: 6**

## INGREDIENTS

- » 2 pounds Brussels sprouts, halved
- » 2 tablespoons olive oil
- » A pinch of black pepper
- » 1 tablespoon sesame oil
- » 2 garlic cloves, minced
- » ½ cup coconut aminos
- » 2 teaspoons apple cider vinegar
- » 1 tablespoon coconut sugar
- » 2 teaspoons chili sauce
- » A pinch of red pepper flakes
- » Sesame seeds for serving

## DIRECTIONS

1. Spread the sprouts on a lined baking dish, add the olive oil, the sesame oil, black pepper, garlic, aminos, vinegar, coconut sugar, chili sauce, and pepper flakes, toss well, introduce in the oven and bake within 20 minutes at 425 degrees F. Divide the sprouts between plates, sprinkle sesame seeds on top and serve as a side dish.

**NUTRITIONS:** Calories: 64, Carbs: 13g, Fat: 0g, Protein: 4g, Sodium: 314 mg

# 176. BAKED CAULIFLOWER WITH CHILI

**COOKING: 30'**          **PREPARATION: 10'**          **SERVINGS: 4**

## INGREDIENTS

- » 3 tablespoons olive oil
- » 2 tablespoons chili sauce
- » Juice of 1 lime
- » 3 garlic cloves, minced
- » 1 cauliflower head, florets separated
- » A pinch of black pepper
- » 1 teaspoon cilantro, chopped

## DIRECTIONS

1. In a bowl, combine the oil with the chili sauce, lime juice, garlic, and black pepper and whisk. Add cauliflower florets, toss, spread on a lined baking sheet, introduce in the oven and bake at 425 degrees F for 30 minutes. Divide the cauliflower between plates, sprinkle cilantro on top, and serve as a side dish.

**NUTRITIONS:** Calories: 31, Carbs: 3g, Fat: 0g, Protein: 3g, Sodium: 4 mg

# 177. BAKED BROCCOLI

**COOKING: 15'**          **PREPARATION: 10'**          **SERVINGS: 4**

## INGREDIENTS

- » 1 tablespoon olive oil
- » 1 broccoli head, florets separated
- » 2 garlic cloves, minced
- » ½ cup coconut cream
- » ½ cup low-fat mozzarella, shredded
- » ¼ cup low-fat parmesan, grated
- » A pinch of pepper flakes, crushed

## DIRECTIONS

1. In a baking dish, combine the broccoli with oil, garlic, cream, pepper flakes, mozzarella, and toss. Sprinkle the parmesan on top, introduce in the oven and bake at 375 degrees F for 15 minutes. Serve.

**NUTRITIONS:** Calories: 90, Carbs: 6g, Fat: 7g, Protein: 3g, Sodium: 30 mg

# 178. SLOW COOKED POTATOES WITH CHEDDAR

**COOKING: 6 H**          **PREPARATION: 10'**          **SERVINGS: 6**

## INGREDIENTS

- » Cooking spray
- » 2 pounds baby potatoes, quartered
- » 3 cups low-fat cheddar cheese, shredded
- » 2 garlic cloves, minced
- » 8 bacon slices, cooked and chopped
- » ¼ cup green onions, chopped
- » 1 tablespoon sweet paprika
- » A pinch of black pepper

## DIRECTIONS

1. Spray a slow cooker with the cooking spray, add baby potatoes, cheddar, garlic, bacon, green onions, paprika, and black pepper, toss, cover, and cook on High for 6 hours. Serve.

**NUTRITIONS:** Calories: 112, Carbs: 26g, Fat: 4g, Protein: 8g, Sodium: 234 mg

# 179. SQUASH SALAD WITH ORANGE

**COOKING: 30'**          **PREPARATION: 10'**          **SERVINGS: 6**

## INGREDIENTS

- » 1 cup of orange juice
- » 3 tablespoons coconut sugar
- » 1 and ½ tablespoons mustard
- » 1 tablespoon ginger, grated
- » 1 and ½ pounds butternut squash, peeled and roughly cubed
- » Cooking spray
- » A pinch of black pepper
- » 1/3 cup olive oil
- » 6 cups salad greens
- » 1 radicchio, sliced
- » ½ cup pistachios, roasted

## DIRECTIONS

1. Mix the orange juice with the sugar, mustard, ginger, black pepper, squash in a bowl, toss well, spread on a lined baking sheet, spray everything with cooking oil, and bake for 30 minutes 400 degrees F.

2. In a salad bowl, combine the squash with salad greens, radicchio, pistachios, and oil, toss well, then serve.

**NUTRITIONS:** Calories: 17, Carbs: 2g, Fat: 0g, Protein: 0g, Sodium: 0 mg

# 180. COLORED ICEBERG SALAD

**COOKING: 0'**     **PREPARATION: 10'**     **SERVINGS: 4**

## INGREDIENTS

- » 1 iceberg lettuce head, leaves torn
- » 6 bacon slices, cooked and halved
- » 2 green onions, sliced
- » 3 carrots, shredded
- » 6 radishes, sliced
- » ¼ cup red vinegar
- » ¼ cup olive oil
- » 3 garlic cloves, minced
- » A pinch of black pepper

## DIRECTIONS

1. Mix the lettuce leaves with the bacon, green onions, carrots, radishes, vinegar, oil, garlic, and black pepper in a large salad bowl, toss, divide between plates and serve as a side dish.

**NUTRITIONS:** Calories: 15, Carbs: 3g, Fat: 0g, Protein: 1g, Sodium: 15 mg

# 181. FENNEL SALAD WITH ARUGULA

**COOKING: 0'**     **PREPARATION: 10'**     **SERVINGS: 4**

## INGREDIENTS

- » 2 fennel bulbs, trimmed and shaved
- » 1 and ¼ cups zucchini, sliced
- » 2/3 cup dill, chopped
- » ¼ cup lemon juice
- » ¼ cup olive oil
- » 6 cups arugula
- » ½ cups walnuts, chopped
- » 1/3 cup low-fat feta cheese, crumbled

## DIRECTIONS

1. Mix the fennel with the zucchini, dill, lemon juice, arugula, oil, walnuts, and cheese in a large bowl, toss, then serve.

**NUTRITIONS:** Calories: 65, Carbs: 6g, Fat: 5g, Protein: 1g, Sodium: 140 mg

# 182. CORN MIX

**COOKING: 0'**     **PREPARATION: 10'**     **SERVINGS: 4**

## INGREDIENTS

- » ½ cup cider vinegar
- » ¼ cup of coconut sugar
- » A pinch of black pepper
- » 4 cups corn
- » ½ cup red onion, chopped
- » ½ cup cucumber, sliced
- » ½ cup red bell pepper, chopped
- » ½ cup cherry tomatoes halved
- » 3 tablespoons parsley, chopped
- » 1 tablespoon basil, chopped
- » 1 tablespoon jalapeno, chopped
- » 2 cups baby arugula leaves

## DIRECTIONS

1. Mix the corn with onion, cucumber, bell pepper, cherry tomatoes, parsley, basil, jalapeno, and arugula in a large bowl. Add vinegar, sugar, and black pepper, toss well, divide between plates and serve as a side dish.

**NUTRITIONS:** Calories: 110, Carbs: 25g, Fat: 0g, Protein: 2g, Sodium: 120 mg

# 183. PERSIMMON SALAD

**COOKING: 0'**     **PREPARATION: 10'**     **SERVINGS: 4**

## INGREDIENTS

- » Seeds from 1 pomegranate
- » 2 persimmons, cored and sliced
- » 5 cups baby arugula
- » 6 tablespoons green onions, chopped
- » 4 navel oranges, cut into segments
- » ¼ cup white vinegar
- » 1/3 cup olive oil
- » 3 tablespoons pine nuts
- » 1 and ½ teaspoons orange zest, grated
- » 2 tablespoons orange juice
- » 1 tablespoon coconut sugar
- » ½ shallot, chopped
- » A pinch of cinnamon powder

## DIRECTIONS

1. In a salad bowl, combine the pomegranate seeds with persimmons, arugula, green onions, and oranges and toss. In another bowl, combine the vinegar with the oil, pine nuts, orange zest, orange juice, sugar, shallot, and cinnamon, whisk well, add to the salad, toss and serve as a side dish.

**NUTRITIONS:** Calories: 310, Carbs: 33g, Fat: 16g, Protein: 7g, Sodium: 320 mg

# 184. AVOCADO SIDE SALAD

**COOKING: 0'**  **PREPARATION: 10'**  **SERVINGS: 4**

## INGREDIENTS

- » 4 blood oranges, slice into segments
- » 2 tablespoons olive oil
- » A pinch of red pepper, crushed
- » 2 avocados, peeled, cut into wedges
- » 1 and ½ cups baby arugula
- » ¼ cup almonds, toasted and chopped
- » 1 tablespoon lemon juice

## DIRECTIONS

1. Mix the oranges with the oil, red pepper, avocados, arugula, almonds, and lemon juice in a bowl, then serve.

**NUTRITIONS:** Calories: 146, Carbs: 8g, Fat: 7g, Protein: 15g, Sodium: 320 mg

# 185. SPICED BROCCOLI FLORETS

**COOKING: 3H**  **PREPARATION: 10'**  **SERVINGS: 10**

## INGREDIENTS

- » 6 cups broccoli florets
- » 1 and ½ cups low-fat cheddar cheese, shredded
- » ½ teaspoon cider vinegar
- » ¼ cup yellow onion, chopped
- » 10 ounces tomato sauce, sodium-free
- » 2 tablespoons olive oil
- » A pinch of black pepper

## DIRECTIONS

1. Grease your slow cooker with the oil, add broccoli, tomato sauce, cider vinegar, onion, and black pepper, cook on High within 2 hours, and 30 minutes. Sprinkle the cheese all over, cover, cook on High for 30 minutes more, divide between plates, and serve as a side dish.

**NUTRITIONS:** Calories 119, Fat 8.7g, Sodium 272mg, Carbohydrate 5.7g, Fiber 1.9g, Sugars 2.3g, Protein 6.2g

# 186. LIMA BEANS DISH

**COOKING: 5 H**  **PREPARATION: 10'**  **SERVINGS: 10**

## INGREDIENTS

- » 1 green bell pepper, chopped
- » 1 sweet red pepper, chopped
- » 1 and ½ cups tomato sauce, salt-free
- » 1 yellow onion, chopped
- » ½ cup of water
- » 16 ounces canned kidney beans, no-salt-added, drained and rinsed
- » 16 ounces canned black-eyed peas, no-salt-added, drained and rinsed
- » 15 ounces corn
- » 15 ounces canned lima beans, no-salt-added, drained and rinsed
- » 15 oz canned black beans, no-salt-added, drained
- » 2 celery ribs, chopped
- » 2 bay leaves
- » 1 teaspoon ground mustard
- » 1 tablespoon cider vinegar

## DIRECTIONS

1. In your slow cooker, mix the tomato sauce with the onion, celery, red pepper, green bell pepper, water, bay leaves, mustard, vinegar, kidney beans, black-eyed peas, corn, lima beans, and black beans, cook on Low within 5 hours. Discard bay leaves, divide the whole mix between plates, and serve.

**NUTRITIONS:** Calories 602, Fat 4.8g, Sodium 255mg, Carbohydrate 117.7g, Fiber 24.6g, Sugars 13.4g, Protein 33g

# 187. SOY SAUCE GREEN BEANS

**COOKING: 2H**  **PREPARATION: 10'**  **SERVINGS: 12**

## INGREDIENTS

- » 3 tablespoons olive oil
- » 16 ounces green beans
- » ½ teaspoon garlic powder
- » ½ cup of coconut sugar
- » 1 teaspoon low-sodium soy sauce

## DIRECTIONS

1. In your slow cooker, mix the green beans with the oil, sugar, soy sauce, and garlic powder, cover, and cook on Low for 2 hours. Toss the beans, divide them between plates, and serve as a side dish.

**NUTRITIONS:** Calories 46, Fat 3.6g, Sodium 29mg, Carbohydrate 3.6g, Fiber 1.3g, Sugars 0.6g, Protein 0.8g

# 188. BUTTER CORN

**COOKING: 4 H**　　　**PREPARATION: 10'**　　　**SERVINGS: 12**

## INGREDIENTS

- » 20 ounces fat-free cream cheese
- » 10 cups corn
- » ½ cup low-fat butter
- » ½ cup fat-free milk
- » A pinch of black pepper
- » 2 tablespoons green onions, chopped

## DIRECTIONS

1. In your slow cooker, mix the corn with cream cheese, milk, butter, black pepper, and onions, cook on Low within 4 hours. Toss one more time, divide between plates and serve as a side dish.

**NUTRITIONS:** Calories 279, Fat 18g, Cholesterol 52mg, Sodium 165mg, Carbohydrate 26g, Fiber 3.5g, Sugars 4.8g, Protein 8.1g

# 189. STEVIA PEAS WITH MARJORAM

**COOKING: 5H**　　　**PREPARATION: 10'**　　　**SERVINGS: 12**

## INGREDIENTS

- » 1-pound carrots, sliced
- » 1 yellow onion, chopped
- » 16 ounces peas
- » 2 tablespoons stevia
- » 2 tablespoons olive oil
- » 4 garlic cloves, minced
- » ¼ cup of water
- » 1 teaspoon marjoram, dried
- » A pinch of white pepper

## DIRECTIONS

1. In your slow cooker, mix the carrots with water, onion, oil, stevia, garlic, marjoram, white pepper, peas, toss, cover, and cook on High for 5 hours. Divide between plates and serve as a side dish.

**NUTRITIONS:** Calories 71, Fat 2.5g, Sodium 29mg, Carbohydrate 12.1g, Fiber 3.1g, Sugars 4.4g, Protein 2.5g, Potassium 231mg

# 190. PILAF WITH BELLA MUSHROOMS

**COOKING: 3H**       **PREPARATION: 10'**       **SERVINGS: 6**

## INGREDIENTS

- » 1 cup wild rice
- » 6 green onions, chopped
- » ½ pound baby Bella mushrooms
- » 2 cups of water
- » 2 tablespoons olive oil
- » 2 garlic cloves, minced

## DIRECTIONS

1. In your slow cooker, mix the rice with garlic, onions, oil, mushrooms, water, toss, cover, and cook on Low for 3 hours. Stir the pilaf one more time, divide between plates and serve.

**NUTRITIONS:** Calories 151, Fat 5.1g, Sodium 9mg, Carbohydrate 23.3g, Fiber 2.6g, Sugars 1.7g, Protein 5.2g

# 191. PARSLEY FENNEL

**COOKING: 2H 30'**       **PREPARATION: 10'**       **SERVINGS: 4**

## INGREDIENTS

- » 2 fennel bulbs, sliced
- » Juice and zest of 1 lime
- » 2 teaspoons avocado oil
- » ½ teaspoon turmeric powder
- » 1 tablespoon parsley, chopped
- » ¼ cup veggie stock, low-sodium

## DIRECTIONS

1. In a slow cooker, combine the fennel with the lime juice, zest, and the other ingredients, cook on Low within 2 hours and 30 minutes. Serve.

**NUTRITIONS:** Calories 47, Fat 0.6g, Sodium 71mg, Carbohydrate 10.8g, Protein 1.7g

# 192. SWEET BUTTERNUT

**COOKING: 4H**       **PREPARATION: 10'**       **SERVINGS: 8**

## INGREDIENTS

- » 1 cup carrots, chopped
- » 1 tablespoon olive oil
- » 1 yellow onion, chopped
- » ½ teaspoon stevia
- » 1 garlic clove, minced
- » ½ teaspoon curry powder
- » 1 butternut squash, cubed
- » 2 and ½ cups low-sodium veggie stock
- » ½ cup basmati rice
- » ¾ cup of coconut milk
- » ½ teaspoon cinnamon powder
- » ¼ teaspoon ginger, grated

## DIRECTIONS

1. Heat-up, a pan with the oil over medium-high heat, add the oil, onion, garlic, stevia, carrots, curry powder, cinnamon, ginger, stir, and cook 5 minutes and transfer to your slow cooker.

2. Add squash, stock, and coconut milk, stir, cover, and cook on Low for 4 hours. Divide the butternut mix between plates and serve as a side dish.

**NUTRITIONS:** Calories 134, Fat 7.2g, Sodium 59mg, Carbohydrate 16.5g, Fiber 1.7g, Sugars 2.7g, Protein 1.8g

# 193. MUSHROOM SAUSAGES

**COOKING: 10'**       **PREPARATION: 2H**       **SERVINGS: 12**

## INGREDIENTS

- » 6 celery ribs, chopped
- » 1 pound no-sugar, beef sausage, chopped
- » 2 tablespoons olive oil
- » ½ pound mushrooms, chopped
- » ½ cup sunflower seeds, peeled
- » 1 cup low-sodium veggie stock
- » 1 cup cranberries, dried
- » 2 yellow onions, chopped
- » 2 garlic cloves, minced
- » 1 tablespoon sage, dried
- » 1 whole-wheat bread loaf, cubed

## DIRECTIONS

1. Heat-up a pan with the oil over medium-high heat, add beef, stir and brown for a few minutes. Add mushrooms, onion, celery, garlic, and sage, stir, cook for a few more minutes and transfer to your slow cooker.

2. Add stock, cranberries, sunflower seeds, and the bread cubes; cover and cook on High for 2 hours. Stir the whole mix, divide between plates and serve as a side dish.

**NUTRITIONS:** Calories 188, Fat 13.8g, Sodium 489mg, Carbohydrate 8.2g, Fiber 1.9g, Protein 7.6g

# 194. PARSLEY RED POTATOES

**COOKING: 6H**　　　**PREPARATION: 10'**　　　**SERVINGS: 8**

## INGREDIENTS

- » 16 baby red potatoes, halved
- » 2 cups low-sodium chicken stock
- » 1 carrot, sliced
- » 1 celery rib, chopped
- » ¼ cup yellow onion, chopped
- » 1 tablespoon parsley, chopped
- » 2 tablespoons olive oil
- » A pinch of black pepper
- » 1 garlic clove minced

## DIRECTIONS

1. In your slow cooker, mix the potatoes with the carrot, celery, onion, stock, parsley, garlic, oil, and black pepper, toss, cover, and cook on Low for 6 hours. Serve.

**NUTRITIONS:** Calories 257, Fat 9.5g, Sodium 845mg, Carbohydrate 43.4g, Protein 4.4g

# 195. JALAPENO BLACK-EYED PEAS MIX

**COOKING: 5H**　　　**PREPARATION: 10'**　　　**SERVINGS: 12**

## INGREDIENTS

- » 17 ounces black-eyed peas
- » 1 sweet red pepper, chopped
- » ½ cup sausage, chopped
- » 1 yellow onion, chopped
- » 1 jalapeno, chopped
- » 2 garlic cloves minced
- » 6 cups of water
- » ½ teaspoon cumin, ground
- » A pinch of black pepper
- » 2 tablespoons cilantro, chopped

## DIRECTIONS

1. In your slow cooker, mix the peas with the sausage, onion, red pepper, jalapeno, garlic, cumin, black pepper, water, cilantro, cover, and cook low for 5 hours. Serve.

**NUTRITIONS:** Calories 75, Fat 3.5g, Sodium 94mg, Carbohydrate 7.2g, Fiber 1.7g, Sugars 0.9g, Protein 4.3g

# 196. SOUR CREAM GREEN BEANS

**COOKING: 4H** | **PREPARATION: 10'** | **SERVINGS: 8**

## INGREDIENTS

- » 15 ounces green beans
- » 14 ounces corn
- » 4 ounces mushrooms, sliced
- » 11 ounces cream of mushroom soup, low-fat and sodium-free
- » ½ cup low-fat sour cream
- » ½ cup almonds, chopped
- » ½ cup low-fat cheddar cheese, shredded

## DIRECTIONS

1. In your slow cooker, mix the green beans with the corn, mushrooms soup, mushrooms, almonds, cheese, sour cream, toss, cover, and cook on Low for 4 hours. Stir one more time, divide between plates and serve as a side dish.

**NUTRITIONS:** Calories 360, Fat 12.7g, Sodium 220mg, Carbohydrate 58.3g, Fiber 10g, Sugars 10.3g, Protein 14g

# 197. CUMIN BRUSSELS SPROUTS

**COOKING: 3H** | **PREPARATION: 10'** | **SERVINGS: 4**

## INGREDIENTS

- » 1 cup low-sodium veggie stock
- » 1-pound Brussels sprouts, trimmed and halved
- » 1 teaspoon rosemary, dried
- » 1 teaspoon cumin, ground
- » 1 tablespoon mint, chopped

## DIRECTIONS

1. In your slow cooker, combine the sprouts with the stock and the other ingredients, cook on Low within 3 hours. Serve.

**NUTRITIONS:** Calories 56, Fat 0.6g, Sodium 65mg, Carbohydrate 11.4g, Fiber 4.5g, Sugars 2.7g, Protein 4g

# 198. PEACH AND CARROTS

**COOKING: 6 H**          **PREPARATION: 10'**          **SERVINGS: 6**

## INGREDIENTS

- » 2 pounds small carrots, peeled
- » ½ cup low-fat butter, melted
- » ½ cup canned peach, unsweetened
- » 2 tablespoons cornstarch
- » 3 tablespoons stevia
- » 2 tablespoons water
- » ½ teaspoon cinnamon powder
- » 1 teaspoon vanilla extract
- » A pinch of nutmeg, ground

## DIRECTIONS

1. In your slow cooker, mix the carrots with the butter, peach, stevia, cinnamon, vanilla, nutmeg, and cornstarch mixed with water, toss, cover, and cook on Low for 6 hours. Toss the carrots one more time, divide between plates and serve as a side dish.

**NUTRITIONS:** Calories139, Fat 10.7g, Sodium 199mg, Carbohydrate 35.4g, Fiber 4.2g, Sugars 6.9g, Protein 3.8g

# 199. BABY SPINACH AND GRAINS MIX

**COOKING: 4H**          **PREPARATION: 10'**          **SERVINGS: 12**

## INGREDIENTS

- » 1 butternut squash, peeled and cubed
- » 1 cup whole-grain blend, uncooked
- » 12 ounces low-sodium veggie stock
- » 6 ounces baby spinach
- » 1 yellow onion, chopped
- » 3 garlic cloves, minced
- » ½ cup of water
- » 2 teaspoons thyme, chopped
- » A pinch of black pepper

## DIRECTIONS

1. In your slow cooker, mix the squash with whole grain, onion, garlic, water, thyme, black pepper, stock, spinach, cover, and cook on Low for 4 hours. Serve.

**NUTRITIONS:** Calories78, Fat 0.6g, Sodium 259mg, Carbohydrate 16.4g, Fiber 1.8g, Sugars 2g, Protein 2.5g

# 200. QUINOA CURRY

**COOKING: 4H**  **PREPARATION: 15'**  **SERVINGS: 8**

## INGREDIENTS

- » 1 chopped Sweet Potato
- » 2 cups Green Beans
- » ½ diced onion (white)
- » 1 diced Carrot
- » 15 oz Chick Peas (organic and drained)
- » 28 oz. Tomatoes (diced)
- » 29 oz Coconut Milk
- » 2 minced cloves of garlic
- » ¼ cup Quinoa
- » 1 tbs. Turmeric (ground)
- » 1 tbsp. Ginger (grated)
- » 1 ½ cups Water
- » 1 tsp. of Chili Flakes
- » 2 tsp. of Tamari Sauce

## DIRECTIONS

1. Put all the listed fixing in the slow cooker. Add 1 cup of water. Stir well. Cook on "high" for 4 hrs. Serve with rice.

**NUTRITIONS:** Calories 297, Fat 18 g, Sodium 364 mg, Carbohydrates 9 mg, Protein 28 g

# 201. LEMON AND CILANTRO RICE

**COOKING: 6H**  **PREPARATION: 15'**  **SERVINGS: 4**

## INGREDIENTS

- » 3 cups Vegetable Broth (low sodium)
- » 1 ½ cups Brown Rice (uncooked)
- » Juice of2 lemons
- » 2 tbsp. chopped cilantro

## DIRECTIONS

1. In a slow cooker, place broth and rice. Cook on "low" for 5 hrs. Check the rice for doneness with a fork. Add the lemon juice and cilantro before serving.

**NUTRITIONS:** Calories 56, Fats 0.3 g, Sodium 174 mg, Carbohydrates 12 g, Protein 1 g

# 202. CHILI BEANS

**COOKING: 4H**　　　**PREPARATION: 15'**　　　**SERVINGS: 5**

## INGREDIENTS

- » 1 ½ cup chopped Bell Pepper
- » 1 ½ cup sliced Mushrooms (white)
- » 1 cup chopped Onion
- » 1 tbsp. Olive Oil
- » 1 tbsp. Chili Powder
- » 2 chopped cloves Garlic
- » 1 tsp. chopped Chipotle Chili
- » ½ tsp. Cumin
- » 15.5 oz drained Black Beans
- » 1 cup diced tomatoes (no salt)
- » 2 tbsp. chopped cilantro

## DIRECTIONS

1. Put all the fixing above in the slow cooker. Cook on "high" for 4 hrs. Serve

**NUTRITIONS:** Calories 343, Fat 11 g, Sodium 308 mg, Carbohydrates 9 mg, Protein 29 g

# 203. BEAN SPREAD

**COOKING: 4H**　　　**PREPARATION: 15'**　　　**SERVINGS: 20**

## INGREDIENTS

- » 30 ounces Cannellini Beans
- » ½ cup Broth (chicken or veg)
- » 1 tbsp. Olive Oil
- » 3 minced cloves Garlic
- » ½ tsp. Marjoram
- » ½ tsp. Rosemary
- » 1/8 tsp. Pepper
- » Pita Chips
- » 1 tbsp Olive Oil

## DIRECTIONS

1. Place olive oil, beans, broth, marjoram, garlic, rosemary, and pepper in the slow cooker. Cook on "low" for 4 hrs. Mash the mixture and transfer to a bowl. Serve with Pita.

**NUTRITIONS:** Calories 298, Fat 18 g, Sodium 298 mg, Carbohydrates 30 mg, Protein 19 g

# 204. STIR-FRIED STEAK, SHIITAKE, AND ASPARAGUS

**COOKING: 2H 20'**    **PREPARATION: 15'**    **SERVINGS: 4**

## INGREDIENTS

- » 1 tbsp. Sherry (dry)
- » 1 tbsp. Vinegar (rice)
- » ½ tbsp. Soy Sauce (low sodium)
- » ½ tbsp. Cornstarch
- » 2 tsp. Canola Oil
- » ¼ tsp. Black Pepper (ground)
- » 1 minced clove Garlic
- » ½ lb. sliced Sirloin Steak
- » 3 oz. Shiitake Mushrooms
- » ½ tbsp. minced Ginger
- » 6 oz. sliced Asparagus
- » 3 oz. Peas (sugar snap)
- » 2 sliced scallions
- » ¼ cup Water

## DIRECTIONS

1. Combine cornstarch, soy sauce, sherry vinegar, broth, and pepper. Place the steaks in 1 tsp hot oil in the slow cooker for 2 mins. Transfer the steaks to a plate. Sauté ginger and garlic in the remaining oil. Add in the mushrooms, peas, and asparagus.

2. Add water and cook on "low" for 1 hr. Add the scallions and cook again for 30 mins on low. Change the heat to "high" and add the vinegar. When the sauce has thickened, transfer the steaks to the slow cooker. Stir well and serve immediately.

**NUTRITIONS:** Calories 182, Fats 7 g, Sodium 157 mg, Carbohydrates 10 mg, Protein 20 g

# 205. CHICKPEAS AND CURRIED VEGGIES

**COOKING: 4H**    **PREPARATION: 15'**    **SERVINGS: 2**

## INGREDIENTS

- » ½ tbsp. Canola Oil
- » 2 sliced Celery Ribs
- » 1/8 tsp. Cayenne Pepper
- » ¼ cup Water
- » 2 sliced Carrots
- » 2 sliced red Potatoes (sliced)
- » ½ tbsp. Curry Powder
- » ½ cup of Coconut Milk (light)
- » ¼ cup drained Chickpeas (low sodium)
- » Chopped Cilantro
- » ¼ cup Yogurt (low fat)

## DIRECTIONS

1. Sauté potatoes for 5 mins in oil. Add the carrots, celery, and onion. Sauté for 5 more mins. Sprinkle on the curry powder and cayenne pepper. Stir well to combine.

2. In a slow cooker, pour water and coconut milk. Add in the potatoes. Cook on "low" for 3 hrs. Add chickpeas and cook for 30 more mins. Serve in bowls along with the yogurt and cilantro garnish.

**NUTRITIONS:** Calories 271, Fats 11 g, Sodium 207 mg, Carbohydrates 39 g, Protein 7 g

# 206. BRUSSELS SPROUTS CASSEROLE

**COOKING: 4H 15'**       **PREPARATION: 15'**       **SERVINGS: 3**

## INGREDIENTS

- » ¾ lb. Brussels Sprouts
- » 1 diced slice Pancetta
- » 1 minced clove Garlic
- » 1 tbsp. chopped Shallot
- » ¼ cup pine nuts (toasted)
- » ¼ tsp. Black Pepper (cracked)
- » 4 tbsp. Water

## DIRECTIONS

1. Slice sprouts and place them in the slow cooker along with the water. Cook on "high" for 1 hr. Drain well. Remove the fat from the pancetta. Sauté the pancetta for 4 mins. Add the shallots, garlic, and 1/8 cup of Pine Nuts to the sauté.

2. Now, add the sprouts. Cook for 3 mins. Transfer the prepared mixture to the slow cooker. Add black pepper. 4 tbsp of water, and cook again on "low" for 2 hrs. Serve immediately.

**NUTRITIONS:** Calories 128, Fats 9 g, Sodium 56 mg, Carbohydrates 5 g, Protein 5 g

# 207. TASTY CAULIFLOWER

**COOKING: 6H 15'**       **PREPARATION: 15'**       **SERVINGS: 4**

## INGREDIENTS

- » 2 minced cloves Garlic
- » 2 cups Cauliflower florets
- » 2 tbsp. Olive Oil
- » Pinch of Sea Salt
- » ¼ tsp. Pepper Flakes (chili)
- » Pinch of Black Pepper (cracked)
- » 4 tbsp. Water
- » Zest of ½ lemon

## DIRECTIONS

1. In a slow cooker, place cauliflower and oil. Add vinegar. Toss well to coat thoroughly. Put in the rest of the ingredients and toss again. Cook on "low" for 2 hrs. Serve immediately.

**NUTRITIONS:** Calories 150, Fats 14 g, Sodium 69 mg, Carbohydrates 6 g, Protein 2.2 g

# 208. ARTICHOKE AND SPINACH DIP

**COOKING: 2H 10'**      **PREPARATION: 15'**      **SERVINGS: 2**

## INGREDIENTS

- » 1/8 tsp. Basil (dried)
- » 14 oz. chopped Artichoke Hearts
- » 1 ½ cups spinach
- » ½ minced clove Garlic
- » ¼ cup Sour Cream (low fat)
- » ¼ cup shredded Cheese (Parmesan)
- » ¼ cup Mozzarella Cheese (shredded)
- » 1/8 tsp. Parsley (dried)
- » ½ cup Yogurt (Greek)
- » Pinch of Black Pepper
- » Pinch of Kosher Salt

## DIRECTIONS

1. Boil spinach in water for 1 min. Drain the water. Set the spinach aside to cool and then chop. Puree all the ingredients, including spinach, in a blender.

2. Transfer the mixture to the slow cooker. Add cheeses and cook for 1 hour on "low." Serve with sliced vegetables.

**NUTRITIONS:** Calories 263, Fats 14 g, Sodium 537 mg, Carbohydrates 18 g, Protein 20 g

# 209. APPLE SALSA

**COOKING: 2H**      **PREPARATION: 15'**      **SERVINGS: 3**

## INGREDIENTS

- » 7 ½ oz. drained Black Beans
- » ¼ cubed Apples (Granny Smith)
- » ¼ chopped Chili Pepper (Serrano)
- » 1/8 cup chopped onion (red)
- » 1 ½ tbsp. chopped cilantro
- » ¼ Lemon
- » ¼ Orange
- » Pinch of Sea Salt
- » Pinch of Black Pepper (cracked)

## DIRECTIONS

1. Mix all the ingredients in the cooker (slow cooker). Cook on "low" for an hour. Transfer to a covered container and allow to cool for 1 hr. Serve.

**NUTRITIONS:** Calories 100, Fats 0.4 g, Sodium 50 mg, Carbohydrates 20 g, Protein 5 g

# CHAPTER 8.
# FISH AND SEAFOOD

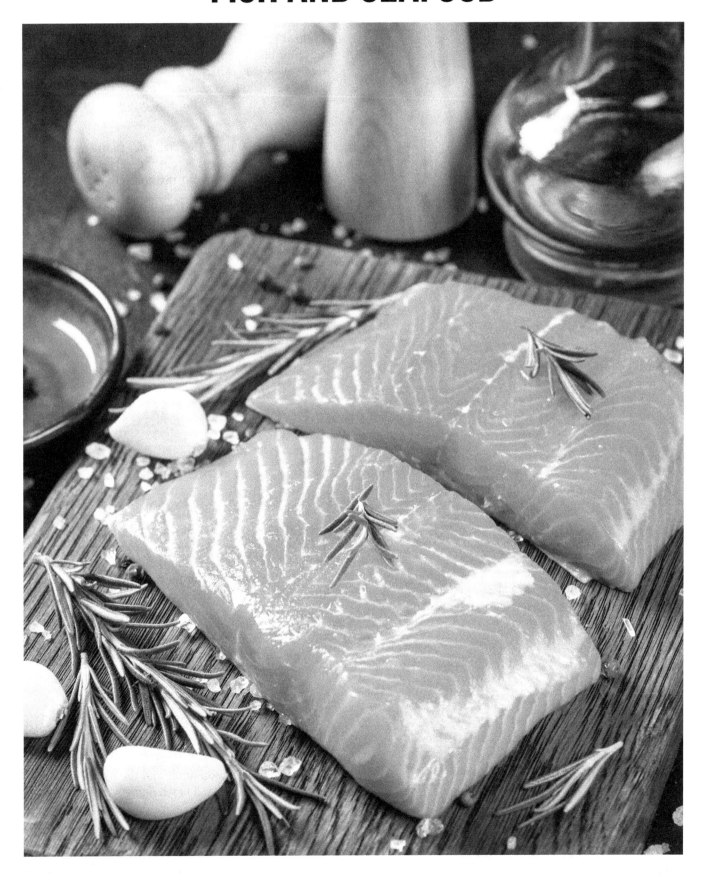

# 210. CITRUS-GLAZED SALMON WITH ZUCCHINI NOODLES

**COOKING: 20'**          **PREPARATION: 15'**          **SERVINGS: 4**

## INGREDIENTS

» 4 (5- to 6-ounce) pieces salmon
» ½ teaspoon kosher salt
» ¼ teaspoon freshly ground black pepper
» 1 tablespoon extra-virgin olive oil
» 1 cup freshly squeezed orange juice
» 1 teaspoon low-sodium soy sauce
» 2 zucchinis (about 16 ounces), spiralized
» 1 tablespoon fresh chives, chopped
» 1 tablespoon fresh parsley, chopped

## DIRECTIONS

1. Preheat the oven to 350°F. Flavor the salmon with salt plus black pepper. Heat-up the olive oil in a large oven-safe skillet or sauté pan over medium-high heat. Add the salmon, skin-side down, and sear for 5 minutes, or until the skin is golden brown and crispy.

2. Flip the salmon over, then transfer to the oven until your desired doneness is reached—about 5 minutes. Place the salmon on a cutting board to rest.

3. Place the same pan on the stove over medium-high heat. Add the orange juice and soy sauce to deglaze the pan. Bring to a simmer, scraping up any brown bits, and simmering 5 to 7 minutes.

4. Split or divide the zucchini noodles into 4 plates and place 1 piece of salmon on each. Pour the orange glaze over the salmon and zucchini noodles. Garnish with the chives and parsley.

**NUTRITIONS:** Calories: 280, Fat: 13g, Sodium: 255mg, Carbohydrates: 11g, Protein: 30g

# 211. SALMON CAKES WITH BELL PEPPER PLUS LEMON YOGURT

**COOKING: 15'**          **PREPARATION: 15'**          **SERVINGS: 4**

## INGREDIENTS

» ¼ cup whole-wheat bread crumbs
» ¼ cup mayonnaise
» 1 large egg, beaten
» 1 tablespoon chives, chopped
» 1 tablespoon fresh parsley, chopped
» Zest of 1 lemon
» ¾ teaspoon kosher salt, divided
» ¼ teaspoon freshly ground black pepper
» 2 (5- to 6-ounce) cans no-salt boneless/skinless salmon, drained and finely flaked
» ½ bell pepper, diced small
» 2 tablespoons extra-virgin olive oil, divided
» 1 cup plain Greek yogurt
» Juice of 1 lemon

## DIRECTIONS

1. Mix the bread crumbs, mayonnaise, egg, chives, parsley, lemon zest, ½ teaspoon of salt, and black pepper in a large bowl. Add the salmon and the bell pepper and stir gently until well combined. Shape the mixture into 8 patties.

2. Heat-up 1 tablespoon of the olive oil in a large skillet over medium-high heat. Cook half the cakes until the bottoms are golden brown, 4 to 5 minutes. Adjust the heat to medium if the bottoms start to burn.

3. Flip the cakes and cook until golden brown, an additional 4 to 5 minutes. Repeat process with the rest of the 1 tablespoon olive oil and the rest of the cakes.

4. Mix the yogurt, lemon juice, and the remaining ¼ teaspoon salt in a small bowl. Serve with the salmon cakes.

**NUTRITIONS:** Calories: 330, Fat: 23g, Sodium: 385mg, Carbohydrates: 9g, Protein: 21g

# 212. HALIBUT IN PARCHMENT WITH ZUCCHINI, SHALLOTS, AND HERBS

**COOKING: 15'**　　　　**PREPARATION: 15'**　　　　**SERVINGS: 4**

## INGREDIENTS

- » ½ cup zucchini, diced small
- » 1 shallot, minced
- » 4 (5-ounce) halibut fillets (about 1 inch thick)
- » 4 teaspoons extra-virgin olive oil
- » ¼ teaspoon kosher salt
- » 1/8 teaspoon freshly ground black pepper
- » 1 lemon, sliced into 1/8 -inch-thick rounds
- » 8 sprigs of thyme

## DIRECTIONS

1. Preheat the oven to 450°F. Combine the zucchini and shallots in a medium bowl. Cut 4 (15-by-24-inch) pieces of parchment paper. Fold each sheet in half horizontally.

2. Draw a large half heart on one side of each folded sheet, with the fold along the heart center. Cut out the heart, open the parchment, and lay it flat.

3. Place a fillet near the center of each parchment heart. Drizzle 1 teaspoon olive oil on each fillet. Sprinkle with salt and pepper. Top each fillet with lemon slices and 2 sprigs of thyme. Sprinkle each fillet with one-quarter of the zucchini and shallot mixture. Fold the parchment over.

4. Starting at the top, fold the parchment edges over, and continue all the way around to make a packet. Twist the end tightly to secure. Arrange the 4 packets on a baking sheet. Bake for about 15 minutes. Place on plates; cut open. Serve immediately.

**NUTRITIONS:** Calories: 190, Fat: 7g, Sodium: 170mg, Carbohydrates: 5g, Protein: 27g

# 213. FLOUNDER WITH TOMATOES AND BASIL

**COOKING: 20'**　　　　**PREPARATION: 15'**　　　　**SERVINGS: 4**

## INGREDIENTS

- » 1-pound cherry tomatoes
- » 4 garlic cloves, sliced
- » 2 tablespoons extra-virgin olive oil
- » 2 tablespoons lemon juice
- » 2 tablespoons basil, cut into ribbons
- » ½ teaspoon kosher salt
- » ¼ teaspoon freshly ground black pepper
- » 4 (5- to 6-ounce) flounder fillets

## DIRECTIONS

1. Preheat the oven to 425°F.

2. Mix the tomatoes, garlic, olive oil, lemon juice, basil, salt, and black pepper in a baking dish. Bake for 5 minutes.

3. Remove, then arrange the flounder on top of the tomato mixture. Bake until the fish is opaque and begins to flake, about 10 to 15 minutes, depending on thickness.

**NUTRITIONS:** Calories: 215, Fat: 9g, Sodium: 261mg, Carbohydrates: 6g, Protein: 28g

# 214. GRILLED MAHI-MAHI WITH ARTICHOKE CAPONATA

**COOKING: 30'**  **PREPARATION: 15'**  **SERVINGS: 4**

## INGREDIENTS

- » 2 tablespoons extra-virgin olive oil
- » 2 celery stalks, diced
- » 1 onion, diced
- » 2 garlic cloves, minced
- » ½ cup cherry tomatoes, chopped
- » ¼ cup white wine
- » 2 tablespoons white wine vinegar
- » 1 can artichoke hearts, drained and chopped
- » ¼ cup green olives, pitted and chopped
- » 1 tablespoon capers, chopped
- » ¼ teaspoon red pepper flakes
- » 2 tablespoons fresh basil, chopped
- » 4 (5- to 6-ounces each) skinless mahi-mahi fillets
- » ½ teaspoon kosher salt
- » ¼ teaspoon freshly ground black pepper
- » Olive oil cooking spray

## DIRECTIONS

1. Warm-up olive oil in a skillet over medium heat, then put the celery and onion, and sauté 4 to 5 minutes. Add the garlic and sauté 30 seconds. Add the tomatoes and cook within 2 to 3 minutes. Add the wine and vinegar to deglaze the pan, increasing the heat to medium-high.

2. Add the artichokes, olives, capers, and red pepper flakes and simmer, reducing the liquid by half, about 10 minutes. Mix in the basil.

3. Season the mahi-mahi with salt and pepper. Heat a grill skillet or grill pan over medium-high heat and coat with olive oil cooking spray. Add the fish and cook within 4 to 5 minutes per side. Serve topped with the artichoke caponata.

**NUTRITIONS:** Calories: 245, Fat: 9g, Sodium: 570mg, Carbohydrates: 10g, Protein: 28g

# 215. COD AND CAULIFLOWER CHOWDER

**COOKING: 40'**  **PREPARATION: 10'**  **SERVINGS: 4**

## INGREDIENTS

- » 2 tablespoons extra-virgin olive oil
- » 1 leek, sliced thinly
- » 4 garlic cloves, sliced
- » 1 medium head cauliflower, coarsely chopped
- » 1 teaspoon kosher salt
- » ¼ teaspoon freshly ground black pepper
- » 2 pints cherry tomatoes
- » 2 cups no-salt-added vegetable stock
- » ¼ cup green olives, pitted and chopped
- » 1 to 1½ pounds cod
- » ¼ cup fresh parsley, minced

## DIRECTIONS

1. Heat-up the olive oil in a Dutch oven or large pot over medium heat. Add the leek and sauté until lightly golden brown, about 5 minutes.

2. Add the garlic and sauté within 30 seconds. Add the cauliflower, salt, and black pepper and sauté 2 to 3 minutes.

3. Add the tomatoes and vegetable stock, increase the heat to high and boil, then turn the heat to low and simmer within 10 minutes.

4. Add the olives and mix. Add the fish, cover, and simmer 20 minutes or until fish is opaque and flakes easily. Gently mix in the parsley.

**NUTRITIONS:** Calories: 270, Fat: 9g, Sodium: 545mg, Potassium: 1475mg, Carbohydrates: 19g, Protein: 30g

# 216. SARDINE BRUSCHETTA WITH FENNEL AND LEMON CREMA

**COOKING: 0'**  **PREPARATION: 15'**  **SERVINGS: 4**

## INGREDIENTS

- » 1/3 cup plain Greek yogurt
- » 2 tablespoons mayonnaise
- » 2 tablespoons lemon juice, divided
- » 2 teaspoons lemon zest
- » ¾ teaspoon kosher salt, divided
- » 1 fennel bulb, cored and thinly sliced
- » ¼ cup parsley, chopped, plus more for garnish
- » ¼ cup fresh mint, chopped2 teaspoons extra-virgin olive oil
- » 1/8 teaspoon freshly ground black pepper
- » 8 slices multigrain bread, toasted
- » 2 (4.4-ounce) cans of smoked sardines

## DIRECTIONS

1. Mix the yogurt, mayonnaise, 1 tablespoon of the lemon juice, the lemon zest, and ¼ teaspoon of the salt in a small bowl.

2. Mix the remaining ½ teaspoon salt, the remaining 1 tablespoon lemon juice, the fennel, parsley, mint, olive oil, and black pepper in a separate small bowl.

3. Spoon 1 tablespoons of the yogurt mixture on each piece of toast. Divide the fennel mixture evenly on top of the yogurt mixture. Divide the sardines among the toasts, placing them on top of the fennel mixture. Garnish with more herbs, if desired.

**NUTRITIONS:** Calories: 400, Fat: 16g, Sodium: 565mg, Carbohydrates: 51g, Protein: 16g

# 217. CHOPPED TUNA SALAD

**COOKING: 0'**  **PREPARATION: 15'**  **SERVINGS: 4**

## INGREDIENTS

- » 2 tablespoons extra-virgin olive oil
- » 2 tablespoons lemon juice
- » 2 teaspoons Dijon mustard
- » ½ teaspoon kosher salt
- » ¼ teaspoon freshly ground black pepper
- » 12 olives, pitted and chopped
- » ½ cup celery, diced
- » ½ cup red onion, diced
- » ½ cup red bell pepper, diced
- » ½ cup fresh parsley, chopped
- » 2 (6-ounce) cans no-salt-added tuna packed in water, drained
- » 6 cups baby spinach

## DIRECTIONS

1. Mix the olive oil, lemon juice, mustard, salt, and black pepper in a medium bowl. Add in the olives, celery, onion, bell pepper, and parsley and mix well. Add the tuna and gently incorporate. Divide the spinach evenly among 4 plates or bowls. Spoon the tuna salad evenly on top of the spinach.

**NUTRITIONS:** Calories: 220, Fat: 11g, Sodium: 396mg, Carbohydrates: 7g, Protein: 25g

# 218. MONKFISH WITH SAUTÉED LEEKS, FENNEL, AND TOMATOES

**COOKING: 35'**       **PREPARATION: 15'**       **SERVINGS: 4**

## INGREDIENTS

- » 1 to 1½ pounds monkfish
- » 3 tablespoons lemon juice, divided
- » 1 teaspoon kosher salt, divided
- » 1/8 teaspoon freshly ground black pepper
- » 2 tablespoons extra-virgin olive oil
- » 1 leek, sliced in half lengthwise and thinly sliced
- » ½ onion, julienned
- » 3 garlic cloves, minced
- » 2 bulbs fennel, cored and thinly sliced, plus ¼ cup fronds for garnish
- » 1 (14.5-ounce) can no-salt-added diced tomatoes
- » 2 tablespoons fresh parsley, chopped
- » 2 tablespoons fresh oregano, chopped
- » ¼ teaspoon red pepper flakes

## DIRECTIONS

1. Place the fish in a medium baking dish and add 2 tablespoons of the lemon juice, ¼ teaspoon of the salt, plus the black pepper. Place in the refrigerator.

2. Warm-up olive oil in a large skillet over medium heat, then put the leek and onion and sauté until translucent, about 3 minutes. Add the garlic and sauté within 30 seconds. Add the fennel and sauté 4 to 5 minutes. Add the tomatoes and simmer for 2 to 3 minutes.

3. Stir in the parsley, oregano, red pepper flakes, the remaining ¾ teaspoon salt, and the remaining 1 tablespoon lemon juice. Put the fish over the leek mixture, cover, and simmer for 20 to 25 minutes. Garnish with the fennel fronds.

**NUTRITIONS:** Calories: 220, Fat: 9g, Sodium: 345mg, Carbohydrates: 11g, Protein: 22g

---

# 219. CARAMELIZED FENNEL AND SARDINES WITH PENNE

**COOKING: 30'**       **PREPARATION: 15'**       **SERVINGS: 4**

## INGREDIENTS

- » 8 ounces whole-wheat penne
- » 2 tablespoons extra-virgin olive oil
- » 1 bulb fennel, cored and thinly sliced, plus ¼ cup fronds
- » 2 celery stalks, thinly sliced, plus ½ cup leaves
- » 4 garlic cloves, sliced
- » ¾ teaspoon kosher salt
- » ¼ teaspoon freshly ground black pepper
- » Zest of 1 lemon
- » Juice of 1 lemon
- » 2 (4.4-ounce) cans boneless/skinless sardines packed in olive oil, undrained

## DIRECTIONS

1. Cook the penne, as stated in the package directions. Drain, reserving 1 cup of pasta water. Warm-up olive oil in a large skillet over medium heat, then put the fennel and celery and cook within 10 to 12 minutes. Add the garlic and cook within 1 minute.

2. Add the penne, reserved pasta water, salt, and black pepper. Adjust the heat to medium-high and cook for 1 to 2 minutes.

3. Remove, then stir in the lemon zest, lemon juice, fennel fronds, and celery leaves. Break the sardines into bite-size pieces and gently mix in, along with the oil they were packed in.

**NUTRITIONS:** Calories: 400, Fat: 15g, Sodium: 530mg, Carbohydrates: 46g, Protein: 22g

---

# 220. CIOPPINO

**COOKING: 35'**  **PREPARATION: 15'**  **SERVINGS: 4**

## INGREDIENTS

- » 2 tablespoons extra-virgin olive oil
- » 1 onion, diced
- » 1 bulb fennel, chopped, plus ½ cup fronds for garnish
- » 1-quart no-salt-added vegetable stock
- » 4 garlic cloves, smashed
- » 8 thyme sprigs
- » 1 teaspoon kosher salt
- » ¼ teaspoon red pepper flakes
- » 1 dried bay leaf
- » 1 bunch kale, stemmed and chopped
- » 1 dozen littleneck clams tightly closed, scrubbed
- » 1-pound fish (cod, halibut, and bass are all good choices)
- » ¼ cup fresh parsley, chopped

## DIRECTIONS

1. Heat-up the olive oil in a large stockpot over medium heat. Add the onion and fennel and sauté for about 5 minutes. Add the vegetable stock, garlic, thyme, salt, red pepper flakes, and bay leaf. Adjust the heat to medium-high, and simmer. Add the kale, cover, and simmer within 5 minutes.

2. Carefully add the clams, cover, and simmer about 15 minutes until they open. Remove the clams and set aside. Discard any clams that do not open.

3. Add the fish, cover, and simmer within 5 to 10 minutes, depending on the fish's thickness, until opaque and easily separated. Gently mix in the parsley. Divide the cioppino among 4 bowls. Place 3 clams in each bowl and garnish with the fennel fronds.

**NUTRITIONS:** Calories: 285, Fat: 9g, Sodium: 570mg, Carbohydrates: 19g, Protein: 32g

# 221. GREEN GODDESS CRAB SALAD WITH ENDIVE

**COOKING: 10'**  **PREPARATION: 15'**  **SERVINGS: 4**

## INGREDIENTS

- » 1 pound lump crabmeat
- » 2/3 cup plain Greek yogurt
- » 3 tablespoons mayonnaise
- » 3 tablespoons fresh chives, chopped, plus additional for garnish
- » 3 tablespoons fresh parsley, chopped, plus extra for garnish
- » 3 tablespoons fresh basil, chopped, plus extra for garnish
- » Zest of 1 lemon
- » Juice of 1 lemon
- » ½ teaspoon kosher salt
- » ¼ teaspoon freshly ground black pepper
- » 4 endives, ends cut off and leaves separated

## DIRECTIONS

1. In a medium bowl, combine the crab, yogurt, mayonnaise, chives, parsley, basil, lemon zest, lemon juice, salt, plus black pepper and mix until well combined.

2. Place the endive leaves on 4 salad plates. Divide the crab mixture evenly on top of the endive. Garnish with additional herbs, if desired.

**NUTRITIONS:** Calories: 200, Fat: 9g, Sodium: 570mg, Carbohydrates: 44g, Protein: 25g

# 222. SEARED SCALLOPS WITH BLOOD ORANGE GLAZE

**COOKING: 20'**　　　　**PREPARATION: 15'**　　　　**SERVINGS: 4**

## INGREDIENTS

- » 3 tablespoons extra-virgin olive oil, divided
- » 3 garlic cloves, minced
- » ½ teaspoon kosher salt, divided
- » 4 blood oranges, juiced
- » 1 teaspoon blood orange zest
- » ½ teaspoon red pepper flakes
- » 1-pound scallops, small side muscle removed
- » ¼ teaspoon freshly ground black pepper
- » ¼ cup fresh chives, chopped

## DIRECTIONS

1. Heat-up 1 tablespoon of the olive oil in a small saucepan over medium-high heat. Add the garlic and ¼ teaspoon of the salt and sauté for 30 seconds.

2. Add the orange juice and zest, bring to a boil, reduce the heat to medium-low, and cook within 20 minutes, or until the liquid reduces by half and becomes a thicker syrup consistency. Remove and mix in the red pepper flakes.

3. Pat the scallops dry with a paper towel and season with the remaining ¼ teaspoon salt and the black pepper. Heat-up the remaining 2 tablespoons of olive oil in a large skillet on medium-high heat. Add the scallops gently and sear.

4. Cook on each side within 2 minutes. If cooking in 2 batches, use 1 tablespoon of oil per batch. Serve the scallops with the blood orange glaze and garnish with the chives.

**NUTRITIONS:** Calories: 140, Fat: 4g, Sodium: 570mg, Carbohydrates: 12g, Protein: 15g

# 223. LEMON GARLIC SHRIMP

**COOKING: 10'**　　　　**PREPARATION: 15'**　　　　**SERVINGS: 4**

## INGREDIENTS

- » 2 tablespoons extra-virgin olive oil
- » 3 garlic cloves, sliced
- » ½ teaspoon kosher salt
- » ¼ teaspoon red pepper flakes
- » 1-pound large shrimp, peeled and deveined
- » ½ cup white wine
- » 3 tablespoons fresh parsley, minced
- » Zest of ½ lemon
- » Juice of ½ lemon

## DIRECTIONS

1. Heat-up the olive oil in a wok or large skillet over medium-high heat. Add the garlic, salt, and red pepper flakes and sauté until the garlic starts to brown, 30 seconds to 1 minute.

2. Add the shrimp and cook within 2 to 3 minutes on each side. Pour in the wine and deglaze the wok, scraping up any flavorful brown bits, for 1 to 2 minutes. Turn off the heat; mix in the parsley, lemon zest, and lemon juice.

**NUTRITIONS:** Calories: 200, Fat: 9g, Sodium: 310mg, Carbohydrates: 3g, Protein: 23g

# 224. SHRIMP FRA DIAVOLO

**COOKING: 10'**　　　　**PREPARATION: 15'**　　　　**SERVINGS: 4**

## INGREDIENTS

» 2 tablespoons extra-virgin olive oil
» 1 onion, diced small
» 1 fennel bulb, cored and diced small, plus ¼ cup fronds for garnish
» 1 bell pepper, diced small
» ½ teaspoon dried oregano
» ½ teaspoon dried thyme
» ½ teaspoon kosher salt
» ¼ teaspoon red pepper flakes
» 1 (14.5-ounce) can no-salt-added diced tomatoes
» 1-pound shrimp, peeled and deveined
» Juice of 1 lemon
» Zest of 1 lemon
» 2 tablespoons fresh parsley, chopped, for garnish

## DIRECTIONS

1. Heat-up the olive oil in a large skillet or sauté pan over medium heat. Add the onion, fennel, bell pepper, oregano, thyme, salt, and red pepper flakes and sauté until translucent, about 5 minutes.

2. Drizzle the pan using the canned tomatoes' juice, scraping up any brown bits, and bringing to a boil. Add the diced tomatoes and the shrimp. Lower heat to a simmer within 3 minutes.

3. Turn off the heat. Add the lemon juice and lemon zest, and toss well to combine. Garnish with the parsley and the fennel fronds.

**NUTRITIONS:** Calories: 240, Fat: 9g, Sodium: 335mg, Carbohydrates: 13g, Protein: 25g

# 225. FISH AMANDINE

**COOKING: 15'**　　　　**PREPARATION: 5'**　　　　**SERVINGS: 4**

## INGREDIENTS

» 4-ounce skinless tilapia, trout, or halibut fillets, 1/2- to 1-inch thick
» ¼ cup buttermilk
» ½ teaspoon dry mustard
» 1/8 teaspoon crushed red pepper
» 1 tablespoon butter, melted
» ¼ teaspoon salt
» ½ cup panko bread crumbs
» 2 tbsp chopped fresh parsley
» ¼ cup sliced almonds, coarsely chopped
» 2 tablespoons grated Parmesan cheese

## DIRECTIONS

1. Defrost fish, if frozen. Preheat oven to 450oF. Grease a shallow baking pan; set aside. Rinse fish; pat dry with paper towels.

2. Pour buttermilk into a shallow dish. In an extra shallow dish, mix bread crumbs, dry mustard, parsley, and salt. Soak fish into buttermilk, then into crumb mixture, turning to coat. Put coated fish in the ready baking pan.

3. Flavor the fish with almonds plus Parmesan cheese; drizzle with melted butter. Sprinkle with crinkled red pepper. Bake for 5 minutes per 1/2-inch thickness of fish or until fish flakes easily when checked with a fork.

**NUTRITIONS:** Calories 209, Fat 8.7 g, Sodium 302 mg, Carbohydrates 6.7 g, Protein 26.2 g

# 226. AIR-FRYER FISH CAKES

**COOKING: 10'**  **PREPARATION: 15'**  **SERVINGS: 2**

## INGREDIENTS

- » Cooking spray
- » 10 oz finely chopped white fish
- » 2/3 cup whole-wheat panko breadcrumbs
- » 3 tablespoons finely chopped fresh Cilantro
- » 2 tablespoons Thai sweet chili sauce
- » 2 tablespoons canola mayonnaise
- » 1 large egg
- » 1/8 teaspoon salt
- » ¼ teaspoon ground pepper
- » 2 lime wedges

## DIRECTIONS

1. Oiled the basket of an air fryer with cooking spray. Put fish, cilantro, panko, chili sauce, egg, mayonnaise, pepper, and salt in a medium bowl; stir until well mixed. Shape the mixture into four 3-inch-diameter cakes.

2. Oiled the cakes with cooking spray; place in the basket. Cook at 400oF until the cakes are browned for 9 to 10 minutes. Serve with lime wedges.

**NUTRITIONS:** Calories 399, Fat 15.5 g, Sodium 537 mg, Carbohydrates 27.9 g, Protein 34.6 g

# 227. PESTO SHRIMP PASTA

**COOKING: 12'**  **PREPARATION: 15'**  **SERVINGS: 4**

## INGREDIENTS

- » 1/8 teaspoon freshly cracked pepper
- » 1 cup dried orzo
- » 4 tsp packaged pesto sauce mix
- » 1 lemon, halved
- » 1/8 teaspoon coarse salt
- » 1-pound medium shrimp, thawed
- » 1 medium zucchini, halved lengthwise and sliced
- » 2 tablespoons olive oil, divided
- » 1-ounce shaved Parmesan cheese

## DIRECTIONS

1. Prepare orzo pasta concerning package directions. Drain; reserving ¼ cup of the pasta cooking water. Mix 1 teaspoon of the pesto mix into the kept cooking water and set aside.

2. Mix 3 teaspoons of the pesto mix plus 1 tablespoon of the olive oil in a large plastic bag. Seal and shake to mix. Put the shrimp in the bag; seal and turn to coat. Set aside.

3. Sauté zucchini in a big skillet over moderate heat for 1 to 2 minutes, stirring repeatedly. Put the pesto-marinated shrimp in the skillet and cook for 5 minutes or until shrimp is dense.

4. Put the cooked pasta in the skillet with the zucchini and shrimp combination. Stir in the kept pasta water until absorbed, grating up any seasoning in the bottom of the pan. Season with pepper and salt. Squeeze the lemon over the pasta. Top with Parmesan, then serve.

**NUTRITIONS:** Calories 361, Fat 10.1 g, Sodium 502 mg, Carbohydrates 35.8 g, Protein 31.6 g

# 228. QUICK SHRIMP SCAMPI

**COOKING: 10'**     **PREPARATION: 5'**     **SERVINGS: 4**

## INGREDIENTS

- » 2 tablespoons olive oil
- » ½ cup (120 ml) dry white wine
- » 3 garlic cloves, minced
- » 1 1/2 pound (680 g) large shrimp, peeled and stroked dry
- » Large pinch of crushed red pepper flakes
- » 1 lemon, zested, one half cut into slices
- » 1/8 Salt
- » 1/8 pepper
- » 4 tbsp unsalted butter, slice into 4 pieces
- » Large handful of fresh chopped flat-leaf parsley.

**NUTRITIONS:** Calories 316, Fat 20.3 g, Sodium 1039 mg, Carbohydrates 4 g, Protein 23.5 g

## DIRECTIONS

1. In a large skillet, warm up the oil over moderate heat. Flavor the shrimp with salt plus pepper, then put them in the skillet in a single coating. Cook, without interruption, until the shrimp's bottoms begin to turn pink, about 1 minute after.

2. Turnover the shrimp and cook until almost cooked through, about 1 minute more. Keep the shrimp on a plate and set aside.

3. Adjust to medium, add the pepper flakes, garlic, and a little more oil if the pan seems dry; cook, repeatedly stirring until the garlic just begins to turn golden, about 1 minute. Add the wine, scraping up any burnt bits from the bottom of the pan, and simmer until most of the wine has vanished.

4. Mix in the butter, then season the sauce with lemon juice and salt from one lemon half. Add the cooked shrimp, the lemon zest, any juices accrued on the plate, and parsley and heave until the shrimp is warmed through, about 1 minute. Serve with lemon wedges, if you wish.

# 229. POACHED SALMON WITH CREAMY PICCATA SAUCE

**COOKING: 15'**     **PREPARATION: 5'**     **SERVINGS: 4**

## INGREDIENTS

- » 1 pound center-cut salmon fillet skinned and cut into 4 portions
- » 2 tablespoons lemon juice
- » 2 teaspoons extra-virgin olive oil
- » ¼ cup reduced-fat sour cream
- » 1 large shallot, minced
- » 1 cup dry white wine, divided
- » 1 tablespoon chopped fresh dill
- » 4 teaspoons capers, rinsed
- » ¼ teaspoon salt

## DIRECTIONS

1. Place salmon in a wide skillet and add ½ cup wine and sufficient water to cover the salmon. Bring it to boil over high-temperature heat. Simmer, turn the salmon over, cook within 5 minutes and then remove from the heat.

2. In the meantime, heat-up oil in a medium skillet over moderate heat. Add shallot and cook, stirring, until scented, about 30 seconds. Add the remaining ½ cup wine; boil until slightly condensed, about 1 minute.

3. Stir in lemon juice plus capers; cook 1 minute more. Remove, stir in sour cream and salt. Top the salmon with the sauce and relish it with dill before serving.

**NUTRITIONS:** Calories 229, Fat 8.3 g, Sodium 286 mg, Carbohydrates 3.7 g, Protein 23.3 g

# 230. TUSCAN-STYLE TUNA SALAD

**COOKING: 0'**　　　　**PREPARATION: 15'**　　　　**SERVINGS: 4**

## INGREDIENTS

- » 2 6-ounce cans chunk light tuna, drained.
- » ¼ teaspoon salt
- » 10 cherry tomatoes
- » 2 tablespoons lemon juice
- » 4 scallions, trimmed and sliced
- » 2 tablespoons extra-virgin olive oil
- » 1 15-ounce can small white beans
- » Freshly ground pepper

## DIRECTIONS

1. Mix tuna, beans, scallions, tomatoes, juice, oil, lemon, pepper, and salt in a medium bowl. Stir gently. Refrigerate until ready to serve.

**NUTRITIONS:** Calories 199, Fat 8.8 g, Sodium 555 mg, Carbohydrates 19.8 g, Protein 16.5 g

# 231. TUNA SALAD-STUFFED TOMATOES WITH ARUGULA

**COOKING: 15'**　　　　**PREPARATION: 5'**　　　　**SERVINGS: 4**

## INGREDIENTS

- » 1 teaspoon dried thyme
- » 3 tablespoons sherry vinegar
- » 3 tablespoons extra-virgin olive oil
- » 1/3 cup chopped celery
- » ¼ teaspoon freshly ground pepper
- » 4 large tomatoes
- » 8 cups baby arugula
- » ¼ cup finely chopped red onion
- » ¼ teaspoon salt
- » ¼ cup chopped Kalamata olives
- » 2 5-oz cans chunk light tuna in olive oil, drained
- » 1 can great northern beans, rinsed

## DIRECTIONS

1. Whisk oil, salt, vinegar, and pepper in an average-sized bowl. Put 3 tablespoons of the dressing in a big bowl and set aside.

2. Slice enough off the top of each tomato to remove the core, chop enough of the tops to equal ½ cup and add to the average-sized bowl. Scoop out the soft tomato tissue using a teaspoon or melon baller and discard the pulp

3. Add tuna, onion, thyme, olives, and celery to the average-sized bowl; gently toss to mix. Fill the scooped tomatoes with the tuna mixture. Add beans and arugula to the gauze in the large bowl and toss to combine. Divide the salad into four plates and top each with a stuffed tomato.

**NUTRITIONS:** Calories 353, Fat 17.6 g, Sodium 501 mg, Carbohydrates 29.9 g, Protein 19.7 g

# 232. HERBED SEAFOOD CASSEROLE

**COOKING: 50'**  **PREPARATION: 15'**  **SERVINGS: 12**

## INGREDIENTS

- » 1 ½ cups uncooked long grain rice
- » 2 tablespoons butter
- » ¼ teaspoon pepper
- » 2 tablespoons minced fresh parsley
- » 1 medium onion, finely chopped
- » 3 garlic cloves, minced
- » 1 medium carrot, shredded
- » ½ teaspoon salt
- » 3 celery ribs, thinly sliced
- » 1 ½ teaspoon snipped fresh dill or ½ teaspoon dill weed

### Seafood:
- » pound uncooked medium shrimp, peeled and deveined
- » 1 can crab meat, drained, flaked, and cartilage removed
- » ¼ cup all-purpose flour
- » pound bay scallops
- » ½ teaspoon salt
- » 1 package (8 ounces) cream cheese, cubed
- » 5 tablespoons butter, cubed
- » 1 ½ cups half-and-half cream
- » 1 ½ teaspoon snipped fresh dill or ½ teaspoon dill weed
- » ¼ teaspoon dried thyme
- » ¼ teaspoon pepper

### Topping:
- » 2 tablespoons butter, melted
- » 1 ½ cups soft bread crumbs

## DIRECTIONS

1. Preheat oven to 325°F. Cook rice according to package directions. In the meantime, in a big skillet, heat butter over moderate heat. Add onion, celery, and carrot; cook and stir until crisp-tender. Add garlic, pepper, and salt; cook 1 minute longer. Add to the cooked rice. Stir in parsley and dill. Transfer to a greased baking dish.

2. Fill a large saucepan with 2/3 full with water and bring to a boil. Reduce heat to medium. Add shrimp; simmer, uncovered, for 30 seconds. Add scallops; simmer for 3 minutes or just until shrimp turn pink and scallops are firm and dense. Reserve 1 cup of cooking liquid. Put the seafood in a large bowl; stir in crab.

3. Dissolve the butter over medium heat in a small saucepan. Stir in flour until mixed; slowly stir in cream and kept cooking liquid. Boil within 2 minutes or until condensed and foamy. Reduce heat. Stir in cream cheese, dill and season until smooth. Stir into the seafood blend.

4. Pour over rice mixture. Mix the bread crumbs with melted butter; sprinkle over the top. Bake, uncovered, 50 minutes or until it turns golden brown. Stand 10 minutes before dishing.

**NUTRITIONS:** Calories 404, Fat 20g, Sodium 616mg, Carbohydrate 29g, Protein 26g

# 233. LEMON HERB BAKED SALMON

**COOKING: 20'**       **PREPARATION: 15'**       **SERVINGS: 8**

## INGREDIENTS

» 1 salmon fillet 3-4lbs
» salt & pepper
» 1 lemon divided
» 2 tablespoons butter melted

**Topping:**
» ¾ cup Panko bread crumbs
» 3 tablespoons butter melted
» 2 tablespoons parmesan cheese shredded
» 1 tablespoon fresh dill minced
» zest from one lemon
» 2 tablespoons fresh parsley minced
» 3 cloves garlic minced

## DIRECTIONS

1. Preheat the oven to 4000F. Put all ingredients in a small bowl. Streak a pan with foil and spray with cooking spray. Put salmon on the pan and brush with melted butter.

2. Season with salt and pepper and crush ½ of the lemon over the top. Sprinkle crumb mixture over salmon. Bake exposed for 15 minutes or until salmon flakes easily and is cooked.

**NUTRITIONS:** Calories: 377, Carbohydrates: 5g, Protein: 40g, Fat: 20g, Sodium: 212mg

---

# 234. BAKED SALMON FOIL PACKETS WITH VEGETABLES

**COOKING: 15'**       **PREPARATION: 15'**       **SERVINGS: 4**

## INGREDIENTS

» 1 lb. Salmon (cut into 4 6-oz fillets)
» 1/2 lb. Asparagus (trimmed, then cut in half)
» 1/2 tsp Sea salt
» 1 tbsp Fresh dill (chopped)
» 1/4 cup Olive oil
» 2 cloves Garlic (minced)
» 10 oz Grape tomatoes
» 1/4 tsp Black pepper
» 1 tbsp lemon juice and ½ tbsp zest
» 10 oz Zucchini (sliced into half-moons)
» 1 tbsp Fresh parsley (chopped)

## DIRECTIONS

1. Preheat the oven to 4000F or preheat the grill to medium. Layout 4 large squares of foil [at least 12x12 inches (30x30 cm)]. Put a salmon fillet in the center of each piece of foil. Divide the veggies squarely among the foil around the salmon.

2. Mix the olive oil, black pepper, parsley, sea salt, lemon juice, minced garlic, lemon zest, and dill in a small bowl. Put half of the oil mixture to skirmish the salmon, getting most of the garlic onto the salmon.

3. Pour the residual oil mixture on the veggies. Put more salt plus pepper on the salmon and veggies. Fold the foil and seal to form packets. Place onto a baking sheet. Bake within 15-20 minutes, or grill (enclosed) within 13-18 minutes.

**NUTRITIONS:** Calories 400, Fat 24g, Protein 36g, Sodium: 212mg, Carbs 8g

# 235. BAKED FISH & POTATOES

**COOKING: 20'**     **PREPARATION: 15'**     **SERVINGS: 4**

## INGREDIENTS

- » 1/2 lb. small red potato es (about 4)
- » 4 RITZ Reduced Fat Crackers, finely crushed
- » 2 tbsp. KRAFT Sun-Dried Tomato Vinaigrette Dressing
- » 2 tbsp. KRAFT Grated Parmesan Cheese, divided
- » 1/2 lb. cod fillet
- » 2 lemon wedges
- » 2 tbsp. KRAFT Light Mayo Reduced Fat Mayonnaise
- » 2 cups fresh broccoli florets, steamed

## DIRECTIONS

1. Heat the oven to 400°F. Slice each potato into 6 pieces and put it in a large bowl. Add dressing; toss to coat. Put, cut sides down, on a rimmed baking sheet sprayed with cooking spray and bake for 10 mins.

2. In the meantime, mix cracker crumbs and 1 tbsp cheese in a shallow dish. Slice the fish crosswise into 1-inch-wide sticks; spread tops and sides with mayo. Roll in crumb mixture until evenly covered.

3. Turn potatoes and move to ends of pan. Put the fish, coated sides up, in the middle of the pan, and bake for 8 to 10 minutes. Sprinkle remaining cheese over potatoes. Serve fish with lemon wedges, broccoli, and potatoes.

**NUTRITIONS:** Calories 330, Fat 11g, Sodium 560mg, Carbohydrates 33g, Protein 28g

# 236. STEAMED SALMON TERIYAKI

**COOKING: 15'**     **PREPARATION:15'**     **SERVINGS: 4**

## INGREDIENTS

- » 3 green onions, minced
- » 2 packet Stevia
- » 1 tbsp freshly grated ginger
- » 1 clove garlic, minced
- » 2 tsp sesame seeds
- » 1 tbsp sesame oil
- » ¼ cup mirin
- » 2 tbsp low sodium soy sauce
- » 1/2-lb salmon filet

## DIRECTIONS

1. Mix stevia, ginger, garlic, oil, mirin, and soy sauce in a heat-proof dish that fits inside a saucepan. Add salmon and cover generously with sauce.

2. Put sesame seeds and green onions on top of the salmon. Cover dish with foil. Place on top of the trivet. Cover and steam for 15 minutes. Let it rest for 5 minutes in the pan. Serve and enjoy.

**NUTRITIONS:** Calories: 242.7, Carbs: 1.2g, Protein: 35.4g, Fats: 10.7g, Sodium: 285mg

# 237. EASY STEAMED ALASKAN COD

**COOKING: 15'**　　　　**PREPARATION: 15'**　　　　**SERVINGS: 3**

## INGREDIENTS

»　2 tbsp butter
»　Pepper to taste
»　1 cup cherry tomatoes, halved
»　1 large Wild Alaskan cod filet, cut into 3 smaller pieces

## DIRECTIONS

1. In a heat-proof dish that fits inside a saucepan, add all ingredients. Cover dish with foil. Place on trivet and steam for 15 minutes. Serve and enjoy.

**NUTRITIONS:** Calories: 132.9, Carbs: 1.9g, Protein: 12.2g, Fats: 8.5g, Sodium: 296mg

# 238. DILL AND LEMON COD PACKETS

**COOKING: 10'**　　　　**PREPARATION: 15'**　　　　**SERVINGS: 12**

## INGREDIENTS

»　2 tsp olive oil, divided
»　4 slices lemon, divided
»　2 sprigs fresh dill, divided
»　½ tsp garlic powder, divided
»　Pepper to taste
»　1/2-lb cod filets

## DIRECTIONS

1. Cut two pieces of 15-inch lengths foil. Put one filet in the middle in one foil. Season with pepper to taste. Sprinkle ¼ tsp garlic. Add a tsp of oil on top of the filet. Top with 2 slices of lemon and a sprig of dill.

2. Fold over the foil and seal the filet inside. Repeat process for the rest of the fish. Place packet on the trivet. Cover and steam for 10 minutes. Serve.

**NUTRITIONS:** Calories: 164.8, Carbs: 9.4g, Protein: 18.3g, Fats: 6g, Sodium: 347mg

# 239. STEAMED FISH MEDITERRANEAN STYLE

**COOKING: 15'**     **PREPARATION: 15'**     **SERVINGS: 4**

## INGREDIENTS

- » Pepper to taste
- » 1 clove garlic, smashed
- » 2 tsp olive oil
- » 1 bunch fresh thyme
- » 2 tbsp pickled capers
- » 1 cup black salt-cured olives
- » 1-lb cherry tomatoes halved
- » 1 ½-lbs. cod filets

## DIRECTIONS

1. In a heat-proof dish that fits inside a saucepan, layer half of the halved cherry tomatoes. Season with pepper.

2. Add filets on top of tomatoes and season with pepper. Drizzle oil. Sprinkle 3/4s of thyme on top and the smashed garlic.

3. Cover top of fish with remaining cherry tomatoes, then place the dish on the trivet. Cover it with foil, then steam for 15 minutes. Serve and enjoy.

**NUTRITIONS:** Calories: 263.2, Carbs: 21.8g, Protein: 27.8g, Fats: 7.2g, Sodium: 264mg

# 240. STEAMED VEGGIE AND LEMON PEPPER SALMON

**COOKING: 15'**     **PREPARATION: 15'**     **SERVINGS: 4**

## INGREDIENTS

- » 1 carrot, peeled and julienned
- » 1 red bell pepper, julienned
- » 1 zucchini, julienned
- » ½ lemon, sliced thinly
- » 1 tsp pepper
- » ½ tsp salt
- » 1/2-lb salmon filet with skin on
- » A dash of tarragon

## DIRECTIONS

1. In a heat-proof dish that fits inside a saucepan, add salmon with skin side down. Season with pepper. Add slices of lemon on top.

2. Place the julienned vegetables on top of salmon and season with tarragon. Cover top of fish with remaining cherry tomatoes and place dish on the trivet. Cover dish with foil. Cover pan and steam for 15 minutes. Serve and enjoy.

**NUTRITIONS:** Calories: 216.2, Carbs: 4.1g, Protein: 35.1g, Fats: 6.6g, Sodium: 332mg

# 241. STEAMED FISH WITH SCALLIONS AND GINGER

**COOKING: 15'**      **PREPARATION: 15'**      **SERVINGS: 3**

## INGREDIENTS

- ¼ cup chopped cilantro
- ¼ cup julienned scallions
- 2 tbsp julienned ginger
- 1 tbsp peanut oil
- 1-lb Tilapia filets
- 1 tsp garlic
- 1 tsp minced ginger
- 2 tbsp rice wine
- 1 tbsp low sodium soy sauce

## DIRECTIONS

1. Mix garlic, minced ginger, rice wine, and soy sauce in a heat-proof dish that fits inside a saucepan. Add the Tilapia filet and marinate for half an hour while turning over at the half time.

2. Cover dish of fish with foil and place on a trivet. Cover pan and steam for 15 minutes. Serve and enjoy.

**NUTRITIONS:** Calories: 219, Carbs: 4.5g, Protein: 31.8g, Fats: 8.2g, Sodium: 252mg

# 242. STEAMED TILAPIA WITH GREEN CHUTNEY

**COOKING: 10'**      **PREPARATION: 15'**      **SERVINGS: 3**

## INGREDIENTS

- 1-pound tilapia fillets, divided into 3
- ½ cup green commercial chutney

## DIRECTIONS

1. Cut 3 pieces of 15-inch lengths foil. In one foil, place one filet in the middle and 1/3 of chutney. Fold over the foil and seal the filet inside. Repeat process for remaining fish. Put packet on the trivet. Steam for 10 minutes. Serve and enjoy.

**NUTRITIONS:** Calories: 151.5, Carbs: 1.1g, Protein: 30.7g, Fats: 2.7g, Sodium: 79mg

# 243. CREAMY HADDOCK WITH KALE

**COOKING: 10'**    **PREPARATION: 15'**    **SERVINGS: 5**

## INGREDIENTS

- » 1 tbsp olive oil
- » 1 onion, chopped
- » 2 cloves of garlic, minced
- » 2 cups chicken broth
- » 1 teaspoon crushed red pepper flakes
- » 1-pound wild Haddock fillets
- » ½ cup heavy cream
- » 1 tablespoon basil
- » 1 cup kale leaves, chopped
- » Pepper to taste

## DIRECTIONS

1. Place a pot on medium-high fire within 3 minutes. Put oil, then sauté the onion and garlic for 5 minutes. Put the rest of the fixing, except for basil, and mix well. Boil on lower fire within 5 minutes. Serve with a sprinkle of basil.

**NUTRITIONS:** Calories: 130.5, Carbs: 5.5g, Protein: 35.7g, Fats: 14.5g, Sodium: 278mg

# 244. COCONUT CURRY SEA BASS

**COOKING: 15'**    **PREPARATION: 15'**    **SERVINGS: 3**

## INGREDIENTS

- » 1 can coconut milk
- » Juice of 1 lime, freshly squeezed
- » 1 tablespoon red curry paste
- » 1 teaspoon coconut aminos
- » 1 teaspoon honey
- » 2 teaspoons sriracha
- » 2 cloves of garlic, minced
- » 1 teaspoon ground turmeric
- » 1 tablespoon curry powder
- » ¼ cup fresh cilantro
- » Pepper

## DIRECTIONS

1. Place a heavy-bottomed pot on medium-high fire. Mix in all ingredients, then simmer on lower fire to a simmer and simmer for 5 minutes. Serve and enjoy.

**NUTRITIONS:** Calories: 241.8, Carbs: 12.8g, Protein: 3.1g, Fats: 19.8g, Sodium: 19mg

# 245. STEWED COD FILET WITH TOMATOES

**COOKING: 15'**        **PREPARATION: 15'**        **SERVINGS: 6**

## INGREDIENTS

- » 1 tbsp olive oil
- » 1 onion, sliced
- » 1 ½ pound fresh cod fillets
- » Pepper
- » 1 lemon juice, freshly squeezed
- » 1 can diced tomatoes

## DIRECTIONS

1. Sauté the onion for 2 minutes in a pot on medium-high fire. Stir in diced tomatoes and cook for 5 minutes. Add cod filet and season with pepper. Simmer on lower fire within 5 minutes. Serve with freshly squeezed lemon juice.

**NUTRITIONS:** Calories: 106.4, Carbs: 2.5g, Protein: 17.8g, Fats: 2.8g, Sodium: 381mg

# 246. LEMONY PARMESAN SHRIMPS

**COOKING: 15'**        **PREPARATION: 15'**        **SERVINGS: 4**

## INGREDIENTS

- » 1 tablespoon olive oil
- » ½ cup onion, chopped
- » 3 cloves of garlic, minced
- » 1-pound shrimps, peeled and deveined
- » ½ cup parmesan cheese, low fat
- » 1 cup spinach, shredded
- » ½ cup chicken broth, low sodium
- » ¼ cup of water
- » Pepper

## DIRECTIONS

1. Sauté the onion and garlic within 5 minutes in a pot with oil on a medium-high fire. Stir in shrimps and cook for 2 minutes.

2. Add remaining ingredients, except for parmesan. Cover, bring to a boil, lower fire to a simmer, and simmer for 5 minutes. Serve and enjoy with a sprinkle of parmesan.

**NUTRITIONS:** Calories: 252.6, Carbs: 5.4g, Protein: 33.9g, Fats: 10.6g, Sodium: 344mg

# 247. TUNA AND CARROTS CASSEROLE

**COOKING: 12'**  **PREPARATION: 15'**  **SERVINGS: 4**

## INGREDIENTS

- » 2 carrots, peeled and chopped
- » ¼ cup diced onions
- » 1 cup frozen peas
- » ¾ cup milk
- » 2 cans tuna in water, drained
- » 1 can cream of celery soup
- » 1 tbsp olive oil
- » ½ cup of water
- » 2 eggs beaten
- » Pepper

## DIRECTIONS

1. Place a heavy-bottomed pot on medium-high fire and heat pot for 3 minutes. Once hot, add oil and stir around to coat pot with oil. Sauté the onion and carrots for 3 minutes.

2. Add remaining ingredients and mix well. Bring to a boil while constantly stirring, cook until thickened around 5 minutes. Serve and enjoy.

**NUTRITIONS:** Calories: 281.3, Carbs: 14.3g, Protein: 24.3g, Fats: 14.1g, Sodium: 275mg

# 248. SWEET-GINGER SCALLOPS

**COOKING: 15'**  **PREPARATION: 15'**  **SERVINGS: 3**

## INGREDIENTS

- » 1-pound sea scallops, shells removed
- » ½ cup coconut aminos
- » 3 tablespoons maple syrup
- » ½ teaspoon garlic powder
- » ½ teaspoon ground ginger

## DIRECTIONS

1. In a heat-proof dish that fits inside a saucepan, add all ingredients. Mix well. Cover dish of scallops with foil and place on a trivet. Cover pan and steam for 10 minutes. Let it stand in the pan for another 5 minutes. Serve and enjoy.

**NUTRITIONS:** Calories: 233.4, Carbs: 23.7g, Protein: 31.5g, Fats: 1.4g, Sodium: 153mg

# 249. SAVORY LOBSTER ROLL

**COOKING: 20'**  **PREPARATION: 15'**  **SERVINGS: 6**

## INGREDIENTS

- » 1 ½ cups chicken broth, low sodium
- » 2 teaspoon old bay seasoning
- » 2 pounds lobster tails, raw and in the shell
- » 1 lemon, halved
- » 3 scallions, chopped
- » 1 teaspoon celery seeds

## DIRECTIONS

1. Place a heavy-bottomed pot on medium-high fire and add all ingredients and ½ of the lemon. Cover, bring to a boil, lower fire to a simmer, and simmer for 15 minutes. Let it rest for another 5 minutes. Serve and enjoy with freshly squeezed lemon juice.

**NUTRITIONS:** Calories: 209, Carbs: 1.9g, Protein: 38.2g, Fats: 5.4g, Sodium: 288mg

# 250. GARLIC AND TOMATOES ON MUSSELS

**COOKING: 15'**  **PREPARATION: 15'**  **SERVINGS: 6**

## INGREDIENTS

- » ¼ cup white wine
- » ½ cup of water
- » 3 Roma tomatoes, chopped
- » 2 cloves of garlic, minced
- » 1 bay leaf
- » 2 pounds mussels, scrubbed
- » ½ cup fresh parsley, chopped
- » 1 tbsp oil
- » Pepper

## DIRECTIONS

1. Warm a pot on medium-high fire within 3 minutes. Put oil and stir around to coat pot with oil. Sauté the garlic, bay leaf, and tomatoes for 5 minutes.

2. Add remaining ingredients except for parsley and mussels. Mix well. Add mussels. Cover, and boil for 5 minutes. Serve with a sprinkle of parsley and discard any unopened mussels.

**NUTRITIONS:** Calories: 172.8, Carbs: 10.2g, Protein: 19.5g, Fats: 6g, Sodium: 261mg

# 251. LEMON SALMON WITH KAFFIR LIME

**COOKING: 30'**         **PREPARATION: 15'**         **SERVINGS: 8**

## INGREDIENTS

» A whole side of salmon fillet
» 1 thinly sliced lemon
» 2 kaffir torn lime leaves
» 1 quartered and bruised lemongrass stalk
» 1 ½ cups fresh coriander leaves

## DIRECTIONS

1. Warm-up oven to 350 F. Covers a baking pan with foil sheets, overlapping the sides (enough to fold over the fish).

2. Put the salmon on the foil, top with the lemon, lime leaves, the lemongrass, and 1 cup of the coriander leaves. Option: season with salt and pepper.

3. Bring the long side of the foil to the center before folding the seal. Roll the ends to close up the salmon. Bake for 30 minutes. Transfer the cooked fish to a platter. Top with fresh coriander. Serve with white or brown rice.

**NUTRITIONS:** Calories 103, Protein 18g, Carbohydrates 43.5g, Fat 11.8g, Sodium 170mg

# 252. BAKED FISH SERVED WITH VEGETABLES

**COOKING: 30'**         **PREPARATION: 15'**         **SERVINGS: 4**

## INGREDIENTS

» 4 haddock or cod fillets, skinless
» 2 Zucchinis, sliced into thick pieces
» 2 red onions, sliced into thick pieces
» 3 large tomatoes, cut in wedges
» ¼ cup black olives pitted
» ¼ cup flavorless oil (olive, canola, or sunflower)
» 1 Tablespoon lemon juice
» 1 Tablespoon Dijon mustard
» 2 garlic cloves, minced
» Salt and pepper to season
» ½ cup chopped parsley

## DIRECTIONS

1. Warm oven to 400 F. In a large baking dish, drizzle some oil over the bottom. Place the fish in the middle. Surround the fish with the zucchini, tomato, onion, and olives. Drizzle more oil over the vegetables and fish. Season with salt and pepper.

2. Place the baking dish in the oven. Bake within 30 minutes, or until the fish is flaky and vegetables are tender. In another bowl, whisk the lemon juice, garlic, mustard, and remaining oil. Set aside.

3. Split the cooked vegetables onto plates, then top with the fish. Drizzle the dressing over the vegetables, fish. Garnish with parsley.

**NUTRITIONS:** Calories 91, Protein 18.7g, Carbohydrates 41g, Fat 7.6g, Sodium 199mg

# 253. FISH IN A VEGETABLE PATCH

**COOKING: 20'**  **PREPARATION: 15'**  **SERVINGS: 3**

## INGREDIENTS

- » 1-pound halibut fillet, skinless
- » 1 Tablespoon flavorless oil (olive, canola, or sunflower)
- » 1 cup tomato sauce
- » 1 ½ Tablespoons Worcestershire sauce
- » 2 large lemons, juiced
- » 1 celery stick, diced
- » ½ green pepper, chopped
- » 1 large carrot, diced
- » ½ an onion, diced
- » 1 lemon, sliced

## DIRECTIONS

1. Warm oven to 400 F. In a small saucepan, combine the tomato sauce, Worcestershire sauce, and lemon juice. Heat for 5 minutes.

2. In a shallow baking dish, drizzle oil along the bottom. Place the vegetables along the bottom and lay the fish over the vegetables. Pour the sauce over the fish. Cover with foil.

3. Bake fillet for 15 minutes, or until the fish is cooked and flaky. Dish out the vegetables, place the fish over the top. Garnish the fish with the lemon slices. Serve with white or brown rice.

**NUTRITIONS:** Calories 80, Protein 18.9g, Carbohydrates 62g, Fat 9g, Sodium 276mg

# 254. SPICY COD

**COOKING: 30'**  **PREPARATION: 15'**  **SERVINGS: 4**

## INGREDIENTS

- » 2 pounds cod fillets
- » 1 Tablespoon flavorless oil (olive, canola, or sunflower)
- » 2 cups low sodium salsa
- » 2 tablespoons fresh chopped parsley

## DIRECTIONS

1. Warm oven to 350 F. In a large, deep baking dish, drizzle the oil along the bottom. Place the cod fillets in the dish. Pour the salsa over the fish.

2. Cover with foil for 20 minutes. Remove the foil last 10 minutes of cooking. Bake in the oven for 20 – 30 minutes, until the fish is flaky. Serve with white or brown rice. Garnish with parsley.

**NUTRITIONS:** Calories 110, Protein 16.5g, Carbohydrates 83g, Fat 11g, Sodium 186mg

# 255. EASY SHRIMP

**COOKING: 10'**　　**PREPARATION: 15'**　　**SERVINGS: 4**

## INGREDIENTS

- » 1-pound cooked shrimp
- » 1 pack mixed frozen vegetables
- » 1 garlic clove, minced
- » 1 teaspoon butter or margarine
- » ¼ cup of water
- » 1 package shrimp-flavored instant noodles
- » 3 teaspoons low sodium soy sauce
- » ½ teaspoon ground ginger

## DIRECTIONS

1. In a large skillet, melt the butter. Add the minced garlic, sweat it for 1 minute. Add the shrimp and vegetables to the skillet. Season with salt and pepper. Cover and simmer for 5 - 10 minutes, until the shrimp turns pink and the vegetables are tender.

2. Boil water in a separate pot. Add the noodles. Turn off the heat, cover the pot. Let it stand for 3 minutes. (Keep the water.)

3. Using a scoop or tongs, transfer the noodles to the skillet with the shrimp and vegetables. Stir in the seasoning packet. Mix, then serve immediately.

**NUTRITIONS:** Calories 80, Protein 18.9g, Carbohydrates 62g, Fat 9g, Sodium 276mg

# 256. STEAMED BLUE CRABS

**COOKING: 10'**　　**PREPARATION: 15'**　　**SERVINGS: 6**

## INGREDIENTS

- » 30 live blue crabs
- » ½ cup seafood seasoning
- » ¼ cup of salt
- » 3 cups beer
- » 3 cups distilled white vinegar

## DIRECTIONS

1. In a large stockpot, combine the seasoning, salt, beer, and white vinegar. Bring it to a boil. Put each crab upside down, then stick a knife into the shell just before cooking them. Cover the lid, leaving a crack for the steam to vent.

2. Steam the crabs until they turn bright orange and float to the top. Allow them to cook for another 2 - 3 minutes. Serve immediately.

**NUTRITIONS:** Calories 77, Protein 9.8g, Carbohydrates 31g, Fat 7g, Sodium 119mg

# 257. GINGER SESAME SALMON

**COOKING: 5'**     **PREPARATION: 15'**     **SERVINGS: 2**

## INGREDIENTS

- » 4 ounces salmon
- » ¼ cup low-sodium soy sauce
- » 2 Tablespoons Balsamic vinegar
- » ½ teaspoon sesame oil
- » 2-inch chunk ginger, peeled and grated
- » 1 garlic clove, minced
- » 1 teaspoon flavorless oil (olive, canola, or sunflower)
- » 1 teaspoon sesame seeds
- » 1 teaspoon green onion, minced

## DIRECTIONS

1. In a glass dish, combine the soy sauce, balsamic vinegar, sesame oil, garlic, and ginger. Place the salmon in the dish. Cover, marinate for 15 - 60 minutes in the fridge.

2. In a nonstick skillet, heat 1 teaspoon of oil. Sauté the fish until it becomes firm and golden on each side. Sprinkle the sesame seeds in the pan. Heat for 1 minute. Serve immediately. Garnish with green onion.

**NUTRITIONS:** Calories 422, Protein 10.8g, Carbohydrates 5.7g, Fat 18g, Sodium 300mg

# 258. SICILIAN SPAGHETTI WITH TUNA

**COOKING: 10'**     **PREPARATION: 5'**     **SERVINGS: 2**

## INGREDIENTS

- » ½ cup fresh Tuna, cut into ½ inch pieces
- » 85 grams whole wheat pasta
- » ½ medium yellow onion, diced
- » 1 garlic clove, minced
- » ½ teaspoon anchovy paste
- » ½ chipotle chili, minced
- » 1 cup fresh tomatoes, chopped
- » 1 teaspoon capers, drained and rinsed
- » 1 cup fresh spinach, chopped
- » ½ tablespoon fresh or dried marjoram
- » 1 teaspoon flavorless oil (olive, canola, or sunflower)

## DIRECTIONS

1. In a large skillet, drizzle oil over the bottom. Sweat the onion for 1 minute. Add the garlic, anchovy paste, and chipotle chili. Cook for 2 minutes.

2. Add the chopped tomatoes and capers. Sauté 2 minutes. Add the fresh spinach and tuna. Cover and cook for 2 - 5 minutes until the tuna is cooked. Turn off the heat. Sprinkle the mixture with the marjoram. Serve over cooked spaghetti.

**NUTRITIONS:** Calories 166, Protein 11g, Carbohydrates 112g, Fat 17.8g, Sodium 304mg

# CHAPTER 9.
# POULTRY

# 259. PARMESAN AND CHICKEN SPAGHETTI SQUASH

**COOKING: 20'**     **PREPARATION: 15'**     **SERVINGS: 6**

## INGREDIENTS

- » 16 oz. mozzarella
- » 1 spaghetti squash piece
- » 1 lb. cooked cube chicken
- » 1 c. Marinara sauce

## DIRECTIONS

1. Split up the squash in halves and remove the seeds. Arrange or put one cup of water in your pot, then put a trivet on top.

2. Add the squash halves to the trivet. Cook within 20 minutes at HIGH pressure. Remove the squashes and shred them using a fork into spaghetti portions

3. Pour sauce over the squash and give it a nice mix. Top them up with the cubed-up chicken and top with mozzarella. Broil for 1-2 minutes and broil until the cheese has melted

**NUTRITIONS:** Calories: 237, Fat:10 g, Carbs:32 g, Protein:11 g, Sodium: 500 mg

# 260. APRICOT CHICKEN

**COOKING: 6'**     **PREPARATION: 15'**     **SERVINGS: 4**

## INGREDIENTS

- » 1 bottle creamy French dressing
- » ¼ c. flavorless oil
- » White cooked rice
- » 1 large jar Apricot preserve
- » 4 lbs. boneless and skinless chicken
- » 1 package onion soup mix

## DIRECTIONS

1. Rinse and pat dry the chicken. Dice into bite-size pieces. In a large bowl, mix the apricot preserve, creamy dressing, and onion soup mix. Stir until thoroughly combined. Place the chicken in the bowl. Mix until coated.

2. In a large skillet, heat the oil. Place the chicken in the oil gently. Cook 4 – 6 minutes on each side, until golden brown. Serve over rice.

**NUTRITIONS:** Calories: 202, Fat:12 g, Carbs:75 g, Protein:20 g, Sugars:10 g, Sodium: 630 mg

# 261. OVEN-FRIED CHICKEN BREASTS

**COOKING: 30'**    **PREPARATION: 15'**    **SERVINGS: 8**

## INGREDIENTS

» ½ pack Ritz crackers
» 1 c. plain non-fat yogurt
» 8 boneless, skinless, and halved chicken breasts

## DIRECTIONS

1. Preheat the oven to 350 oF. Rinse and pat dry the chicken breasts. Pour the yogurt into a shallow bowl. Dip the chicken pieces in the yogurt, then roll in the cracker crumbs. Place the chicken in a single layer in a baking dish. Bake within 15 minutes per side. Serve.

**NUTRITIONS:** Calories: 200, Fat:13 g, Carbs:98 g, Protein:19 g, Sodium:217 mg

# 262. ROSEMARY ROASTED CHICKEN

**COOKING: 20'**    **PREPARATION: 15'**    **SERVINGS: 8**

## INGREDIENTS

» 8 rosemary springs
» 1 minced garlic clove
» Black pepper
» 1 tbsp. chopped rosemary
» 1 chicken
» 1 tbsp. organic olive oil

## DIRECTIONS

1. In a bowl, mix garlic with rosemary, rub the chicken with black pepper, the oil and rosemary mix, place it inside roasting pan, introduce inside the oven at 350 oF, and roast for sixty minutes and 20 min. Carve chicken, divide between plates and serve using a side dish. Enjoy!

**NUTRITIONS:** Calories: 325, Fat:5 g, Carbs:15 g, Protein:14 g, Sodium: 950 mg

# 263. ARTICHOKE AND SPINACH CHICKEN

**COOKING: 5'**        **PREPARATION: 15'**        **SERVINGS: 4**

## INGREDIENTS

- » 10 oz baby spinach
- » ½ tsp. crushed red pepper flakes
- » 14 oz. chopped artichoke hearts
- » 28 oz. no-salt-added tomato sauce
- » 2 tbsps. Essential olive oil
- » 4 boneless and skinless chicken breasts

## DIRECTIONS

1. Heat-up a pan with the oil over medium-high heat, add chicken and red pepper flakes and cook for 5 minutes on them. Add spinach, artichokes, and tomato sauce, toss, cook for ten minutes more, divide between plates and serve. Enjoy!

**NUTRITIONS:** Calories: 212, Fat:3 g, Carbs:16 g, Protein:20 g, Sugars:5 g, Sodium:418 mg

# 264. PUMPKIN AND BLACK BEANS CHICKEN

**COOKING: 25'**        **PREPARATION: 15'**        **SERVINGS: 4**

## INGREDIENTS

- » 1 tbsp. essential olive oil
- » 1 tbsp. Chopped cilantro
- » 1 c. coconut milk
- » 15 oz canned black beans, drained
- » 1 lb. skinless and boneless chicken breasts
- » 2 c. water
- » ½ c. pumpkin flesh

## DIRECTIONS

1. Heat a pan when using oil over medium-high heat, add the chicken and cook for 5 minutes. Add the river, milk, pumpkin, and black beans toss, cover the pan, reduce heat to medium and cook for 20 mins. Add cilantro, toss, divide between plates and serve. Enjoy!

**NUTRITIONS:** Calories: 254, Fat:6 g, Carbs:16 g, Protein:22 g, Sodium:92 mg

# 265. CHICKEN THIGHS AND APPLES MIX

**COOKING: 60'**  **PREPARATION: 15'**  **SERVINGS: 4**

## INGREDIENTS

- » 3 cored and sliced apples
- » 1 tbsp apple cider vinegar treatment
- » ¾ c. natural apple juice
- » ¼ tsp. pepper and salt
- » 1 tbsp. grated ginger
- » 8 chicken thighs
- » 3 tbsps. Chopped onion

## DIRECTIONS

1. In a bowl, mix chicken with salt, pepper, vinegar, onion, ginger, and apple juice, toss well, cover, keep within the fridge for ten minutes, transfer with a baking dish, and include apples. Introduce inside the oven at 400 oF for just 1 hour. Divide between plates and serve. Enjoy!

**NUTRITIONS:** Calories: 214, Fat:3 g, Carbs:14 g, Protein:15 g, Sodium:405 mg

# 266. THAI CHICKEN THIGHS

**COOKING: 1H 5'**  **PREPARATION: 15'**  **SERVINGS: 6**

## INGREDIENTS

- » ½ c. Thai chili sauce
- » 1 chopped green onions bunch
- » 4 lbs. chicken thighs

## DIRECTIONS

1. Heat a pan over medium-high heat. Add chicken thighs, brown them for 5 minutes on both sides Transfer to some baking dish, then add chili sauce and green onions and toss.

2. Introduce within the oven and bake at 400oF for 60 minutes. Divide everything between plates and serve. Enjoy!

**NUTRITIONS:** Calories: 220, Fat:4 g, Carbs:12 g, Protein:10 g, Sodium: 870 mg

# 267. FALLING "OFF" THE BONE CHICKEN

**COOKING: 40'**　　　　**PREPARATION: 15'**　　　　**SERVINGS: 4**

## INGREDIENTS

- » 6 peeled garlic cloves
- » 1 tbsp. organic extra virgin coconut oil
- » 2 tbsps. Lemon juice
- » 1 ½ c. pacific organic bone chicken broth
- » ¼ tsp freshly ground black pepper
- » ½ tsp. sea flavored vinegar
- » 1 whole organic chicken piece
- » 1 tsp. paprika
- » 1 tsp. dried thyme

## DIRECTIONS

1. Take a small bowl and toss in the thyme, paprika, pepper, and flavored vinegar and mix them. Use the mixture to season the chicken properly. Pour down the oil in your instant pot and heat it to shimmering; toss in the chicken with breast downward and let it cook for about 6-7 minutes

2. After the 7 minutes, flip over the chicken pour down the broth, garlic cloves, and lemon juice. Cook within 25 minutes on a high setting. Remove the dish from the cooker and let it stand for about 5 minutes before serving.

**NUTRITIONS:** Calories: 664, Fat:44 g, Carbs:44 g, Protein:27 g, Sugars:0.1 g, Sodium:800 mg

# 268. FEISTY CHICKEN PORRIDGE

**COOKING: 30'**　　　　**PREPARATION: 15'**　　　　**SERVINGS: 4**

## INGREDIENTS

- » 1 ½ c. fresh ginger
- » 1 lb. cooked chicken legs
- » Green onions
- » Toasted cashew nuts
- » 5 c. chicken broth
- » 1 cup jasmine rice
- » 4 c. water

## DIRECTIONS

1. Place the rice in your fridge and allow it to chill 1 hour before cooking. Take the rice out and add them to your Instant Pot. Pour broth and water. Lock up the lid and cook on Porridge mode.

2. Separate the meat from the chicken legs and add the meat to your soup. Stir well over sauté mode. Season with a bit of flavored vinegar and enjoy with a garnish of nuts and onion

**NUTRITIONS:** Calories: 206, Fat:8 g, Carbs:8 g, Protein:23 g, Sugars:0 g, Sodium:950 mg

# 269. THE ULTIMATE FAUX-TISSERIE CHICKEN

**COOKING: 35'**     **PREPARATION: 15'**     **SERVINGS: 5**

## INGREDIENTS

- » 1 c. low sodium broth
- » 2 tbsps. Olive oil
- » ½ quartered medium onion
- » 2 tbsps. Favorite seasoning
- » 2 ½ lbs. whole chicken
- » Black pepper
- » 5 large fresh garlic cloves

## DIRECTIONS

1. Massage the chicken with 1 tablespoon of olive oil and sprinkle pepper on top. Place onion wedges and garlic cloves inside the chicken. Take a butcher's twin and secure the legs

2. Set your pot to Sauté mode. Put olive oil in your pan on medium heat, allow the oil to heat up. Add chicken and sear both sides for 4 minutes per side. Sprinkle your seasoning over the chicken, remove the chicken and place a trivet at the bottom of your pot

3. Sprinkle seasoning over the chicken, making sure to rub it. Transfer the chicken to the trivet with the breast side facing up, lock up the lid. Cook on HIGH pressure for 25 minutes. Allow it to rest and serve!

**NUTRITIONS:** Calories: 1010, Fat:64 g, Carbs:47 g, Protein:60 g, Sodium:209 mg

# 270. OREGANO CHICKEN THIGHS

**COOKING: 20'**     **PREPARATION: 15'**     **SERVINGS: 6**

## INGREDIENTS

- » 12 chicken thighs
- » 1 tsp dried parsley
- » ¼ tsp. pepper and salt.
- » ½ c. extra virgin essential olive oil
- » 4 minced garlic cloves
- » 1 c. chopped oregano
- » ¼ c. low-sodium veggie stock

## DIRECTIONS

1. In your food processor, mix parsley with oregano, garlic, salt, pepper, and stock and pulse. Put chicken thighs within the bowl, add oregano paste, toss, cover, and then leave aside within the fridge for 10 minutes.

2. Heat the kitchen grill over medium heat, add chicken pieces, close the lid and cook for twenty or so minutes with them. Divide between plates and serve!

**NUTRITIONS:** Calories: 254, Fat:3 g, Carbs:7 g, Protein:17 g, Sugars:0.9 g, Sodium:730 mg

# 271. PESTO CHICKEN BREASTS WITH SUMMER SQUASH

**COOKING: 10'**          **PREPARATION: 15'**          **SERVINGS: 4**

## INGREDIENTS

» 4 medium boneless, skinless chicken breast halves
» 1 tbsp. olive oil
» 2 tbsps. Homemade pesto
» 2 c. finely chopped zucchini
» 2 tbsps. Finely shredded Asiago

## DIRECTIONS

1. Cook your chicken in hot oil on medium heat within 4 minutes in a large nonstick skillet. Flip the chicken then put the zucchini.

2. Cook within 4 to 6 minutes more or until the chicken is tender and no longer pink (170 F), and squash is crisp-tender, stirring squash gently once or twice. Transfer chicken and squash to 4 dinner plates. Spread pesto over chicken; sprinkle with Asiago.

**NUTRITIONS:** Calories: 230, Fat:9 g, Carbs:8 g, Protein:30 g, Sodium:578 mg

# 272. CHICKEN, TOMATO AND GREEN BEANS

**COOKING: 25'**          **PREPARATION: 15'**          **SERVINGS: 4**

## INGREDIENTS

» 6 oz. low-sodium canned tomato paste
» 2 tbsps. Olive oil
» ¼ tsp. black pepper
» 2 lbs. trimmed green beans
» 2 tbsps. Chopped parsley
» 1 ½ lbs. boneless, skinless, and cubed chicken breasts
» 25 oz. no-salt-added canned tomato sauce

## DIRECTIONS

1. Heat a pan with 50 % with the oil over medium heat, add chicken, stir, cover, cook within 5 minutes on both sides and transfer to a bowl. Heat inside the same pan while using rest through the oil over medium heat, add green beans, stir and cook for 10 minutes.

2. Return chicken for that pan, add black pepper, tomato sauce, tomato paste, and parsley, stir, cover, cook for 10 minutes more, divide between plates and serve. Enjoy!

**NUTRITIONS:** Calories: 190, Fat:4 g, Carbs:12 g, Protein:9 g, Sodium:168 mg

# 273. CHICKEN TORTILLAS

**COOKING: 5'**　　　**PREPARATION: 15'**　　　**SERVINGS: 4**

## INGREDIENTS

- » 6 oz. boneless, skinless, and cooked chicken breasts
- » Black pepper
- » 1/3 c. fat-free yogurt
- » 4 heated up whole-wheat tortillas
- » 2 chopped tomatoes

## DIRECTIONS

1. Heat-up a pan over medium heat, add one tortilla during those times, heat up, and hang them on the working surface. Spread yogurt on each tortilla, add chicken and tomatoes, roll, divide between plates and serve. Enjoy!

**NUTRITIONS:** Calories:190, Fat:2 g, Carbs:12 g, Protein:6 g, Sodium:300 mg

# 274. CHICKEN WITH POTATOES OLIVES & SPROUTS

**COOKING: 35'**　　　**PREPARATION: 15'**　　　**SERVINGS: 4**

## INGREDIENTS

- » 1 lb. chicken breasts, skinless, boneless, and cut into pieces
- » ¼ cup olives, quartered
- » 1 tsp oregano
- » 1 ½ tsp Dijon mustard
- » 1 lemon juice
- » 1/3 cup vinaigrette dressing
- » 1 medium onion, diced
- » 3 cups potatoes cut into pieces
- » 4 cups Brussels sprouts, trimmed and quartered
- » ¼ tsp pepper
- » ¼ tsp salt

## DIRECTIONS

1. Warm-up oven to 400 F. Place chicken in the center of the baking tray, then place potatoes, sprouts, and onions around the chicken.

2. In a small bowl, mix vinaigrette, oregano, mustard, lemon juice, and salt and pour over chicken and veggies. Sprinkle olives and season with pepper.

3. Bake in preheated oven for 20 minutes. Transfer chicken to a plate. Stir the vegetables and roast for 15 minutes more. Serve and enjoy.

**NUTRITIONS:** Calories: 397, Fat: 13g, Protein: 38.3g, Carbs: 31.4g, Sodium 175 mg

# 275. GARLIC MUSHROOM CHICKEN

**COOKING: 15'**          **PREPARATION: 15'**          **SERVINGS: 4**

## INGREDIENTS

- » 4 chicken breasts, boneless and skinless
- » 3 garlic cloves, minced
- » 1 onion, chopped
- » 2 cups mushrooms, sliced
- » 1 tbsp olive oil
- » ½ cup chicken stock
- » ¼ tsp pepper
- » ½ tsp salt

## DIRECTIONS

1. Season chicken with pepper and salt. Warm oil in a pan on medium heat, then put season chicken in the pan and cook for 5-6 minutes on each side. Remove and place on a plate.

2. Add onion and mushrooms to the pan and sauté until tender, about 2-3 minutes. Add garlic and sauté for a minute. Add stock and bring to boil. Stir well and cook for 1-2 minutes. Pour over chicken and serve.

**NUTRITIONS:** Calories: 331, Fat: 14.5g, Protein: 43.9g, Carbs: 4.6g, Sodium 420 mg

# 276. GRILLED CHICKEN

**COOKING: 15'**          **PREPARATION: 5'**          **SERVINGS: 4**

## INGREDIENTS

- » 4 chicken breasts, skinless and boneless
- » 1 ½ tsp dried oregano
- » 1 tsp paprika
- » 5 garlic cloves, minced
- » ½ cup fresh parsley, minced
- » ½ cup olive oil
- » ½ cup fresh lemon juice
- » Pepper
- » Salt

## DIRECTIONS

1. Add lemon juice, oregano, paprika, garlic, parsley, and olive oil to a large zip-lock bag. Season chicken with pepper and salt and add to bag. Seal bag and shake well to coat chicken with marinade. Let sit chicken in the marinade for 20 minutes.

2. Remove chicken from marinade and grill over medium-high heat for 5-6 minutes on each side. Serve and enjoy.

**NUTRITIONS:** Calories: 512, Fat: 36.5g, Protein: 43.1g, Carbs: 3g, Sodium 110mg

# 277. DELICIOUS LEMON CHICKEN SALAD

**COOKING: 5'**          **PREPARATION: 15'**          **SERVINGS: 4**

## INGREDIENTS

- » 1 lb. chicken breast, cooked and diced
- » 1 tbsp fresh dill, chopped
- » 2 tsp olive oil
- » 1/4 cup low-fat yogurt
- » 1 tsp lemon zest, grated
- » 2 tbsp onion, minced
- » ¼ tsp pepper
- » ¼ tsp salt

## DIRECTIONS

1. Put all your fixing into the large mixing bowl and toss well. Season with pepper and salt. Cover and place in the refrigerator. Serve chilled and enjoy.

**NUTRITIONS:** Calories: 165, Fat: 5.4g, Protein: 25.2g, Carbs: 2.2g, Sodium 153mg

# 278. HEALTHY CHICKEN ORZO

**COOKING: 15'**          **PREPARATION: 15'**          **SERVINGS: 4**

## INGREDIENTS

- » 1 cup whole wheat orzo
- » 1 lb. chicken breasts, sliced
- » ½ tsp red pepper flakes
- » ½ cup feta cheese, crumbled
- » ½ tsp oregano
- » 1 tbsp fresh parsley, chopped
- » 1 tbsp fresh basil, chopped
- » ¼ cup pine nuts
- » 1 cup spinach, chopped
- » ¼ cup white wine
- » ½ cup olives, sliced
- » 1 cup grape tomatoes, cut in half
- » ½ tbsp garlic, minced
- » 2 tbsp olive oil
- » ½ tsp pepper
- » ½ tsp salt

## DIRECTIONS

1. Add water in a small saucepan and bring to boil. Heat 1 tablespoon of olive oil in a pan over medium heat. Season chicken with pepper and salt and cook in the pan for 5-7 minutes on each side. Remove from pan and set aside.

2. Add orzo in boiling water and cook according to the packet directions. Heat remaining olive oil in a pan on medium heat, then put garlic in the pan and sauté for a minute. Stir in white wine and cherry tomatoes and cook on high for 3 minutes.

3. Add cooked orzo, spices, spinach, pine nuts, and olives and stir until well combined. Add chicken on top of orzo and sprinkle with feta cheese. Serve and enjoy.

**NUTRITIONS:** Calories: 518, Fat: 27.7g, Protein: 40.6g, Carbs: 26.2g, Sodium 121mg

# 279. LEMON GARLIC CHICKEN

**COOKING: 12'**　　　**PREPARATION: 15'**　　　**SERVINGS: 3**

## INGREDIENTS

- » 3 chicken breasts, cut into thin slices
- » 2 lemon zest, grated
- » ¼ cup olive oil
- » 4 garlic cloves, minced
- » Pepper
- » Salt

## DIRECTIONS

1. Warm-up olive oil in a pan over medium heat. Add garlic to the pan and sauté for 30 seconds. Put the chicken in the pan and sauté within 10 minutes. Add lemon zest and lemon juice and bring to boil. Remove from heat and season with pepper and salt. Serve and enjoy.

**NUTRITIONS:** Calories: 439, Fat: 27.8g, Protein: 42.9g, Carbs: 4.9g, Sodium 306 mg

# 280. SIMPLE MEDITERRANEAN CHICKEN

**COOKING: 15'**　　　**PREPARATION: 15'**　　　**SERVINGS: 12**

## INGREDIENTS

- » 2 chicken breasts, skinless and boneless
- » 1 ½ cup grape tomatoes, cut in half
- » ½ cup olives
- » 2 tbsp olive oil
- » 1 tsp Italian seasoning
- » ¼ tsp pepper
- » ¼ tsp salt

## DIRECTIONS

1. Season chicken with Italian seasoning, pepper, and salt. Warm-up olive oil in a pan over medium heat. Add season chicken to the pan and cook for 4-6 minutes on each side. Transfer chicken on a plate.

2. Put tomatoes plus olives in the pan and cook for 2-4 minutes. Pour olive and tomato mixture on top of the chicken and serve.

**NUTRITIONS:** Calories: 468, Fat: 29.4g, Protein: 43.8g, Carbs: 7.8g, Sodium 410 mg

# 281. ROASTED CHICKEN THIGHS

**COOKING: 55'**     **PREPARATION: 15'**     **SERVINGS: 4**

## INGREDIENTS

- » 8 chicken thighs
- » 3 tbsp fresh parsley, chopped
- » 1 tsp dried oregano
- » 6 garlic cloves, crushed
- » ¼ cup capers, drained
- » 10 oz roasted red peppers, sliced
- » 2 cups grape tomatoes
- » 1 ½ lbs. potatoes, cut into small chunks
- » 4 tbsp olive oil
- » Pepper
- » Salt

## DIRECTIONS

1. Warm oven to 200 400 F. Season chicken with pepper and salt. Heat-up 2 tablespoons of olive oil in a pan over medium heat. Add chicken to the pan and sear until lightly golden brown from all the sides.

2. Transfer chicken onto a baking tray. Add tomato, potatoes, capers, oregano, garlic, and red peppers around the chicken. Season with pepper and salt and drizzle with remaining olive oil. Bake in preheated oven for 45-55 minutes. Garnish with parsley and serve.

**NUTRITIONS:** Calories: 848, Fat: 29.1g, Protein: 91.3g, Carbs: 45.2g, Sodium 110 mg

# 282. MEDITERRANEAN TURKEY BREAST

**COOKING: 4H 30'**     **PREPARATION: 15'**     **SERVINGS: 4**

## INGREDIENTS

- » 4 lbs. turkey breast
- » 3 tbsp flour
- » ¾ cup chicken stock
- » 4 garlic cloves, chopped
- » 1 tsp dried oregano
- » ½ fresh lemon juice
- » ½ cup sun-dried tomatoes, chopped
- » ½ cup olives, chopped
- » 1 onion, chopped
- » ¼ tsp pepper
- » ½ tsp salt

## DIRECTIONS

1. Add turkey breast, garlic, oregano, lemon juice, sun-dried tomatoes, olives, onion, pepper, and salt to the slow cooker. Add half stock. Cook on high within 4 hours.

2. Whisk remaining stock and flour in a small bowl and add to slow cooker. Cover and cook for 30 minutes more. Serve and enjoy.

**NUTRITIONS:** Calories: 537, Fat: 9.7g, Protein: 79.1g, Carbs: 29.6g, Sodium 330 mg

# 283. OLIVE CAPERS CHICKEN

**COOKING: 16'**         **PREPARATION: 15'**         **SERVINGS: 4**

## INGREDIENTS

- » 2 lbs. chicken
- » 1/3 cup chicken stock
- » 3.5 oz Capers
- » 6 oz olives
- » 1/4 cup fresh basil
- » 1 tbsp olive oil
- » 1 tsp oregano
- » 2 garlic cloves, minced
- » 2 tbsp red wine vinegar
- » 1/8 tsp pepper
- » 1/4 tsp salt

## DIRECTIONS

1. Put olive oil in your instant pot and set the pot on sauté mode. Add chicken to the pot and sauté for 3-4 minutes. Add remaining ingredients and stir well. Seal pot with the lid and select manual, and set timer for 12 minutes. Serve and enjoy.

**NUTRITIONS:** Calories: 433, Fat: 15.2g, Protein: 66.9g, Carbs: 4.8g, Sodium 244 mg

# 284. CHICKEN WITH MUSHROOMS

**COOKING: 6H 10'**         **PREPARATION: 15'**         **SERVINGS: 2**

## INGREDIENTS

- » 2 chicken breasts, skinless and boneless
- » 1 cup mushrooms, sliced
- » 1 onion, sliced
- » 1 cup chicken stock
- » 1/2 tsp thyme, dried
- » Pepper
- » Salt

## DIRECTIONS

1. Add all ingredients to the slow cooker. Cook on low within 6 hours. Serve and enjoy.

**NUTRITIONS:** Calories: 313, Fat: 11.3g, Protein: 44.3g, Carbs: 6.9g, Sodium 541 mg

# 285. BAKED CHICKEN

**COOKING: 35'**     **PREPARATION: 15'**     **SERVINGS: 4**

## INGREDIENTS

- » 2 lbs. chicken tenders
- » 1 large zucchini
- » 1 cup grape tomatoes
- » 2 tbsp olive oil
- » 3 dill sprigs

**For topping:**
- » 2 tbsp feta cheese, crumbled
- » 1 tbsp olive oil
- » 1 tbsp fresh lemon juice
- » 1 tbsp fresh dill, chopped

## DIRECTIONS

1. Warm oven to 200 C/ 400 F. Drizzle the olive oil on a baking tray, then place chicken, zucchini, dill, and tomatoes on the tray. Season with salt. Bake chicken within 30 minutes.

2. Meanwhile, in a small bowl, stir all topping ingredients. Place chicken on the serving tray, then top with veggies and discard dill sprigs. Sprinkle topping mixture on top of chicken and vegetables. Serve and enjoy.

**NUTRITIONS:** Calories: 557, Fat: 28.6g, Protein: 67.9g, Carbs: 5.2g, Sodium 760 mg

# 286. GARLIC PEPPER CHICKEN

**COOKING: 25'**     **PREPARATION: 15'**     **SERVINGS: 2**

## INGREDIENTS

- » 2 chicken breasts, cut into strips
- » 2 bell peppers, cut into strips
- » 5 garlic cloves, chopped
- » 3 tbsp water
- » 2 tbsp olive oil
- » 1 tbsp paprika
- » 2 tsp black pepper
- » 1/2 tsp salt

## DIRECTIONS

1. Warm-up olive oil in a large saucepan over medium heat. Add garlic and sauté for 2-3 minutes. Add peppers and cook for 3 minutes. Add chicken and spices and stir to coat. Add water and stir well. Bring to boil. Cover and simmer for 10-15 minutes. Serve and enjoy.

**NUTRITIONS:** Calories: 462, Fat: 25.7g, Protein: 44.7g, Carbs: 14.8g, Sodium 720 mg

# 287. MUSTARD CHICKEN TENDERS

**COOKING: 20'**　　　**PREPARATION: 15'**　　　**SERVINGS: 4**

## INGREDIENTS

- » 1 lb. chicken tenders
- » 2 tbsp fresh tarragon, chopped
- » 1/2 cup whole grain mustard
- » 1/2 tsp paprika
- » 1 garlic clove, minced
- » 1/2 oz fresh lemon juice
- » 1/2 tsp pepper
- » 1/4 tsp kosher salt

## DIRECTIONS

1. Warm oven to 425 F. Add all ingredients except chicken to the large bowl and mix well. Put the chicken in the bowl, then stir until well coated. Place chicken on a baking dish and cover. Bake within 15-20 minutes. Serve and enjoy.

**NUTRITIONS:** Calories: 242, Fat: 9.5g, Protein: 33.2g, Carbs: 3.1g, Sodium 240 mg

# 288. SALSA CHICKEN CHILI

**COOKING: 20'**　　　**PREPARATION: 15'**　　　**SERVINGS: 8**

## INGREDIENTS

- » 2 1/2 lbs. chicken breasts, skinless and boneless
- » 1/2 tsp cumin powder
- » 3 garlic cloves, minced
- » 1 onion, diced
- » 16 oz salsa
- » 1 tsp oregano
- » 1 tbsp olive oil

## DIRECTIONS

1. Add oil into the instant pot and set the pot on sauté mode. Add onion to the pot and sauté until softened, about 3 minutes. Add garlic and sauté for a minute. Add oregano and cumin and sauté for a minute. Add half salsa and stir well. Place chicken and pour remaining salsa over chicken.

2. Seal pot with the lid and select manual, and set timer for 10 minutes. Remove chicken and shred. Move it back to the pot, then stir well to combine. Serve and enjoy.

**NUTRITIONS:** Calories: 308, Fat: 12.4g, Protein: 42.1g, Carbs: 5.4g, Sodium 656 mg

# 289. HONEY CRUSTED CHICKEN

**COOKING: 25'**　　　**PREPARATION: 10'**　　　**SERVINGS: 2**

## INGREDIENTS

- » 1 teaspoon paprika
- » 8 saltine crackers, 2 inches square
- » 2 chicken breasts, each 4 ounces
- » 4 tsp honey

## DIRECTIONS

1. Set the oven to heat at 375 degrees F. Grease a baking dish with cooking oil. Smash the crackers in a Ziplock bag and toss them with paprika in a bowl. Brush chicken with honey and add it to the crackers.

2. Mix well and transfer the chicken to the baking dish. Bake the chicken for 25 minutes until golden brown. Serve.

**NUTRITIONS:** Calories 219, Fat 17 g, Sodium 456 mg, Carbs 12.1 g, Protein 31 g

# 290. PAELLA WITH CHICKEN, LEEKS, AND TARRAGON

**COOKING: 20'**　　　**PREPARATION: 10'**　　　**SERVINGS: 2**

## INGREDIENTS

- » 1 teaspoon extra-virgin olive oil
- » 1 small onion, sliced
- » 2 leeks (whites only), thinly sliced
- » 3 garlic cloves, minced
- » 1-pound boneless, skinless chicken breast, cut into strips 1/2-inch-wide and 2 inches long
- » 2 large tomatoes, chopped
- » 1 red pepper, sliced
- » 2/3 cup long-grain brown rice
- » 1 teaspoon tarragon, or to taste
- » 2 cups fat-free, unsalted chicken broth
- » 1 cup frozen peas
- » 1/4 cup chopped fresh parsley
- » 1 lemon, cut into 4 wedges

## DIRECTIONS

1. Preheat a nonstick pan with olive oil over medium heat. Toss in leeks, onions, chicken strips, and garlic. Sauté for 5 minutes. Stir in red pepper slices and tomatoes. Stir and cook for 5 minutes.

2. Add tarragon, broth, and rice. Let it boil, then reduce the heat to a simmer. Continue cooking for 10 minutes, then add peas and continue cooking until the liquid is thoroughly cooked. Garnish with parsley and lemon. Serve.

**NUTRITIONS:** Calories 388, Fat 15.2 g, Sodium 572 mg, Carbs 5.4 g, Protein 27 g

# 291. SOUTHWESTERN CHICKEN AND PASTA

**COOKING: 10'**　　　**PREPARATION: 10'**　　　**SERVINGS: 2**

## INGREDIENTS

- » 1 cup uncooked whole-wheat rigatoni
- » 2 chicken breasts, cut into cubes
- » 1/4 cup of salsa
- » 1 1/2 cups of canned unsalted tomato sauce
- » 1/8 tsp garlic powder
- » 1 tsp cumin
- » 1/2 tsp chili powder
- » 1/2 cup canned black beans, drained
- » 1/2 cup fresh corn
- » 1/4 cup Monterey Jack and Colby cheese, shredded

## DIRECTIONS

1. Fill a pot with water up to ¾ full and boil it. Add pasta to cook until it is al dente, then drain the pasta while rinsing under cold water. Preheat a skillet with cooking oil, then cook the chicken for 10 minutes until golden from both sides.

2. Add tomato sauce, salsa, cumin, garlic powder, black beans, corn, and chili powder. Cook the mixture while stirring, then toss in the pasta. Serve with 2 tablespoons cheese on top. Enjoy.

**NUTRITIONS:** Calories 245, Fat 16.3 g, Sodium 515 mg, Carbs 19.3 g, Protein 33.3 g

# 292. STUFFED CHICKEN BREASTS

**COOKING: 30'**　　　**PREPARATION: 15'**　　　**SERVINGS: 4**

## INGREDIENTS

- » 3 tbsp seedless raisins
- » 1/2 cup of chopped onion
- » 1/2 cup of chopped celery
- » 1/4 tsp garlic, minced
- » 1 bay leaf
- » 1 cup apple with peel, chopped
- » 2 tbsp chopped water chestnuts
- » 4 large chicken breast halves, 5 ounces each
- » 1 tablespoon olive oil
- » 1 cup fat-free milk
- » 1 teaspoon curry powder
- » 2 tablespoons all-purpose (plain) flour
- » 1 lemon, cut into 4 wedges

## DIRECTIONS

1. Set the oven to heat at 425 degrees F. Grease a baking dish with cooking oil. Soak raisins in warm water until they swell. Grease a heated skillet with cooking spray.

2. Add celery, garlic, onions, and bay leaf. Sauté for 5 minutes. Discard the bay leaf, then toss in apples. Stir cook for 2 minutes. Drain the soaked raisin and pat them dry to remove excess water.

3. Add raisins and water chestnuts to the apple mixture. Pull apart the chicken's skin and stuff the apple raisin mixture between the skin and the chicken. Preheat olive oil in another skillet and sear the breasts for 5 minutes per side.

4. Place the chicken breasts in the baking dish and cover the dish. Bake for 15 minutes until temperature reaches 165 degrees F. Prepare sauce by mixing milk, flour, and curry powder in a saucepan.

5. Stir cook until the mixture thickens, about 5 minutes. Pour this sauce over the baked chicken. Bake again in the covered dish for 10 minutes. Serve.

**NUTRITIONS:** Calories 357, Fat 32.7 g, Sodium 277 mg, Carbs 17.7 g, Protein 31.2 g

# 293. BUFFALO CHICKEN SALAD WRAP

**COOKING: 10'**          **PREPARATION: 10'**          **SERVINGS: 4**

## INGREDIENTS

- » 3-4 ounces chicken breasts
- » 2 whole chipotle peppers
- » 1/4 cup white wine vinegar
- » 1/4 cup low-calorie mayonnaise
- » 2 stalks celery, diced
- » 2 carrots, cut into matchsticks
- » 1 small yellow onion, diced
- » 1/2 cup thinly sliced rutabaga or another root vegetable
- » 4 ounces spinach, cut into strips
- » 2 whole-grain tortillas (12-inch diameter)

## DIRECTIONS

1. Set the oven or a grill to heat at 375 degrees F. Bake the chicken first for 10 minutes per side. Blend chipotle peppers with mayonnaise and wine vinegar in the blender. Dice the baked chicken into cubes or small chunks.

2. Mix the chipotle mixture with all the ingredients except tortillas and spinach. Spread 2 ounces of spinach over the tortilla and scoop the stuffing on top. Wrap the tortilla and cut it into half. Serve.

**NUTRITIONS:** Calories 300, Fat 16.4 g, Sodium 471 mg, Carbs 8.7 g, Protein 38.5 g

# 294. CHICKEN SLIDERS

**COOKING: 10'**          **PREPARATION: 10'**          **SERVINGS: 4**

## INGREDIENTS

- » 10 ounces ground chicken breast
- » 1 tablespoon black pepper
- » 1 tablespoon minced garlic
- » 1 tablespoon balsamic vinegar
- » 1/2 cup minced onion
- » 1 fresh chili pepper, minced
- » 1 tablespoon fennel seed, crushed
- » 4 whole-wheat mini buns
- » 4 lettuce leaves
- » 4 tomato slices

## DIRECTIONS

1. Combine all the ingredients except the wheat buns, tomato, and lettuce. Mix well and refrigerate the mixture for 1 hour. Divide the mixture into 4 patties.

2. Broil these patties in a greased baking tray until golden brown. Place the chicken patties in the wheat buns along with lettuce and tomato. Serve.

**NUTRITIONS:** Calories 224, Fat 4.5 g, Sodium 212 mg, Carbs 10.2 g, Protein 67.4 g

# 295. WHITE CHICKEN CHILI

**COOKING: 15'**     **PREPARATION: 20'**     **SERVINGS: 4**

## INGREDIENTS

- » 1 can white chunk chicken
- » 2 cans low-sodium white beans, drained
- » 1 can low-sodium diced tomatoes
- » 4 cups of low-sodium chicken broth
- » 1 medium onion, chopped
- » 1/2 medium green pepper, chopped
- » 1 medium red pepper, chopped
- » 2 garlic cloves, minced
- » 2 teaspoons chili powder
- » 1 teaspoon ground cumin
- » 1 teaspoon dried oregano
- » Cayenne pepper, to taste
- » 8 tablespoons shredded reduced-fat Monterey Jack cheese
- » 3 tablespoons chopped fresh cilantro

## DIRECTIONS

1. In a soup pot, add beans, tomatoes, chicken, and chicken broth. Cover this soup pot and let it simmer over medium heat. Meanwhile, grease a nonstick pan with cooking spray. Add peppers, garlic, and onions. Sauté for 5 minutes until soft.

2. Transfer the mixture to the soup pot. Add cumin, chili powder, cayenne pepper, and oregano. Cook for 10 minutes, then garnish the chili with cilantro and 1 tablespoon cheese. Serve.

**NUTRITIONS:** Calories 225, Fat 12.9 g, Sodium 480 mg, Carbs 24.7 g, Protein 25.3g

# 296. SWEET POTATO-TURKEY MEATLOAF

**COOKING: 25'**     **PREPARATION: 15'**     **SERVINGS: 4**

## INGREDIENTS

- » 1 large sweet potato, peeled and cubed
- » 1-pound ground turkey (breast)
- » 1 large egg
- » 1 small sweet onion, finely chopped
- » 2 cloves garlic, minced
- » 2 slices whole-wheat bread, crumbs
- » ¼ cup honey barbecue sauce
- » ¼ cup ketchup
- » 2 Tablespoons Dijon Mustard
- » 1 Tablespoon fresh ground pepper
- » ½ Tablespoon salt

## DIRECTIONS

1. Warm oven to 350 F. Grease a baking dish. In a large pot, boil a cup of lightly salted water, add the sweet potato. Cook until tender. Drain the water. Mash the potato.

2. Mix the honey barbecue sauce, ketchup, and Dijon mustard in a small bowl. Mix thoroughly. In a large bowl, mix the turkey and the egg. Add the sweet onion, garlic. Pour in the combined sauces. Add the bread crumbs. Season the mixture with salt and pepper.

3. Add the sweet potato. Combine thoroughly with your hands. If the mixture feels wet, add more bread crumbs. Shape the mixture into a loaf. Place in the loaf pan. Bake for 25 – 35 minutes until the meat is cooked through. Broil for 5 minutes. Slice and serve.

**NUTRITIONS:** Calories - 133, Protein - 85g, Carbohydrates - 50g, Fat - 34g, Sodium - 202mg

# 297. OAXACAN CHICKEN

**COOKING: 28'**          **PREPARATION: 15'**          **SERVINGS: 2**

## INGREDIENTS

- » 1 4-ounce chicken breast, skinned and halved
- » ½ cup uncooked long-grain rice
- » 1 teaspoon of extra-virgin olive oil
- » ½ cup low-sodium salsa
- » ½ cup chicken stock, mixed with 2 Tablespoons water
- » ¾ cup baby carrots
- » 2 tablespoons green olives, pitted and chopped
- » 2 Tablespoons dark raisins
- » ½ teaspoon ground Cinnamon
- » 2 Tablespoons fresh cilantro or parsley, coarsely chopped

## DIRECTIONS

1. Warm oven to 350 F. In a large saucepan that can go in the oven, heat the olive oil. Add the rice. Sauté the rice until it begins to pop, approximately 2 minutes.

2. Add the salsa, baby carrots, green olives, dark raisins, halved chicken breast, chicken stock, and ground cinnamon. Bring the mix to a simmer, stir once.

3. Cover the mixture tightly, bake in the oven until the chicken stock has been completely absorbed, approximately 25 minutes. Sprinkle fresh cilantro or parsley, mix. Serve immediately.

**NUTRITIONS:** Calories - 143, Protein - 102g, Carbohydrates - 66g, Fat - 18g, Sodium - 97mg

# 298. SPICY CHICKEN WITH MINTY COUSCOUS

**COOKING: 28'**          **PREPARATION: 15'**          **SERVINGS: 2**

## INGREDIENTS

- » 2 small chicken breasts, sliced
- » 1 red chili pepper, finely chopped
- » 1 garlic clove, crushed
- » ginger root, 2 cm long peeled and grated
- » 1 teaspoon ground cumin
- » ½ teaspoon turmeric
- » 2 Tablespoons extra-virgin olive oil
- » 1 pinch sea salt
- » ¾ cup couscous
- » Small bunch mint leaves, finely chopped
- » 2 lemons, grate the rind and juice them

## DIRECTIONS

1. In a large bowl, place the chicken breast slices and chopped chili pepper. Sprinkle with the crushed garlic, ginger, cumin, turmeric, and a pinch of salt. Add the grated rind of both lemons and the juice from 1 lemon. Pour 1 tablespoon of the olive oil over the chicken, coat evenly.

2. Cover the dish with plastic and refrigerate within 1 hour. After 1 hour, coat a skillet with olive oil and fry the chicken. As the chicken is cooking, pour the couscous into a bowl and pour hot water over it, let it absorb the water (approximately 5 minutes).

3. Fluff the couscous. Add some chopped mint, the other tablespoon of olive oil, and juice from the second lemon. Top the couscous with the chicken. Garnish with chopped mint. Serve immediately.

**NUTRITIONS:** Calories - 166, Protein - 106g, Carbohydrates - 52g, Sugars - 0.1g, Fat - 17g, Sodium - 108mg

# 299. CHICKEN, PASTA AND SNOW PEAS

**COOKING: 20'**      **PREPARATION: 15'**      **SERVINGS: 2**

## INGREDIENTS

- » 1-pound chicken breasts
- » 2 ½ cups penne pasta
- » 1 cup snow peas, trimmed and halved
- » 1 teaspoon olive oil
- » 1 standard jar Tomato and Basil pasta sauce
- » Fresh ground pepper

## DIRECTIONS

1. In a medium frying pan, heat the olive oil. Flavor the chicken breasts with salt and pepper. Cook the chicken breasts until cooked through (approximately 5 – 7 minutes each side).

2. Cook the pasta, as stated in the instruction of the package. Cook the snow peas with the pasta. Scoop 1 cup of the pasta water. Drain the pasta and peas, set aside.

3. Once the chicken is cooked, slice diagonally. Return back the chicken in the frying pan. Add the pasta sauce. If the mixture seems dry, add some of the pasta water to the desired consistency. Heat, then divide into bowls. Serve immediately.

**NUTRITIONS:** Calories - 140, Protein - 34g, Carbohydrates - 52g, Fat - 17g, Sodium - 118mg

---

# 300. CHICKEN WITH NOODLES

**COOKING: 30'**      **PREPARATION: 15'**      **SERVINGS: 6**

## INGREDIENTS

- » 4 chicken breasts, skinless, boneless
- » 1-pound pasta (angel hair, or linguine, or ramen)
- » ½ teaspoon sesame oil
- » 1 Tablespoon canola oil
- » 2 Tablespoons chili paste
- » 1 onion, diced
- » 2 garlic cloves, chopped coarsely
- » ½ cup of soy sauce
- » ½ medium cabbage, sliced
- » 2 carrots, chopped coarsely

## DIRECTIONS

1. Cook your pasta in a large pot. Mix the canola oil, sesame oil, and chili paste and heat for 25 seconds in a large pot. Add the onion, cook for 2 minutes. Put the garlic and fry within 20 seconds. Add the chicken, cook on each side 5 - 7 minutes, until cooked through.

2. Remove the mix from the pan, set aside. Add the cabbage, carrots, cook until the vegetables are tender. Pour everything back into the pan. Add the noodles. Pour in the soy sauce and combine thoroughly. Heat for 5 minutes. Serve immediately.

**NUTRITIONS:** Calories - 110, Protein - 30g, Carbohydrates - 32g, Sugars - 0.1g, Fat - 18g, Sodium - 121mg

# 301. TERIYAKI CHICKEN WINGS

**COOKING: 30'**     **PREPARATION: 15'**     **SERVINGS: 6**

## INGREDIENTS

- » 3 pounds of chicken wings (15 – 20)
- » 1/3 cup lemon juice
- » ¼ cup of soy sauce
- » ¼ cup of vegetable oil
- » 3 tablespoons chili sauce
- » 1 garlic clove, finely chopped
- » ¼ teaspoon fresh ground pepper
- » ¼ teaspoon celery seed
- » Dash liquid mustard

## DIRECTIONS

1. Prepare the marinade. Combine lemon juice, soy sauce, chili sauce, oil, celery seed, garlic, pepper, and mustard. Stir well, set aside. Rinse and dry the chicken wings.

2. Pour marinade over the chicken wings. Coat thoroughly. Refrigerate for 2 hours. After 2 hours. Preheat the broiler in the oven. Drain off the excess sauce.

3. Place the wings on a cookie sheet with parchment paper. Broil on each side for 10 minutes. Serve immediately.

**NUTRITIONS:** Calories - 96, Protein - 15g, Carbohydrates - 63g, Fat - 15g, Sodium- 145mg

# 302. HOT CHICKEN WINGS

**COOKING: 25'**     **PREPARATION: 15'**     **SERVINGS: 4**

## INGREDIENTS

- » 10 - 20 chicken wings
- » ½ stick margarine
- » 1 bottle Durkee hot sauce
- » 2 Tablespoons honey
- » 10 shakes Tabasco sauce
- » 2 Tablespoons cayenne pepper

## DIRECTIONS

1. Warm canola oil in a deep pot. Deep-fry the wings until cooked, approximately 20 minutes. Mix the hot sauce, honey, Tabasco, and cayenne pepper in a medium bowl. Mix well.

2. Place the cooked wings on paper towels. Drain the excess oil. Mix the chicken wings in the sauce until coated evenly.

**NUTRITIONS:** Calories - 102, Protein - 23g, Carbohydrates - 55g, Sugars - 0.1g, Fat - 14g, Sodium- 140mg

# 303. CRISPY CASHEW CHICKEN

**COOKING: 30'**      **PREPARATION: 15'**      **SERVINGS: 5**

## INGREDIENTS

- » 2 chicken breasts, skinless, boneless
- » 2 egg whites
- » 1 cup cashew nuts
- » ¼ cup bread crumbs
- » 2 cups of peanut oil or vegetable oil
- » ¼ cup of corn starch
- » 1 teaspoon brown sugar
- » 2 teaspoons salt
- » 1 teaspoon dry sherry

**NUTRITIONS:** Calories - 86, Protein - 21g, Carbohydrates - 50g, Sugars - 0.1g, Fat - 16g, Sodium- 139mg

## DIRECTIONS

1. Warm oven to 400 F. Put the cashews in a blender. Pulse until they are finely chopped. Place in a shallow bowl and stir in the bread crumbs.

2. Wash the chicken breasts. Pat them dry. Cut into small cubes. In a separate shallow bowl, mix the salt, corn starch, brown sugar, and sherry. In a separate bowl, beat the egg white.

3. Put the oil into a large, deep pot. Heat to high temp. Place the chicken pieces on a plate. Arrange the bowls in a row; flour, eggs, cashews & bread crumbs. Prepare a baking tray with parchment paper.

4. Dunk the chicken pieces in the flour, then the egg, and then the cashew mixture. Shake off the excess mixture. Gently place the chicken in the oil. Fry on each side for 2 minutes. Place on the baking tray.

5. Once done, slide the baking tray into the oven. Cook for an additional 4 minutes, flip, cook for an additional 4 minutes, until golden brown. Serve immediately, or cold, with your favorite low-fat dip.

# 304. CHICKEN TORTELLINI SOUP

**COOKING: 30'**      **PREPARATION: 15'**      **SERVINGS: 5**

## INGREDIENTS

- » 2 chicken breasts, boneless, skinless; diced into cubes
- » 1 Tablespoon flavorless oil (olive oil, canola, sunflower)
- » 1 teaspoon butter
- » 2 cups cheese tortellini
- » 2 cups frozen broccoli
- » 2 cans cream of chicken soup
- » 4 cups of water
- » 1 large onion, diced
- » 2 garlic cloves, minced
- » 2 large carrots, sliced
- » 1 celery stick, sliced
- » 1 teaspoon Oregano
- » ½ teaspoon Basil

## DIRECTIONS

1. Pull the broccoli out of the freezer. Set in a bowl. Rinse and pat dry the chicken breasts. Dice into cubes. In a large pot, heat the oil. Fry the cubes of chicken breast. Pull from the pot, place on paper to drain off the oil.

2. Add the teaspoon of butter to the hot pot. Sauté the onion, garlic, carrots, and celery, broccoli. Once the vegetable el dente, add the chicken soup and water. Stir the ingredients until they are combined. Bring it to a simmer.

3. Add the chicken and tortellini back to the pot. Cook on low within 10 minutes, or until the tortellini is cooked. Serve immediately.

**NUTRITIONS:** Calories - 79, Protein - 15g, Carbohydrates - 55g, Sugars - 0g, Fat - 13g, Sodium- 179mg

# 305. CHICKEN DIVAN

**COOKING: 30'**     **PREPARATION: 15'**     **SERVINGS: 4**

## INGREDIENTS

»   1/2-pound cooked chicken, boneless, skinless, diced in bite-size pieces
»   1 cup broccoli, cooked, diced into bite-size pieces
»   1 cup extra sharp cheddar cheese, grated
»   1 can mushroom soup
»   ½ cup of water
»   1 cup croutons

## DIRECTIONS

1. Warm oven to 350 F. In a large pot, heat the soup and water. Add the chicken, broccoli, and cheese. Combine thoroughly. Pour into a greased baking dish. Place the croutons over the mixture. Bake within 30 minutes or until the casserole is bubbling, and the croutons are golden brown.

**NUTRITIONS:** Calories - 380, Protein - 25g, Carbohydrates - 10g, Sugars - 1g, Fat - 22g, Sodium- 397mg

# 306. CREAMY CHICKEN FRIED RICE

**COOKING: 45'**     **PREPARATION: 15'**     **SERVINGS: 4**

## INGREDIENTS

»   2 pounds of chicken; white and dark meat (diced into cubes)
»   2 Tablespoons butter or margarine
»   1 ½ cups instant rice
»   1 cup mixed frozen vegetables
»   1 can condensed cream of chicken soup
»   1 cup of water
»   1 cube instant chicken bouillon
»   Salt and pepper to taste

## DIRECTIONS

1. Take the vegetables out of the freezer. Set aside. Warm large, deep skillet over medium heat, add the butter or margarine. Place the chicken in the skillet, season with salt and pepper. Fry until both sides are brown.

2. Remove the chicken, then adjust the heat and add the rice. Add the water and bouillon. Cook the rice, then add the chicken, the vegetables. Mix in the soup, then simmer until the vegetables are tender. Serve immediately.

**NUTRITIONS:** Calories - 119, Protein - 22g, Carbohydrates - 63g, Fat - 18g, Sodium - 180mg

# 307. CHICKEN TIKKA

**COOKING: 20'**　　　　**PREPARATION: 15'**　　　　**SERVINGS: 6**

## INGREDIENTS

- » 4 chicken breasts, skinless, boneless; cubed
- » 2 large onion, cubed
- » 10 Cherry tomatoes
- » 1/3 cup plain non-fat yogurt
- » 4 garlic cloves, crushed
- » 1 ½ inch fresh ginger, peeled and chopped
- » 1 small onion, grated
- » 1 ½ teaspoon chili powder
- » 1 Tablespoon ground coriander
- » 1 teaspoon salt
- » 2 tablespoons of coriander leaves

## DIRECTIONS

1. In a large bowl, combine the non-fat yogurt, crushed garlic, ginger, chili powder, coriander, salt, and pepper. Add the cubed chicken, stir until the chicken is coated. Cover with plastic film, place in the fridge. Marinate 2 – 4 hours. Heat the broiler or barbecue.

2. After marinating the chicken, get some skewers ready. Alternate pieces of chicken cubes, cherry tomatoes, and cubed onions onto the skewers.

3. Grill within 6 – 8 minutes on each side. Once the chicken is cooked through, pull the meat and vegetables off the skewers onto plates. Garnish with coriander. Serve immediately.

**NUTRITIONS:** Calories - 117, Protein - 19g, Carbohydrates - 59g, Fat - 19g, Sodium - 203mg

# 308. HONEY SPICED CAJUN CHICKEN

**COOKING: 20'**　　　　**PREPARATION: 15'**　　　　**SERVINGS: 4**

## INGREDIENTS

- » 2 chicken breasts, skinless, boneless
- » 1 Tablespoon butter or margarine
- » 1 pound of linguini
- » 3 large mushrooms, sliced
- » 1 large tomato, diced
- » 2 Tablespoons regular mustard
- » 4 Tablespoons honey
- » 3 ounces low-fat table cream
- » Parsley, roughly chopped

## DIRECTIONS

1. Wash and dry the chicken breasts. Warm 1 tablespoon of butter or margarine in a large pan. Add the chicken breasts. Season with salt and pepper. Cook on each side 6 – 10 minutes, until cooked thoroughly. Pull the chicken breasts from the pan. Set aside.

2. Cook the linguine as stated to instructions on the package in a large pot. Save 1 cup of the pasta water. Drain the linguine. Add the mushrooms, tomatoes to the pan from cooking the chicken. Heat until they are tender.

3. Add the honey, mustard, and cream. Combine thoroughly. Add the chicken and linguine to the pan. Stir until coated. Garnish with parsley. Serve immediately.

**NUTRITIONS:** Calories - 112, Protein - 12g, Carbohydrates - 56g, Fat - 20g, Sodium - 158mg

# 309. ITALIAN CHICKEN

**COOKING: 35'**     **PREPARATION: 15'**     **SERVINGS: 4**

## INGREDIENTS

- » 4 chicken breasts, skinless boneless
- » 1 large jar of pasta sauce, low sodium
- » 1 Tablespoon flavorless oil (olive, canola, or sunflower)
- » 1 large onion, diced
- » 1 large green pepper, diced
- » ½ teaspoon garlic salt
- » Salt and pepper to taste
- » 1 cup low-fat mozzarella cheese, grated
- » Spinach leaves, washed, dried, rough chop

## DIRECTIONS

1. Wash the chicken breasts, pat dry. In a large pot, heat the oil. Add the onion, cook, until it sweats and becomes translucent. Add the chicken. Season with salt, pepper, and garlic salt. Cook the chicken. 6 – 10 minutes on each side.

2. Add the peppers. Cook for 2 minutes. Pour the pasta sauce over the chicken. Mix well. Simmer on low for 20 minutes. Serve on plates, sprinkle the cheese over each piece. Garnish with spinach.

**NUTRITIONS:** Calories - 142, Protein - 17g, Carbohydrates - 51g, Fat - 15g, Sodium - 225mg

# 310. LEMON-PARSLEY CHICKEN BREAST

**COOKING: 15'**     **PREPARATION: 15'**     **SERVINGS: 2**

## INGREDIENTS

- » 2 chicken breasts, skinless, boneless
- » 1/3 cup white wine
- » 1/3 cup lemon juice
- » 2 garlic cloves, minced
- » 3 Tablespoons bread crumbs
- » 2 Tablespoons flavorless oil (olive, canola, or sunflower)
- » ¼ cup fresh parsley

## DIRECTIONS

1. Mix the wine, lemon juice, plus garlic in a measuring cup. Pound each chicken breast until they are ¼ inch thick. Coat the chicken with bread crumbs, and heat the oil in a large skillet.

2. Fry the chicken within 6 minutes on each side, until they turn brown. Stir in the wine mixture over the chicken. Simmer for 5 minutes. Pour any extra juices over the chicken. Garnish with parsley.

**NUTRITIONS:** Calories - 117, Protein - 14g, Carbohydrates - 74 g, Fat - 12g, Sodium - 189mg

# CHAPTER 10.
# VEGETABLES

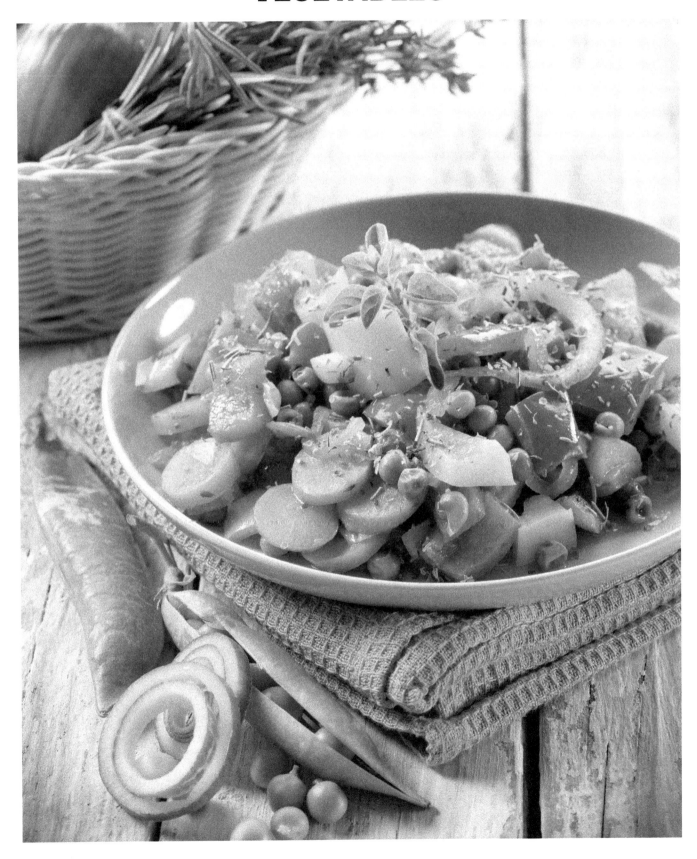

# 311. MOROCCAN-INSPIRED TAGINE WITH CHICKPEAS & VEGETABLES

**COOKING: 45'**  **PREPARATION: 15'**  **SERVINGS: 3**

## INGREDIENTS

» 2 teaspoons olive oil
» 1 cup chopped carrots
» ½ cup finely chopped onion
» 1 sweet potato, diced
» 1 cup low-sodium vegetable broth
» ¼ teaspoon ground cinnamon
» 1/8 teaspoon salt
» 1½ cups chopped bell peppers, any color
» 3 ripe plum tomatoes, chopped
» 1 tablespoon tomato paste
» 1 garlic clove, pressed or minced
» 1 (15-ounce) can chickpeas, drained and rinsed
» ½ cup chopped dried apricots
» 1 teaspoon curry powder
» ½ teaspoon paprika
» ½ teaspoon turmeric

## DIRECTIONS

1. Warm-up oil over medium heat in a large Dutch oven or saucepan. Add the carrots and onion and cook until the onion is translucent about 4 minutes. Add the sweet potato, broth, cinnamon, and salt and cook for 5 to 6 minutes, until the broth is slightly reduced.

2. Add the peppers, tomatoes, tomato paste, and garlic. Stir and cook for another 5 minutes. Add the chickpeas, apricots, curry powder, paprika, and turmeric to the pot. Bring all to a boil, then reduce the heat to low, cover, simmer for about 30 minutes, and serve.

**NUTRITIONS:** Calories: 469, Fat: 9g, Carbohydrates: 88g, Protein: 16g, Sodium: 256mg

# 312. SPAGHETTI SQUASH WITH MAPLE GLAZE & TOFU CRUMBLES

**COOKING: 22'**     **PREPARATION: 15'**     **SERVINGS: 3**

## INGREDIENTS

- » 2 ounces firm tofu, well-drained
- » 1 small spaghetti squash, halved lengthwise
- » 2½ teaspoons olive oil, divided
- » 1/8 teaspoon salt
- » ½ cup chopped onion
- » 1 teaspoon dried rosemary
- » ¼ cup dry white wine
- » 2 tablespoons maple syrup
- » ½ teaspoon garlic powder
- » ¼ cup shredded Gruyère cheese

## DIRECTIONS

1. Put the tofu in a large mesh colander and place over a large bowl to drain. Score the squash using a paring knife so the steam can vent while it cooks. Place the squash in a medium microwave-safe dish and microwave on high for 5 minutes. Remove the squash from the microwave and allow it to cool.

2. Cut the cooled squash in half on a cutting board. Remove the seeds, then put the squash halves into a 9-by-11-inch baking dish.

3. Drizzle the squash with half a teaspoon of olive oil and season it with the salt, then wrap it using wax paper and put it back in the microwave for 5 more minutes on high. Once it's cooked, scrape the squash strands with a fork into a small bowl and cover it to keep it warm.

4. While the squash is cooking, heat 1 teaspoon of oil in a large skillet over medium-high heat. Put the onion and sauté for within minutes. Add the rosemary and stir for 1 minute, until fragrant.

5. Put the rest of the oil in the same skillet. Crumble the tofu into the skillet, stir fry until lightly browned, about 4 minutes, and transfer it to a small bowl.

6. Add the wine, maple syrup, and garlic powder to the skillet and stir to combine. Cook for 2 minutes until slightly reduced and thickened. Remove from the heat. Evenly divide the squash between two plates, then top it with the tofu mixture. Drizzle the maple glaze over the top, then add the grated cheese.

**NUTRITIONS:** Calories: 330, Fat: 15g, Carbohydrates: 36g, Fiber: 5g, Protein: 12g, Sodium: 326mg, Potassium: 474mg

# 313. STUFFED TEX-MEX BAKED POTATOES

**COOKING: 45'**     **PREPARATION: 15'**     **SERVINGS: 2**

## INGREDIENTS

- » 2 large Idaho potatoes
- » ½ cup black beans, rinsed and drained
- » ¼ cup store-bought salsa
- » 1 avocado, diced
- » 1 teaspoon freshly squeezed lime juice
- » ½ cup nonfat plain Greek yogurt
- » ¼ teaspoon reduced-sodium taco seasoning
- » ¼ cup shredded sharp cheddar cheese

## DIRECTIONS

1. Preheat the oven to 400°F. Scrub the potatoes, then slice an "X" into the top of each using a paring knife. Put the potatoes on the oven rack, then bake for 45 minutes until they are tender.

2. In a small bowl, stir the beans and salsa and set aside. In another small bowl, mix the avocado and lime juice and set aside. In a third small bowl, stir the yogurt and the taco seasoning until well blended.

3. When the potatoes are baked, carefully open them up. Top each potato with the bean and salsa mixture, avocado, seasoned yogurt, and cheddar cheese, evenly dividing each component, and serve.

**NUTRITIONS:** Calories: 624, Fat: 21g, Carbohydrates: 91g, Fiber: 21g, Protein: 24g, Sodium: 366mg, Potassium: 2134mg

# 314. LENTIL-STUFFED ZUCCHINI BOATS

**COOKING: 45'**     **PREPARATION: 15'**     **SERVINGS: 2**

## INGREDIENTS

- » 2 medium zucchinis, halved lengthwise and seeded
- » 2¼ cups water, divided
- » 1 cup green or red lentils, dried & rinsed
- » 2 teaspoons olive oil
- » 1/3 cup diced onion
- » 2 tablespoons tomato paste
- » ½ teaspoon oregano
- » ¼ teaspoon garlic powder
- » Pinch salt
- » ¼ cup grated part-skim mozzarella cheese

## DIRECTIONS

1. Preheat the oven to 375°F. Line a baking sheet with parchment paper. Place the zucchini, hollow sides up, on the baking sheet, and set aside.

2. Boil 2 cups of water to a boil over high heat in a medium saucepan and add the lentils. Lower the heat, then simmer within 20 to 25 minutes. Drain and set aside.

3. Heat-up the olive oil in a medium skillet over medium-low heat. Sauté the onions until they are translucent, about 4 minutes. Lower the heat and add the cooked lentils, tomato paste, oregano, garlic powder, and salt.

4. Add the last quarter cup of water and simmer for 3 minutes, until the liquid reduces and forms a sauce. Remove from heat.

5. Stuff each zucchini half with the lentil mixture, dividing it evenly, top with cheese, bake for 25 minutes and serve. The zucchini should be fork-tender, and the cheese should be melted.

**NUTRITIONS:** Calories: 479, Fat: 9g, Carbohydrates: 74g, Fiber: 14g, Protein: 31g, Sodium: 206mg, Potassium: 1389mg

# 315. BAKED EGGPLANT PARMESAN

**COOKING: 35'**          **PREPARATION: 15'**          **SERVINGS: 4**

## INGREDIENTS

- » 1 small to medium eggplant, cut into ¼-inch slices
- » ½ teaspoon salt-free Italian seasoning blend
- » 1 tablespoon olive oil
- » ¼ cup diced onion
- » ½ cup diced yellow or red bell pepper
- » 2 garlic cloves, pressed or minced
- » 1 (8-ounce) can tomato sauce
- » 3 ounces fresh mozzarella, cut into 6 pieces
- » 1 tablespoon grated Parmesan cheese, divided
- » 5 to 6 fresh basil leaves, chopped

**NUTRITIONS:** Calories: 213, Fat: 12g, Carbohydrates: 20g, Fiber: 7g, Protein: 10g, Sodium: 222mg, Potassium: 763mg

## DIRECTIONS

1. Preheat an oven-style air fryer to 400°F.

2. Working in two batches, place the eggplant slices onto the air-fryer tray and sprinkle them with Italian seasoning. Bake for 7 minutes. Repeat with the remaining slices, then set them aside on a plate.

3. In a medium skillet, heat the oil over medium heat and sauté the onion and peppers until softened about 5 minutes. Add the garlic and sauté for 1 to 2 more minutes. Add the tomato sauce and stir to combine. Remove the sauce from the heat.

4. Spray a 9-by-6-inch casserole dish with cooking spray. Spread one-third of the sauce into the bottom of the dish. Layer eggplant slices onto the sauce. Sprinkle with half of the Parmesan cheese.

5. Continue layering the sauce and eggplant, ending with the sauce. Place the mozzarella pieces on the top. Sprinkle the remaining Parmesan evenly over the entire dish. Bake in the oven for 20 minutes. Garnish with fresh basil, cut into four servings, and serve.

# 316. SWEET POTATO RICE WITH SPICY PEANUT SAUCE

**COOKING: 25'**          **PREPARATION: 15'**          **SERVINGS: 2**

## INGREDIENTS

- » ½ cup basmati rice
- » 2 teaspoons olive oil, divided
- » 1 (8-ounce) can chickpeas, drained and rinsed
- » 2 medium sweet potatoes, small cubes
- » ¼ teaspoon ground cumin
- » 1 cup of water
- » 1/8 teaspoon salt
- » 2 tablespoons chopped cilantro
- » 3 tablespoons peanut butter
- » 1 tablespoon sriracha
- » 2 teaspoons reduced-sodium soy sauce
- » ½ teaspoon garlic powder
- » ¼ teaspoon ground ginger

**NUTRITIONS:** Calories: 667, Fat: 22g, Carbohydrates: 100g, Fiber: 14g, Protein: 20g, Sodium: 563mg, Potassium: 963mg

## DIRECTIONS

1. Heat-up 1 teaspoon of oil in a large nonstick skillet over medium-high heat. Add the chickpeas and heat for 3 minutes. Stir and cook until lightly browned. Transfer the chickpeas to a small bowl.

2. Put the rest of the 1 teaspoon of oil to the skillet, then add the potatoes and cumin, distributing them evenly. Cook the potatoes until they become lightly browned before turning them.

3. While the potatoes are cooking, boil the water with the salt in a large saucepan over medium-high heat. Put the rice in the boiling water, adjust the heat to low, cover, and simmer for 20 minutes.

4. When the potatoes have fully cooked, about 10 minutes in total, remove the skillet from the heat. Transfer the potatoes and chickpeas to the rice, folding all gently. Add the chopped cilantro.

5. In a small bowl, whisk the peanut butter, sriracha, soy sauce, garlic powder, and ginger until well blended. Divide the rice mixture between two serving bowls. Drizzle with the sauce and serve.

# 317. VEGETABLE RED CURRY

**COOKING: 25'**     **PREPARATION: 15'**     **SERVINGS: 2**

## INGREDIENTS

- » 2 teaspoons olive oil
- » 1 cup sliced carrots
- » ½ cup chopped onion
- » 1 garlic clove, pressed or minced
- » 2 bell peppers, seeded and thinly sliced
- » 1 cup chopped cauliflower
- » 2/3 cup light coconut milk
- » ½ cup low-sodium vegetable broth
- » 1 tablespoon tomato paste
- » 1 teaspoon curry powder
- » ½ teaspoon ground cumin
- » ½ teaspoon ground coriander
- » ¼ teaspoon turmeric
- » 2 cups fresh baby spinach
- » 1 cup quick-cooking brown rice

**NUTRITIONS:** Calories: 584, Fat: 16g, Carbohydrates: 101g, Fiber: 10g, Protein: 13g, Sodium: 102mg, Potassium: 1430mg

## DIRECTIONS

1. Heat-up oil in a large nonstick skillet over medium heat. Add the carrots, onion, and garlic and cook for 2 to 3 minutes. Reduce the heat to medium-low, add the peppers and cauliflower to the skillet, cover, and cook within 5 minutes.

2. Add the coconut milk, broth, tomato paste, curry powder, cumin, coriander, and turmeric, stirring to combine. Simmer, covered (vent the lid slightly), for 10 to 15 minutes until the curry is slightly reduced and thickened.

3. Uncover, add the spinach, and stir for 2 minutes until it is wilted and mixed into the vegetables. Remove from the heat. Cook the rice as stated to the package instructions. Serve the curry over the rice.

# 318. BLACK BEAN BURGERS

**COOKING: 20'**     **PREPARATION: 15'**     **SERVINGS: 4**

## INGREDIENTS

- » ½ cup quick-cooking brown rice
- » 2 teaspoons canola oil, divided
- » ½ cup finely chopped carrots
- » ¼ cup finely chopped onion
- » 1 can black beans, drained
- » 1 tablespoon salt-free mesquite seasoning blend
- » 4 small, hard rolls

**NUTRITIONS:** Calories: 368, Fat: 6g, Carbohydrates: 66g, Fiber: 8g, Protein: 13g, Sodium: 322mg, Potassium: 413mg

## DIRECTIONS

1. Cook the rice as stated in the package directions and set aside. Heat-up 1 teaspoon of oil in a large nonstick skillet over medium heat. Add the carrots and onions and cook until the onions are translucent about 4 minutes. Adjust the heat to low, and cook again for 5 to 6 minutes, until the carrots are tender.

2. Add the beans and seasoning to the skillet and continue cooking for 2 to 3 more minutes. Pulse bean mixture in a food processor within 3 to 4 times or until the mixture is coarsely blended. Put the batter in a medium bowl and fold in the brown rice until well combined.

3. Divide the mixture evenly and form it into 4 patties with your hands. Heat the remaining oil in the skillet. Cook the patties within 4 to 5 minutes per side, turning once. Serve the burgers on the rolls with your choice of toppings.

# 319. SUMMER BARLEY PILAF WITH YOGURT DILL SAUCE

**COOKING: 30'**          **PREPARATION: 15'**          **SERVINGS: 3**

## INGREDIENTS

- » 2 2/3 cups low-sodium vegetable broth
- » 2 teaspoons avocado oil
- » 1 small zucchini, diced
- » 1/3 cup slivered almonds
- » 2 scallions, sliced
- » 1 cup barley
- » ½ cup plain nonfat Greek yogurt
- » 2 teaspoons grated lemon zest
- » ¼ teaspoon dried dill

**NUTRITIONS:** Calories: 545, Fat: 15g, Carbohydrates: 87g, Fiber: 19g, Protein: 21g, Sodium: 37mg, Potassium: 694mg

## DIRECTIONS

1. Boil the broth in a large saucepan. Heat-up the oil in a skillet. Add the zucchini and sauté 3 to 4 minutes. Add the almonds and the white parts of the scallions and sauté for 2 minutes. Remove, and transfer it to a small bowl.

2. Add the barley to the skillet and sauté for 2 to 3 minutes to toast. Transfer the barley to the boiling broth and reduce the heat to low, cover, and simmer for 25 minutes or until tender. Remove, and let stand within 10 minutes or until the liquid is absorbed.

3. Simultaneously, mix the yogurt, lemon zest, and dill in a small bowl and set aside. Fluff the barley with a fork. Add the zucchini, almond, and onion mixture and mix gently. To serve, divide the pilaf between two bowls and drizzle the yogurt over each bowl.

# 320. LENTIL QUINOA GRATIN WITH BUTTERNUT SQUASH

**COOKING: 1H 15'**          **PREPARATION: 10'**          **SERVINGS: 3**

## INGREDIENTS

**For the Lentils and Squash:**
- » Nonstick cooking spray
- » 2 cups of water
- » ½ cup dried green or red lentils, rinsed
- » Pinch salt
- » 1 teaspoon olive oil, divided
- » ½ cup quinoa
- » ¼ cup diced shallot
- » 2 cups frozen cubed butternut squash
- » ¼ cup low-fat milk
- » 1 teaspoon chopped fresh rosemary
- » Freshly ground black pepper

**For the Gratin Topping:**
- » ¼ cup panko bread crumbs
- » 1 teaspoon olive oil
- » 1/3 cup shredded Gruyère cheese

**NUTRITIONS:** Calories: 576, Fat: 15g, Carbohydrates: 87g, Fiber: 12g, Protein: 28g, Sodium: 329mg, Potassium: 1176mg

## DIRECTIONS

1. Preheat the oven to 400°F. Spray a 1½-quart casserole dish or an 8-by-8-inch baking dish with cooking spray.

2. In a medium saucepan, stir the water, lentils, and salt and boil over medium-high heat. Lower the heat once the water is boiling, cover, and simmer for 20 to 25 minutes. Then drain and transfer the lentils to a large bowl and set aside.

3. In the same saucepan, heat-up ½ teaspoon of oil over medium heat. Add the quinoa and quickly stir for 1 minute to toast it lightly. Cook according to the package directions, about 20 minutes.

4. While the quinoa cooks, heat the remaining olive oil in a medium skillet over medium-low heat, add the shallots, and sauté them until they are translucent, about 3 minutes. Add the squash, milk, and rosemary and cook for 1 to 2 minutes.

5. Remove, then transfer to the lentil bowl. Add in the quinoa and gently toss all. Season with pepper to taste. Transfer the mixture to the casserole dish.

6. For the gratin topping, mix the panko bread crumbs with the olive oil in a small bowl. Put the bread crumbs over the casserole and top them with the cheese. Bake the casserole for 25 minutes and serve.

# 321. BROWN RICE CASSEROLE WITH COTTAGE CHEESE

**COOKING: 45'**   **PREPARATION: 15'**   **SERVINGS: 3**

## INGREDIENTS

- » Nonstick cooking spray
- » 1 cup quick-cooking brown rice
- » 1 teaspoon olive oil
- » ½ cup diced sweet onion
- » 1 (10-ounce) bag of fresh spinach
- » 1½ cups low-fat cottage cheese
- » 1 tablespoon grated Parmesan cheese
- » ¼ cup sunflower seed kernels

## DIRECTIONS

1. Preheat the oven to 375°F. Spray a small 1½-quart casserole dish with cooking spray. Cook the rice, as stated in the package directions. Set aside.

2. Warm-up oil in a large nonstick skillet over medium-low heat. Add the onion and sauté for 3 to 4 minutes. Add the spinach and cover the skillet, cooking for 1 to 2 minutes until the spinach wilts. Remove the skillet from the heat.

3. In a medium bowl, mix the rice, spinach mixture, and cottage cheese. Transfer the mixture to the prepared casserole dish. Top with the Parmesan cheese and sunflower seeds, bake for 25 minutes until lightly browned, and serve.

**NUTRITIONS:** Calories: 334, Fat: 9g, Carbohydrates: 47g, Fiber: 5g, Protein: 19g, Sodium: 425mg, Potassium: 553mg

# 322. QUINOA-STUFFED PEPPERS

**COOKING: 35'**   **PREPARATION: 15'**   **SERVINGS: 2**

## INGREDIENTS

- » 2 large green bell peppers, halved
- » 1½ teaspoons olive oil, divided
- » ½ cup quinoa
- » ½ cup minced onion
- » 1 garlic clove, pressed or minced
- » 1 cup chopped portobello mushrooms
- » 3 tablespoons grated Parmesan cheese, divided
- » 4 ounces tomato sauce

## DIRECTIONS

1. Preheat the oven to 400°F. Put the pepper halves on your prepared baking sheet. Brush the insides of peppers with ½ teaspoon olive oil and bake for 10 minutes.

2. Remove the baking sheet, then set aside. While the peppers bake, cook the quinoa in a large saucepan over medium heat according to the package directions and set aside.

3. Warm-up the rest of the oil in a medium-size skillet over medium heat. Add the onion and sauté until it's translucent about 3 minutes. Put the garlic and cook within 1 minute.

4. Put the mushrooms in the skillet, adjust the heat to medium-low, cover, and cook within 5 to 6 minutes. Uncover, and if there's still liquid in the pan, reduce the heat and cook until the liquid evaporates.

5. Add the mushroom mixture, 1 tablespoon of Parmesan, and the tomato sauce to the quinoa and gently stir to combine. Carefully spoon the quinoa mixture into each pepper half and sprinkle with the remaining Parmesan. Return the peppers to the oven, bake for 10 to 15 more minutes until tender, and serve.

**NUTRITIONS:** Calories: 292, Fat: 9g, Carbohydrates: 45g, Fiber: 8g, Protein: 12g, Sodium: 154mg, Potassium: 929mg

# 323. GREEK FLATBREAD WITH SPINACH, TOMATOES & FETA

**COOKING: 9'**    **PREPARATION: 15'**    **SERVINGS: 2**

## INGREDIENTS

- » 2 cups fresh baby spinach, coarsely chopped
- » 2 teaspoons olive oil
- » 2 slices naan, or another flatbread
- » ¼ cup sliced black olives
- » 2 plum tomatoes, thinly sliced
- » 1 teaspoon salt-free Italian seasoning blend
- » ¼ cup crumbled feta

## DIRECTIONS

1. Preheat the oven to 400°F. Heat 3 tablespoons of water in a small skillet over medium heat. Add the spinach, cover, and steam until wilted, about 2 minutes. Drain off any excess water, then put aside.

2. Drizzle the oil evenly onto both flatbreads. Top each evenly with the spinach, olives, tomatoes, seasoning, and feta. Bake the flatbreads within 5 to 7 minutes, or until lightly browned. Cut each into four pieces and serve hot.

**NUTRITIONS:** Calories: 411, Fat: 15g, Carbohydrates: 53g, Fiber: 7g, Protein: 15g, Sodium: 621mg, Potassium: 522mg

# 324. MUSHROOM RISOTTO WITH PEAS

**COOKING: 20'**    **PREPARATION: 15'**    **SERVINGS: 2**

## INGREDIENTS

- » 2 cups low-sodium vegetable or chicken broth
- » 1 teaspoon olive oil
- » 8 ounces baby portobello mushrooms, thinly sliced
- » ½ cup frozen peas
- » 1 teaspoon butter
- » 1 cup arborio rice
- » 1 tablespoon grated Parmesan cheese

## DIRECTIONS

1. Pour the broth into a microwave-proof glass measuring cup. Microwave on high for 1½ minutes or until hot. Warm-up oil over medium heat in a large saucepan. Add the mushrooms and stir for 1 minute. Cover and cook until soft, about 3 more minutes. Stir in the peas and reduce the heat to low.

2. Put the mushroom batter to the saucepan's sides and add the butter to the middle, heating until melted. Put the rice in the saucepan and stir for 1 to 2 minutes to lightly toast. Add the hot broth, ½ cup at a time, and stir gently.

3. As the broth is cooked into the rice, continue adding more broth, ½ cup at a time, stirring after each addition, until all broth is added. Once all of the liquid is absorbed (this should take 15 minutes), remove from the heat. Serve immediately, topped with Parmesan cheese.

**NUTRITIONS:** Calories: 430, Fat: 6g, Carbohydrates: 83g, Fiber: 5g, Protein: 10g, Sodium: 78mg, Potassium: 558mg

# 325. LOADED TOFU BURRITO WITH BLACK BEANS

**COOKING: 20'**  **PREPARATION: 15'**  **SERVINGS: 2**

## INGREDIENTS

»   4 ounces extra-firm tofu, pressed and cut into 2-inch cubes
»   2 teaspoons mesquite salt-free seasoning, divided
»   2 teaspoons canola oil
»   1 cup thinly sliced bell peppers
»   ½ cup diced onions
»   2/3 cup of black beans, drained
»   2 (10-inch) whole-wheat tortillas
»   1 tablespoon sriracha
»   Nonfat Greek yogurt, for serving

## DIRECTIONS

1.  Put the tofu and 1 teaspoon of seasoning in a medium zip-top plastic freezer bag and toss until the tofu is well coated.

2.  Heat-up the oil in a medium skillet over medium-high heat. Put the tofu in the skillet. Don't stir; allow the tofu to brown before turning. When lightly browned, about 6 minutes, transfer the tofu from the skillet to a small bowl and set aside.

3.  Put the peppers plus onions in the skillet and sauté until tender, about 5 minutes. Lower the heat to medium-low, then put the beans and the remaining seasoning. Cook within 5 minutes.

4.  For the burritos, lay each tortilla flat on a work surface. Place half of the tofu in the center of each tortilla, top with half of the pepper-bean mixture, and drizzle with the sriracha.

5.  Fold the bottom portion of each tortilla up and over the tofu mixture. Then fold each side into the middle, tuck in, and tightly roll it up toward the open end. Serve with a dollop of yogurt.

**NUTRITIONS:** Calories: 327, Fat: 12g, Carbohydrates: 41g, Fiber: 11g, Protein: 16g, Sodium: 282mg

# 326. SOUTHWEST TOFU SCRAMBLE

**COOKING: 15'**  **PREPARATION: 15'**  **SERVINGS: 1**

## INGREDIENTS

»   ½ tablespoon olive oil
»   ½ red onion, chopped
»   2 cups chopped spinach
»   8 ounces firm tofu, drained well
»   1 teaspoon ground cumin
»   ½ teaspoon garlic powder
»   Optional for serving: sliced avocado or sliced tomatoes

## DIRECTIONS

1.  Heat-up the olive oil in a medium skillet over medium heat. Put the onion and cook within 5 minutes. Add the spinach and cover to steam for 2 minutes.

2.  Using a spatula, move the veggies to one side of the pan. Crumble the tofu into the open area in the pan, breaking it up with a fork. Add the cumin and garlic to the crumbled tofu and mix well. Sauté for 5 to 7 minutes until the tofu is slightly browned.

3.  Serve immediately with whole-grain bread, fruit, or beans. Top with optional sliced avocado and tomato, if using.

**NUTRITIONS:** Calories: 267, Fat: 17g, Sodium: 75mg, Carbohydrate: 13g, Protein: 23g

# 327. BLACK-BEAN AND VEGETABLE BURRITO

**COOKING: 15'**     **PREPARATION: 15'**     **SERVINGS: 4**

## INGREDIENTS

- » ½ tablespoon olive oil
- » 2 red or green bell peppers, chopped
- » 1 zucchini or summer squash, diced
- » ½ teaspoon chili powder
- » 1 teaspoon cumin
- » Freshly ground black pepper
- » 2cans black beans drained and rinsed
- » 1 cup cherry tomatoes, halved
- » 4 (8-inch) whole-wheat tortillas
- » Optional for serving: spinach, sliced avocado, chopped scallions, or hot sauce

## DIRECTIONS

1. Heat-up the oil in a large sauté pan over medium heat. Add the bell peppers and sauté until crisp-tender, about 4 minutes. Add the zucchini, chili powder, cumin, and black pepper to taste, and continue to sauté until the vegetables are tender, about 5 minutes.

2. Add the black beans and cherry tomatoes and cook within 5 minutes. Divide between 4 burritos and serve topped with optional ingredients as desired. Enjoy immediately.

**NUTRITIONS:** Calories: 311, Fat: 6g, Sodium: 499mg, Carbohydrate: 52g, Protein: 19g

# 328. BAKED EGGS IN AVOCADO

**COOKING: 15'**     **PREPARATION: 15'**     **SERVINGS: 2**

## INGREDIENTS

- » 2 avocados
- » Juice of 2 limes
- » Freshly ground black pepper
- » 4 eggs
- » 2 (8-inch) whole-wheat or corn tortillas, warmed
- » Optional for serving: halved cherry tomatoes and chopped cilantro

## DIRECTIONS

1. Adjust the oven rack to the middle position and preheat the oven to 450°F. Scrape out the center of halved avocado using a spoon about 1½ tablespoons.

2. Press lime juice over the avocados and season with black pepper to taste, and then place it on a baking sheet. Crack an egg into the avocado.

3. Bake within 10 to 15 minutes. Remove from oven and garnish with optional cilantro and cherry tomatoes and serve with warm tortillas.

**NUTRITIONS:** Calories: 534, Fat: 39g, Sodium: 462mg, Potassium: 1,095mg, Carbohydrate: 30g, Fiber: 20g, Sugars: 3g, Protein: 23g

# 329. RED BEANS AND RICE

**COOKING: 45'**          **PREPARATION: 15'**          **SERVINGS: 4**

## INGREDIENTS

- » ½ cup dry brown rice
- » 1 cup water, plus ¼ cup
- » 1 can red beans, drained
- » 1 tablespoon ground cumin
- » Juice of 1 lime
- » 4 handfuls of fresh spinach
- » Optional toppings: avocado, chopped tomatoes, Greek yogurt, onions

## DIRECTIONS

1. Mix rice plus water in a pot and bring to a boil. Cover and reduce heat to a low simmer. Cook within 30 to 40 minutes or according to package directions.

2. Meanwhile, add the beans, ¼ cup of water, cumin, and lime juice to a medium skillet. Simmer within 5 to 7 minutes.

3. Once the liquid is mostly gone, remove from the heat and add the spinach. Cover and let spinach wilt slightly, 2 to 3 minutes. Mix in with the beans. Serve beans with rice. Add toppings, if using.

**NUTRITIONS:** Calories: 232, Fat: 2g, Sodium: 210mg, Carbohydrate: 41g, Protein: 13g

# 330. HEARTY LENTIL SOUP

**COOKING: 30'**          **PREPARATION: 15'**          **SERVINGS: 4**

## INGREDIENTS

- » 1 tablespoon olive oil
- » 2 carrots, peeled and chopped
- » 2 celery stalks, diced
- » 1 onion, chopped
- » 1 teaspoon dried thyme
- » ½ teaspoon garlic powder
- » Freshly ground black pepper
- » 1 (28-ounce) can no-salt diced tomatoes, drained
- » 1 cup dry lentils
- » 5 cups of water
- » Salt

## DIRECTIONS

1. Heat-up the oil in a large Dutch oven or pot over medium heat. Once the oil is simmering, add the carrot, celery, and onion. Cook, often stirring within 5 minutes.

2. Add the thyme, garlic powder, and black pepper. Cook within 30 seconds. Pour in the drained diced tomatoes and cook for a few more minutes, often stirring to enhance their flavor.

3. Put the lentils, water, plus a pinch of salt. Raise the heat and bring to a boil, then partially cover the pot and reduce heat to maintain a gentle simmer.

4. Cook within 30 minutes, or until lentils are tender but still hold their shape. Ladle into serving bowls and serve with a fresh green salad and whole-grain bread.

**NUTRITIONS:** Calories: 168, Fat: 4g, Sodium: 130mg, Carbohydrate: 35g, Protein: 10g

# 331. BLACK-BEAN SOUP

**COOKING: 20'**        **PREPARATION: 15'**        **SERVINGS: 4**

## INGREDIENTS

- » 1 yellow onion
- » 1 tablespoon olive oil
- » 2 cans black beans, drained
- » 1 cup diced fresh tomatoes
- » 5 cups low-sodium vegetable broth
- » ¼ teaspoon freshly ground black pepper
- » ¼ cup chopped fresh cilantro

## DIRECTIONS

1. Cook or sauté the onion in the olive oil within 4 to 5 minutes in a large saucepan over medium heat. Put the black beans, tomatoes, vegetable broth, and black pepper. Boil, then adjust heat to simmer within 15 minutes.

2. Remove, then working in batches, ladle the soup into a blender and process until somewhat smooth. Put it back to the pot, add the cilantro, and heat until warmed through. Serve immediately.

**NUTRITIONS:** Calories: 234, Fat: 5g, Sodium: 363mg, Carbohydrate: 37g, Protein: 11g

# 332. LOADED BAKED SWEET POTATOES

**COOKING: 20'**        **PREPARATION: 15'**        **SERVINGS: 4**

## INGREDIENTS

- » 4 sweet potatoes
- » ½ cup nonfat or low-fat plain Greek yogurt
- » Freshly ground black pepper
- » 1 teaspoon olive oil
- » 1 red bell pepper, cored and diced
- » ½ red onion, diced
- » 1 teaspoon ground cumin
- » 1 (15-ounce) can chickpeas, drained and rinsed

## DIRECTIONS

1. Prick the potatoes using a fork and cook on your microwave's potato setting until potatoes are soft and cooked through, about 8 to 10 minutes for 4 potatoes. If you don't have a microwave, bake at 400°F for about 45 minutes.

2. Combine the yogurt and black pepper in a small bowl and mix well. Heat the oil in a medium pot over medium heat. Add bell pepper, onion, cumin, and additional black pepper to taste.

3. Add the chickpeas, stir to combine, and heat through about 5 minutes. Slice the potatoes lengthwise down the middle and top each half with a portion of the bean mixture followed by 1 to 2 tablespoons of the yogurt. Serve immediately.

**NUTRITIONS:** Calories: 264, Fat: 2g, Sodium: 124mg, Carbohydrate: 51g, Protein: 11g

# 333. WHITE BEANS WITH SPINACH AND PAN-ROASTED TOMATOES

**COOKING: 10'**  **PREPARATION: 15'**  **SERVINGS: 2**

## INGREDIENTS

- » 1 tablespoon olive oil
- » 4 small plum tomatoes, halved lengthwise
- » 10 ounces frozen spinach, defrosted and squeezed of excess water
- » 2 garlic cloves, thinly sliced
- » 2 tablespoons water
- » ¼ teaspoon freshly ground black pepper
- » 1 can white beans, drained
- » Juice of 1 lemon

## DIRECTIONS

1. Heat-up the oil in a large skillet over medium-high heat. Put the tomatoes, cut-side down, and cook within 3 to 5 minutes; turn and cook within 1 minute more. Transfer to a plate.

2. Reduce heat to medium and add the spinach, garlic, water, and pepper to the skillet. Cook, tossing until the spinach is heated through, 2 to 3 minutes.

3. Return the tomatoes to the skillet, put the white beans and lemon juice, and toss until heated through 1 to 2 minutes.

**NUTRITIONS:** Calories: 293, Fat: 9g, Sodium: 267mg, Carbohydrate: 43g, Protein: 15g

# 334. BLACK-EYED PEAS AND GREENS POWER SALAD

**COOKING: 6'**  **PREPARATION: 15'**  **SERVINGS: 2**

## INGREDIENTS

- » 1 tablespoon olive oil
- » 3 cups purple cabbage, chopped
- » 5 cups baby spinach
- » 1 cup shredded carrots
- » 1 can black-eyed peas, drained
- » Juice of ½ lemon
- » Salt
- » Freshly ground black pepper

## DIRECTIONS

1. In a medium pan, add the oil and cabbage and sauté for 1 to 2 minutes on medium heat. Add in your spinach, cover for 3 to 4 minutes on medium heat, until greens are wilted. Remove from the heat and add to a large bowl.

2. Add in the carrots, black-eyed peas, and a splash of lemon juice. Season with salt and pepper, if desired. Toss and serve.

**NUTRITIONS:** Calories: 320, Fat: 9g, Sodium: 351mg, Potassium: 544mg, Carbohydrate: 49g, Protein: 16g

# 335. BUTTERNUT-SQUASH MACARONI AND CHEESE

**COOKING: 20'**          **PREPARATION: 15'**          **SERVINGS: 2**

## INGREDIENTS

- » 1 cup whole-wheat ziti macaroni
- » 2 cups peeled and cubed butternut squash
- » 1 cup nonfat or low-fat milk, divided
- » Freshly ground black pepper
- » 1 teaspoon Dijon mustard
- » 1 tablespoon olive oil
- » ¼ cup shredded low-fat cheddar cheese

## DIRECTIONS

1. Cook the pasta al dente. Put the butternut squash plus ½ cup milk in a medium saucepan and place over medium-high heat. Season with black pepper. Bring it to a simmer. Lower the heat, then cook until fork-tender, 8 to 10 minutes.

2. To a blender, add squash and Dijon mustard. Purée until smooth. Meanwhile, place a large sauté pan over medium heat and add olive oil. Add the squash purée and the remaining ½ cup of milk. Simmer within 5 minutes. Add the cheese and stir to combine.

3. Add the pasta to the sauté pan and stir to combine. Serve immediately.

**NUTRITIONS:** Calories: 373, Fat: 10g, Sodium: 193mg, Carbohydrate: 59g, Protein: 14g

# 336. PASTA WITH TOMATOES AND PEAS

**COOKING: 15'**          **PREPARATION: 15'**          **SERVINGS: 2**

## INGREDIENTS

- » ½ cup whole-grain pasta of choice
- » 8 cups water, plus ¼ for finishing
- » 1 cup frozen peas
- » 1 tablespoon olive oil
- » 1 cup cherry tomatoes, halved
- » ¼ teaspoon freshly ground black pepper
- » 1 teaspoon dried basil
- » ¼ cup grated Parmesan cheese (low-sodium)

## DIRECTIONS

1. Cook the pasta al dente. Add the water to the same pot you used to cook the pasta, and when it's boiling, add the peas. Cook within 5 minutes. Drain and set aside.

2. Heat-up the oil in a large skillet over medium heat. Add the cherry tomatoes, put a lid on the skillet and let the tomatoes soften for about 5 minutes, stirring a few times.

3. Season with black pepper and basil. Toss in the pasta, peas, and ¼ cup of water, stir and remove from the heat. Serve topped with Parmesan.

**NUTRITIONS:** Calories: 266, Fat: 12g, Sodium: 320mg, Carbohydrate: 30g, Protein: 13g

# 337. HEALTHY VEGETABLE FRIED RICE

**COOKING: 10'**     **PREPARATION: 15'**     **SERVINGS: 4**

## INGREDIENTS

**For the sauce:**
- » 1/3 cup garlic vinegar
- » 1½ tablespoons dark molasses
- » 1 teaspoon onion powder

**For the fried rice:**
- » 1 teaspoon olive oil
- » 2 lightly beaten whole eggs + 4 egg whites
- » 1 cup of frozen mixed vegetables
- » 1 cup frozen edamame
- » 2 cups cooked brown rice

## DIRECTIONS

1. Prepare the sauce by combining the garlic vinegar, molasses, and onion powder in a glass jar. Shake well.

2. Heat-up oil in a large wok or skillet over medium-high heat. Add eggs and egg whites, let cook until the eggs set, for about 1 minute.

3. Break up eggs with a spatula or spoon into small pieces. Add frozen mixed vegetables and frozen edamame. Cook for 4 minutes, stirring frequently.

4. Add the brown rice and sauce to the vegetable-and-egg mixture. Cook for 5 minutes or until heated through. Serve immediately.

**NUTRITIONS:** Calories: 210, Fat: 6g, Sodium: 113mg, Carbohydrate: 28g, Protein: 13g

# 338. PORTOBELLO-MUSHROOM CHEESEBURGERS

**COOKING: 10'**     **PREPARATION: 15'**     **SERVINGS: 4**

## INGREDIENTS

- » 4 portobello mushrooms, caps removed and brushed clean
- » 1 tablespoon olive oil
- » ½ teaspoon freshly ground black pepper
- » 1 tablespoon red wine vinegar
- » 4 slices reduced-fat Swiss cheese, sliced thin
- » 4 whole-wheat 100-calorie sandwich thins
- » ½ avocado, sliced thin

## DIRECTIONS

1. Heat-up a skillet or grill pan over medium-high heat. Clean the mushrooms and remove the stems. Brush each cap with olive oil and sprinkle with black pepper. Place in skillet cap-side up and cook for about 4 minutes. Flip and cook for another 4 minutes.

2. Sprinkle with the red wine vinegar and flip. Add the cheese and cook for 2 more minutes. For optimal melting, place a lid loosely over the pan. Meanwhile, toast the sandwich thins. Create your burgers by topping each with sliced avocado. Enjoy immediately.

**NUTRITIONS:** Calories: 245, Fat: 12g, Sodium: 266mg, Carbohydrate: 28g, Protein: 14g

# 339. BAKED CHICKPEA-AND-ROSEMARY OMELET

**COOKING: 15'**     **PREPARATION: 15'**     **SERVINGS: 2**

## INGREDIENTS

- » ½ tablespoon olive oil
- » 4 eggs
- » ¼ cup grated Parmesan cheese
- » 1 (15-ounce) can chickpeas, drained and rinsed
- » 2 cups packed baby spinach
- » 1 cup button mushrooms, chopped
- » 2 sprigs rosemary, leaves picked (or 2 teaspoons dried rosemary)
- » Salt
- » Freshly ground black pepper

## DIRECTIONS

1. Warm oven to 400 F and puts a baking tray on the middle shelf. Line an 8-inch springform pan with baking paper and grease generously with olive oil. If you don't have a springform pan, grease an oven-safe skillet (or cast-iron skillet) with olive oil.

2. Lightly whisk the eggs and Parmesan. Place chickpeas in the prepared pan. Layer the spinach and mushrooms on top of the beans. Pour the egg mixture on top and scatter the rosemary. Season to taste with salt and pepper.

3. Place the pan on the preheated tray and bake until golden and puffy and the center feels firm and springy about 15 minutes. Remove from the oven, slice, and serve immediately.

**NUTRITIONS:** Calories: 418, Fat: 19g, Sodium: 595mg, Carbohydrate: 33g, Protein: 30g

# 340. CHILLED CUCUMBER-AND-AVOCADO SOUP WITH DILL

**COOKING: 30'**     **PREPARATION: 15'**     **SERVINGS: 4**

## INGREDIENTS

- » 2 English cucumbers, peeled and diced, plus ¼ cup reserved for garnish
- » 1 avocado, peeled, pitted, and chopped, plus ¼ cup reserved for garnish
- » 1½ cups nonfat or low-fat plain Greek yogurt
- » ½ cup of cold water
- » 1/3 cup loosely packed dill, plus sprigs for garnish
- » 1 tablespoon freshly squeezed lemon juice
- » ¼ teaspoon freshly ground black pepper
- » ¼ teaspoon salt
- » 1 clove garlic

## DIRECTIONS

1. Purée ingredients in a blender until smooth. If you prefer a thinner soup, add more water until you reach the desired consistency. Divide soup among 4 bowls. Cover with plastic wrap and refrigerate within 30 minutes. Garnish with cucumber, avocado, and dill sprigs, if desired.

**NUTRITIONS:** Calories: 142, Fat: 7g, Sodium: 193mg, Carbohydrate: 12g, Protein: 11g

# 341. SOUTHWESTERN BEAN-AND-PEPPER SALAD

**COOKING: 0'**     **PREPARATION: 6'**     **SERVINGS: 4**

## INGREDIENTS

- » 1 can pinto beans, drained
- » 2 bell peppers, cored and chopped
- » 1 cup corn kernels
- » Salt
- » Freshly ground black pepper
- » Juice of 2 limes
- » 1 tablespoon olive oil
- » 1 avocado, chopped

## DIRECTIONS

1. Mix beans, peppers, corn, salt, plus pepper in a large bowl. Press fresh lime juice, then mix in olive oil. Let the salad stand in the fridge within 30 minutes. Add avocado just before serving.

**NUTRITIONS:** Calories: 245, Fat: 11g, Sodium: 97mg, Carbohydrate: 32g, Protein: 8g

# 342. CAULIFLOWER MASHED POTATOES

**COOKING: 10'**     **PREPARATION: 10'**     **SERVINGS: 4**

## INGREDIENTS

- » 16 cups water (enough to cover cauliflower)
- » 1 head cauliflower (about 3 pounds), trimmed and cut into florets
- » 4 garlic cloves
- » 1 tablespoon olive oil
- » ¼ teaspoon salt
- » 1/8 teaspoon freshly ground black pepper
- » 2 teaspoons dried parsley

## DIRECTIONS

1. Boil a large pot of water, then the cauliflower and garlic. Cook within 10 minutes, then strain. Move it back to the hot pan, and let it stand within 2 to 3 minutes with the lid on.

2. Put the cauliflower plus garlic in a food processor or blender. Add the olive oil, salt, pepper, and purée until smooth. Taste and adjust the salt and pepper.

3. Remove, then put the parsley, and mix until combined. Garnish with additional olive oil, if desired. Serve immediately.

**NUTRITIONS:** Calories: 87g, Fat: 4g, Sodium: 210mg, Carbohydrate: 12g, Protein: 4g

# 343. ROASTED BRUSSELS SPROUTS

**COOKING: 20'**     **PREPARATION: 5'**     **SERVINGS: 4**

## INGREDIENTS

- » 1½ pounds Brussels sprouts, trimmed and halved
- » 2 tablespoons olive oil
- » ¼ teaspoon salt
- » ½ teaspoon freshly ground black pepper

## DIRECTIONS

1. Preheat the oven to 400°f. Combine the Brussels sprouts and olive oil in a large mixing bowl and toss until they are evenly coated.

2. Turn the Brussels sprouts out onto a large baking sheet and flip them over, so they are cut-side down with the flat part touching the baking sheet. Sprinkle with salt and pepper.

3. Bake within 20 to 30 minutes or until the Brussels sprouts are lightly charred and crisp on the outside and toasted on the bottom. The outer leaves will be extra dark, too. Serve immediately.

**NUTRITIONS:** Calories: 134, Fat: 8g, Sodium: 189mg, Carbohydrate: 15g, Protein: 6g

# 344. BROCCOLI WITH GARLIC AND LEMON

**COOKING: 4'**     **PREPARATION: 2'**     **SERVINGS: 4**

## INGREDIENTS

- » 1 cup of water
- » 4 cups broccoli florets
- » 1 teaspoon olive oil
- » 1 tablespoon minced garlic
- » 1 teaspoon lemon zest
- » Salt
- » Freshly ground black pepper

## DIRECTIONS

1. Put the broccoli in the boiling water in a small sauccpan and cook within 2 to 3 minutes. The broccoli should retain its bright-green color. Drain the water from the broccoli.

2. Put the olive oil in a small sauté pan over medium-high heat. Add the garlic and sauté for 30 seconds. Put the broccoli, lemon zest, salt, plus pepper. Combine well and serve.

**NUTRITIONS:** Calories: 38g, Fat: 1g, Sodium: 24mg, Carbohydrate: 5g, Protein: 3g

# 345. BROWN RICE PILAF

**COOKING: 10'**　　　**PREPARATION: 5'**　　　**SERVINGS: 4**

## INGREDIENTS

» 1 cup low-sodium vegetable broth
» ½ tablespoon olive oil
» 1 clove garlic, minced
» 1 scallion, thinly sliced
» 1 tablespoon minced onion flakes
» 1 cup instant brown rice
» 1/8 teaspoon freshly ground black pepper

## DIRECTIONS

1. Mix the vegetable broth, olive oil, garlic, scallion, and minced onion flakes in a saucepan and boil. Put rice, then boil it again, adjust the heat and simmer within 10 minutes. Remove and let stand within 5 minutes. Fluff with a fork and season with black pepper.

**NUTRITIONS:** Calories: 100g, Fat: 2g, Sodium: 35mg, Carbohydrate: 19g, Protein: 2g

# 346. CHUNKY BLACK-BEAN DIP

**COOKING: 1'**　　　**PREPARATION: 5'**　　　**SERVINGS: 2**

## INGREDIENTS

» 1 (15-ounce) can black beans, drained, with liquid reserved
» ½-can of chipotle peppers in adobo sauce
» ¼ cup plain Greek yogurt
» Freshly ground black pepper

## DIRECTIONS

1. Combine beans, peppers, and yogurt in a food processor or blender and process until smooth. Add some of the bean liquid, 1 tablespoon at a time, for a thinner consistency. Season to taste with black pepper. Serve.

**NUTRITIONS:** Calories: 70g, Fat: 1g, Sodium: 159mg, Carbohydrate: 11g, Protein: 5g

# 347. CLASSIC HUMMUS

**COOKING: 0'**      **PREPARATION: 5-8'**      **SERVINGS: 6-8**

## INGREDIENTS

- » 1 (15-ounce) can chickpeas, drained and rinsed
- » 3 tablespoons sesame tahini
- » 2 tablespoons olive oil
- » 3 garlic cloves, chopped
- » Juice of 1 lemon
- » Salt
- » Freshly ground black pepper

## DIRECTIONS

1. Mix all the ingredients until smooth but thick in a food processor or blender. Add water if necessary to produce a smoother hummus. Store covered for up to 5 days.

**NUTRITIONS:** Calories: 147g, Fat: 10g, Sodium: 64mg, Carbohydrate: 11g, Protein: 6g.

# 348. CRISPY POTATO SKINS

**COOKING: 19'**      **PREPARATION: 2'**      **SERVINGS: 2**

## INGREDIENTS

- » 2 russet potatoes
- » Cooking spray
- » 1 teaspoon dried rosemary
- » 1/8 teaspoon freshly ground black pepper

## DIRECTIONS

1. Preheat the oven to 375°f. Prick or pierce the potatoes all over using a fork. Put on a plate. Cook on full power in the microwave within 5 minutes. Flip over, and cook again within 3 to 4 minutes more, or until soft.

2. Carefully—the potatoes will be very hot—scoop out the pulp of the potatoes, leaving a 1/8 inch of potato pulp attached to the skin. Set aside.

3. Spray the inside of each potato with cooking spray. Press in the rosemary and pepper. Place the skins on a baking sheet and bake in a preheated oven for 5 to 10 minutes until slightly browned and crispy. Serve immediately.

**NUTRITIONS:** Calories 114, Fat: 0g, Sodium: 0mg, Carbohydrate: 27g, Protein: 3g

# 349. ROASTED CHICKPEAS

**COOKING: 30'**   **PREPARATION: 5'**   **SERVINGS: 2**

## INGREDIENTS

- » 1 (15-ounce can) chickpeas, drained and rinsed
- » ½ teaspoon olive oil
- » 2 teaspoons of your favorite herbs or spice blend
- » ¼ teaspoon salt

## DIRECTIONS

1. Preheat the oven to 400°f.

2. Wrap a rimmed baking sheet with paper towels, place the chickpeas on it in an even layer, and blot with more paper towels until most of the liquid is absorbed.

3. In a medium bowl, gently toss the chickpeas and olive oil until combined. Sprinkle the mixture with the herbs and salt and toss again.

4. Place the chickpeas back on the baking sheet and spread in an even layer. Bake for 30 to 40 minutes, until crunchy and golden brown. Stir halfway through. Serve.

**NUTRITIONS:** Calories: 175g, Fat: 3g, Sodium: 474mg, Carbohydrate: 29g, Protein: 11g

# 350. CARROT-CAKE SMOOTHIE

**COOKING: 0'**   **PREPARATION: 5'**   **SERVINGS: 2**

## INGREDIENTS

- » 1 frozen banana, peeled and diced
- » 1 cup carrots, diced (peeled if preferred)
- » 1 cup nonfat or low-fat milk
- » ½ cup nonfat or low-fat vanilla Greek yogurt
- » ½ cup ice
- » ¼ cup diced pineapple, frozen
- » ½ teaspoon ground cinnamon
- » Pinch nutmeg
- » Optional toppings: chopped walnuts, grated carrots

## DIRECTIONS

1. Process all of the fixings to a blender. Serve immediately with optional toppings as desired.

**NUTRITIONS:** Calories: 180g, Fat: 1g, Sodium: 114mg, Carbohydrate: 36g, Protein 10g

# 351. VEGETABLE CHEESE CALZONE

**COOKING: 20'**  **PREPARATION: 15'**  **SERVINGS: 4**

## INGREDIENTS

» 3 asparagus stalks, cut into pieces
» 1/2 cup spinach, chopped
» 1/2 cup broccoli, chopped
» 1/2 cup sliced
» 2 tablespoons garlic, minced
» 2 teaspoons olive oil, divided
» 1/2 lb. frozen whole-wheat bread dough, thawed
» 1 medium tomato, sliced
» 1/2 cup mozzarella, shredded
» 2/3 cup pizza sauce

## DIRECTIONS

1. Prepare the oven to 400 degrees F to preheat. Grease a baking sheet with cooking oil and set it aside. Toss asparagus with mushrooms, garlic, broccoli, and spinach in a bowl. Stir in 1 teaspoon olive oil and mix well. Heat a greased skillet on medium heat.

2. Stir in vegetable mixture and sauté for 5 minutes. Set these vegetables aside. Cut the bread dough into quarters.

3. Spread each bread quarter on a floured surface into an oval. Add sautéed vegetables, 2 tbsp cheese, and tomato slice to half of each oval.

4. Wet the edges of each oval and fold the dough over the vegetable filling. Pinch and press the two edges.

5. Place these calzones on the baking sheet. Brush each calzone with foil and bake for 10 minutes. Heat pizza sauce in a saucepan for a minute. Serve the calzone with pizza sauce.

**NUTRITIONS:** Calories 198, Fat 8 g, Sodium 124 mg, Carbs 36 g, Protein 12 g

# 352. MIXED VEGETARIAN CHILI

**COOKING: 36'**  **PREPARATION: 10'**  **SERVINGS: 4**

## INGREDIENTS

» 1 tablespoon olive oil
» 14 oz. canned black beans, rinsed and drained
» ½ cup yellow Onion, chopped
» 12 oz. extra-firm tofu, cut into pieces
» 14 oz. canned kidney beans, rinsed and drained
» 2 cans (14 oz.) diced tomatoes
» 3 tablespoons chili powder
» 1 tablespoon oregano
» 1 tablespoon chopped cilantro (fresh coriander)

## DIRECTIONS

1. Take a soup pot and heat olive oil in it over medium heat. Add onions and sauté for 6 minutes until soft. Add tomatoes, beans, chili powder, oregano, and beans. Boil it first, then reduce the heat to a simmer. Cook for 30 minutes, then add cilantro. Serve warm.

**NUTRITIONS:** Calories 314, Fat 6 g, Sodium 119 mg, Carbs 46g, Protein 19 g

# 353. ZUCCHINI PEPPER KEBABS

**COOKING: 40'**  **PREPARATION: 15'**  **SERVINGS: 2**

## INGREDIENTS

» 1 small zucchini, sliced into 8 pieces
» 1 red onion, cut into 4 wedges
» 1 green bell pepper, cut into 4 chunks
» 8 cherry tomatoes
» 8 button mushrooms
» 1 red bell pepper, cut into 4 chunks
» 1/2 cup Italian dressing, fat-free
» 1/2 cup brown rice
» 1 cup of water
» 4 wooden skewers, soaked and drained

## DIRECTIONS

1. Toss tomatoes with zucchini, onion, peppers, and mushrooms in a bowl. Stir in Italian dressing and mix well to coat the vegetables. Marinate them for 10 minutes. Boil water with rice in a saucepan, then reduce the heat to a simmer.

2. Cover the rice and cook for 30 minutes until rice is done. Meanwhile, prepare the grill and preheat it on medium heat. Grease the grilling rack with cooking spray and place it 4 inches above the heat.

3. Thread 2 mushrooms, 2 tomatoes, and 2 zucchini slices along with 1 onions wedge, 1 green and red pepper slice on each skewer. Grill these kebabs for 5 minutes per side. Serve warm with boiled rice.

**NUTRITIONS:** Calories 335, Fat 8.2 g, Sodium 516 mg, Carbs 67 g, Protein 8.8 g

# 354. ASPARAGUS CHEESE VERMICELLI

**COOKING: 15'**  **PREPARATION: 10'**  **SERVINGS: 4**

## INGREDIENTS

» 2 teaspoons olive oil, divided
» 6 asparagus spears, cut into pieces
» 4 oz. dried whole-grain vermicelli
» 1 medium tomato, chopped
» 1 tablespoon garlic, minced
» 2 tablespoons fresh basil, chopped
» 4 tablespoons Parmesan, freshly grated, divided
» 1/8 teaspoon black pepper, ground

## DIRECTIONS

1. Add 1 tsp oil to a skillet and heat it. Stir in asparagus and sauté until golden brown.

2. Cut the sautéed asparagus into 1-inch pieces. Fill a sauce pot with water up to ¾ full. After boiling the water, add pasta and cook for 10 minutes until it is all done.

3. Drain and rinse the pasta under tap water. Add pasta to a large bowl, then toss in olive oil, tomato, garlic, asparagus, basil, garlic, and parmesan. Serve with black pepper on top.

**NUTRITIONS:** Calories 325, Fat 8 g, Sodium 350 mg, Carbs 48 g, Protein 7.3 g

# 355. CORN STUFFED PEPPERS

**COOKING: 35'**     **PREPARATION: 10'**     **SERVINGS: 4**

## INGREDIENTS

- » 4 red or green bell peppers
- » 1 tablespoon olive oil
- » ¼ cup onion, chopped
- » 1 green bell pepper, chopped
- » 2 1/2 cups fresh corn kernels
- » 1/8 teaspoon chili powder
- » 2 tablespoons chopped fresh parsley
- » 3 egg whites
- » 1/2 cup skim milk
- » 1/2 cup water

## DIRECTIONS

1. Prepare the oven to 350 F to preheat. Layer a baking dish with cooking spray. Cut the bell peppers from the top and remove their seeds from inside. Put the peppers in your prepared baking dish with their cut side up.

2. Add oil to a skillet, then heat it on medium flame. Stir in onion, corn, and green pepper. Sauté for 5 minutes. Add cilantro and chili powder. Switch the heat to low. Mix milk plus egg whites in a bowl. Pour this mixture into the skillet and cook for 5 minutes while stirring.

3. Divide this mixture into each pepper. Add some water to the baking dish. Cover the stuffed peppers with an aluminum sheet. Bake for 15 minutes, then serves warm.

**NUTRITIONS:** Calories 197, Fat 5 g, Sodium 749 mg, Carbs 29 g, Protein 9 g

# 356. STUFFED EGGPLANT SHELLS

**COOKING: 25'**     **PREPARATION: 10'**     **SERVINGS: 2**

## INGREDIENTS

- » 1 medium eggplant
- » 1 cup of water
- » 1 tablespoon olive oil
- » 4 oz. cooked white beans
- » 1/4 cup onion, chopped
- » 1/2 cup red, green, or yellow bell peppers, chopped
- » 1 cup canned unsalted tomatoes
- » 1/4 cup tomatoes liquid
- » 1/4 cup celery, chopped
- » 1 cup fresh mushrooms, sliced
- » 3/4 cup whole-wheat breadcrumbs
- » Freshly ground black pepper, to taste

## DIRECTIONS

1. Prepare the oven to 350 degrees F to preheat. Grease a baking dish with cooking spray and set it aside. Trim and cut the eggplant into half, lengthwise. Scoop out the pulp using a spoon and leave the shell about ¼ inch thick.

2. Place the shells in the baking dish with their cut side up. Add water to the bottom of the dish. Dice the eggplant pulp into cubes and set them aside. Add oil to an iron skillet and heat it over medium heat. Stir in onions, peppers, chopped eggplant, tomatoes, celery, mushrooms, and tomato juice.

3. Cook for 10 minutes on simmering heat, then stirs in beans, black pepper, and breadcrumbs. Divide this mixture into the eggplant shells. Cover the shells with a foil sheet and bake for 15 minutes. Serve warm.

**NUTRITIONS:** Calories 334, Fat 10 g, Sodium 142 mg, Carbs 35 g, Protein 26 g

# 357. SOUTHWESTERN VEGETABLES TACOS

**COOKING: 20'**　　　　**PREPARATION: 10'**　　　　**SERVINGS: 4**

## INGREDIENTS

- » 1 tablespoon olive oil
- » 1 cup red onion, chopped
- » 1 cup yellow summer squash, diced
- » 1 cup green zucchini, diced
- » 3 large garlic cloves, minced
- » 4 medium tomatoes, seeded and chopped
- » 1 jalapeno chili, seeded and chopped
- » 1 cup fresh corn kernels
- » 1 cup canned pinto, rinsed and drained
- » 1/2 cup fresh cilantro, chopped
- » 8 corn tortillas
- » 1/2 cup smoke-flavored salsa

## DIRECTIONS

1. Add olive oil to a saucepan, then heat it over medium heat. Stir in onion and sauté until soft. Add zucchini and summer squash. Cook for 5 minutes.

2. Stir in corn kernels, jalapeno, garlic, beans, and tomatoes. Cook for another 5 minutes. Stir in cilantro, then remove the pan from the heat.

3. Warm each tortilla in a dry nonstick skillet for 20 secs per side. Place the tortilla on the serving plate. Spoon the vegetable mixture in each tortilla. Top the mixture with salsa. Serve.

**NUTRITIONS:** Calories 310, Fat 6 g, Sodium 97 mg, Carbs 54 g, Protein 10g

# CHAPTER 11.
# SOUPS

# 358. CHICKEN AND TORTILLA SOUP

**COOKING: 6 H**          **PREPARATION: 15'**          **SERVINGS: 12**

## INGREDIENTS

- »  3 Chicken Breasts (boneless and skinless)
- »  15 ounces diced Tomatoes
- »  10 ounces Enchilada Sauce
- »  1 chopped onion (med.)
- »  4 ounces chopped Chili Pepper (green)
- »  3 minced cloves Garlic
- »  2 cups Water
- »  14.5-ounces Chicken Broth (fat-free)
- »  1 tbsp. Cumin
- »  1 tbs. Chile Powder
- »  1 tsp. Salt
- »  ¼ tsp. Black Pepper
- »  Bay Leaf
- »  1 tbsp. Cilantro (chopped)
- »  10 ounces Frozen Corn
- »  3 tortillas, cut into thin slices

## DIRECTIONS

1. Put all the listed fixing in the slow cooker. Stir well to mix. Cook on low heat within 8 hrs. or high heat for 6 hrs. Shred the chicken breasts to a plate. Add chicken to other ingredients. Serve hot, garnished with tortilla slices.

**NUTRITIONS:** Calories 93.4, Fat 1.9 g, Cholesterol 18.6, Sodium 841.3 mg, Carbohydrates 11.9 g, Fiber 2.1 g, Protein 8.3 g

# 359. STUFFED PEPPER SOUP

**COOKING: 8H 10'**          **PREPARATION: 15'**          **SERVINGS: 1**

## INGREDIENTS

- »  1 lb. ground Beef (drained)
- »  1 chopped onion (large)
- »  2 cups Tomatoes (diced)
- »  2 chopped Green Peppers
- »  2 cups Tomato Sauce
- »  1 tbs. Beef Bouillon
- »  3 cups of water
- »  Pepper
- »  1 tsp. of Salt
- »  1 cup of cooked rice (white)

## DIRECTIONS

1. Place all ingredients in a cooker. Cook for 8 hours on "low." Serve hot.

**NUTRITIONS:** Calories 216.1, Fat 5.1 g, Cholesterol 43.4 mg, Sodium 480.7 mg, Carbohydrates 21.8 mg, Fiber 2.5 g, Protein 18.8 g

# 360. HAM AND PEA SOUP

**COOKING: 8H**   **PREPARATION: 15'**   **SERVINGS: 8**

## INGREDIENTS

- » 1 lb. Split Peas (dried)
- » 1 cup sliced Celery
- » 1 cup sliced Carrots
- » 1 cup sliced Onion
- » 2 cups chopped ham (cooked)
- » 8 cups of water

## DIRECTIONS

1. Place all the listed fixing in the slow cooker. Cook on "high" within 4 hrs. Serve hot.

**NUTRITIONS:** Calories 118.6, Fat 1.9 g, Cholesterol 15.9 mg, Sodium 828.2 mg, Carbohydrates 14.5 mg, Fiber 5.1 g, Protein 11.1 g

# 361. PEA SOUP

**COOKING: 8H**   **PREPARATION: 15'**   **SERVINGS: 8**

## INGREDIENTS

- » 16 oz. Split Peas (dried)
- » 1 cup chopped Baby Carrots
- » 1chopped onion (white)
- » 3 Bay Leaves
- » 10 oz. cubed Turkey Ham
- » 4 cubes Chicken Bouillon
- » 7 cups of water

## DIRECTIONS

1. Rinse and drain peas. Place all the fixing in the slow cooker. Cook on "low" for 8 hrs. Serve hot.

**NUTRITIONS:** Calories 122.7, Fat 2 g, Cholesterol 24 mg, Sodium 780.6 mg, Carbohydrates 15 mg, Fiber 5.2 g, Protein 11.8 g

# 362. SOUP FOR THE DAY

**COOKING: 10 H 10'**　　　**PREPARATION: 15'**　　　**SERVINGS: 8**

## INGREDIENTS

- » 1 Beef Steak (cubed)
- » 1 chopped onion (med.)
- » 1 tbsp. Olive Oil
- » 5 thinly sliced med. Carrots
- » 4 cups Cabbage
- » 4 diced Red Potatoes
- » 2 diced Celery Stalks
- » 2 cans Tomatoes, diced
- » 2 cans Beef Broth
- » 1 tsp. Sugar
- » 1 can Tomato Soup
- » 1 tsp. Parsley Flakes (dried)
- » 2 tsp. Italian Seasoning

## DIRECTIONS

1. In a skillet, sauté onion, and steak in oil. Transfer the sautéed mixture to the slow cooker. Put the rest of the fixing in the slow cooker. Cook on "low" for 10 hrs. Serve hot.

**NUTRITIONS:** Calories 259.6, Fat 6.7 g, Cholesterol 29.8 mg, Sodium 699.2 mg, Carbohydrates 31.6 mg, Fiber 4.6 g, Protein 18.9 g

# 363. CHIPOTLE SQUASH SOUP

**COOKING: 4H 20'**　　　**PREPARATION: 15'**　　　**SERVINGS: 6**

## INGREDIENTS

- » 6 cups Butternut Squash (cubed)
- » ½ cup chopped Onion
- » 2 tsp. Adobo Chipotle
- » 2 cups Chicken Broth
- » 1 tbsp. Brown Sugar
- » ¼ cup Tart Apple (chopped)
- » 1 cup Yogurt (Greek style)
- » 2 tbsp. Chives (chopped)

## DIRECTIONS

1. Except for yogurt, chives, and apple, place all the ingredients in the slow cooker. Cook on "low" for 4 hrs. Now, in a blender or food processer, puree the cooked ingredients. Transfer puree to slow cooker.

2. Put the yogurt and cook on "Low" within 20 more mins. Garnish with chives and apples. Serve hot in heated bowls.

**NUTRITIONS:** Calories 102, Fat 11 g, Cholesterol 2 mg, Sodium 142 mg, Carbohydrates 22 mg, Fiber 3 g, Protein 4 g

# 364. KALE VERDE

**COOKING: 6H**   **PREPARATION: 15'**   **SERVINGS: 6**

## INGREDIENTS

- » ¼ cup Olive Oil (extra virgin)
- » 1 Yellow Onion (large)
- » 2 cloves Garlic
- » 2 ounces Tomatoes, dried
- » 2 cups Yellow Potatoes (diced)
- » 14-ounce Tomatoes (diced)
- » 6 cups Chicken broth
- » White pepper (ground)
- » 1-pound o chopped Kale

## DIRECTIONS

1. Sauté onion for 5 mins in oil. Add the garlic and sauté again for 1 minute. Transfer the sautéed mixture to the slow cooker. Put rest of the fixing except pepper into the slow cooker. Cook on "low" for 6 hrs. Season with white pepper to taste. Serve hot in heated bowls

**NUTRITIONS:** Calories 257, Fat 22 g, Cholesterol 3 mg, Sodium 239 mg, Carbohydrates 27 mg, Fiber 6 g, Protein 14 g

# 365. ESCAROLE WITH BEAN SOUP

**COOKING: 6H**   **PREPARATION: 15'**   **SERVINGS: 6**

## INGREDIENTS

- » 1 tbsp. Olive Oil
- » 8 crushed cloves Garlic
- » 1 cup chopped Onions
- » 1 diced Carrot
- » 3 tsp. Basil (dried)
- » 3 tsp. Oregano (dried)
- » 4 cups Chicken Broth
- » 3 cups chopped Escarole
- » 1 cup of Northern Beans (dried)
- » Parmesan Cheese (grated)
- » 14 ounces o Tomatoes (diced)

## DIRECTIONS

1. Sauté garlic for 2 mins in oil using a large soup pot. Except for the cheese, broth, and beans, add the rest of the ingredients and cook for 5 mins. Transfer the cooked ingredients to the slow cooker.

2. Mix in the broth and beans. Cook on "low" for 6 hrs. Garnish with cheese. Serve hot in heated bowls.

**NUTRITIONS:** Calories 98, Fat 33 g, Cholesterol 1 mg, Sodium 115 mg, Carbohydrates 14 mg, Fiber 3 g, Protein 8 g

# 366. CHICKEN SQUASH SOUP

**COOKING: 5 H 30'**     **PREPARATION: 5'**     **SERVINGS: 3**

## INGREDIENTS

- » ½ Butternut Squash (large)
- » 1 clove Garlic
- » 1 ¼ quarts broth (vegetable or chicken)
- » 1/8 tsp. Pepper (white)
- » ½ tbsp. chopped Parsley
- » 2 minced Sage leaves
- » 1 tbsp. Olive Oil
- » ¼ chopped onion (white)
- » 1/16 tsp. Black Pepper (cracked)
- » 1/2 tbsp. of Pepper Flakes (chili)
- » ½ tsp. chopped rosemary

## DIRECTIONS

1. Preheat oven to 400 degrees. Grease a baking sheet. Roast the squash in a preheated oven for 30 mins. Transfer it to a plate and let it cool. Sauté onion and garlic in the oil.

2. Now, scoop out the flesh from the roasted squash and add to the sautéed onion & garlic. Mash all of it well. Pour ½ quart of the broth into the slow cooker. Add the squash mixture. Cook on "low" for 4 hrs. Using a blender, make a smooth puree.

3. Transfer the puree to the slow cooker. Add in the rest of the broth and other ingredients. Cook again for 1 hr. on "high". Serve in heated soup bowls.

**NUTRITIONS:** Calories 158, Fats 6 g, Sodium 699 mg, Carbohydrates 24 mg, Fiber 6 g, Protein 3 g

# 367. VEGGIE AND BEEF SOUP

**COOKING: 4H**     **PREPARATION: 15'**     **SERVINGS: 4**

## INGREDIENTS

- » 1 chopped Carrot
- » 1 chopped Celery Rib
- » ¾ l. Sirloin (ground)
- » 1 cup Water
- » ½ Butternut Squash (large)
- » 1 clove Garlic
- » ½ quart Beef broth
- » 7 ounces diced Tomatoes (unsalted)
- » ½ tsp. Kosher Salt
- » 1 tbsp. chopped parsley
- » ¼ tsp. Thyme (dried)
- » ¼ tsp. Black Pepper (ground)
- » ½ Bay Leaf

## DIRECTIONS

1. Sauté all the vegetables in oil. Put the vegetables to the side, then place sirloin in the center. Sauté, using a spoon to crumble the meat. When cooked, combine with the vegetables on the sides of the pan.

2. Now, pour the rest of the ingredients into the slow cooker. Add cooked meat and vegetables. Stir well. Cook on "low" for 3 hrs. Serve in soup bowls.

**NUTRITIONS:** Calories 217, Fats 7 g, Cholesterol 53 mg, Sodium 728 mg, Carbohydrates 17 mg, Fiber 5 g, Protein 22 g

# 368. COLLARD, SWEET POTATO AND PEA SOUP

**COOKING: 4H**     **PREPARATION: 15'**     **SERVINGS: 4**

## INGREDIENTS

- » 3 1/2 oz. Ham Steak, chopped
- » ½ chopped Yellow Onion
- » ½ lb. sliced Sweet Potatoes
- » ¼ tsp. Red Pepper (hot and crushed)
- » ½ cup frozen Peas (black-eyed)
- » ½ tbsp. Canola Oil
- » 1 minced clove of Garlic
- » 1 ½ cup Water
- » ¼ tsp. Salt
- » 2 cups Collard Greens (julienned and without stems)

## DIRECTIONS

1. Sauté ham with garlic and onion in oil. In a slow cooker, place other ingredients except for collard greens and peas.

2. Add in the ham mixture. Cook on "low" for 3 hrs. Now, add collard green and peas and cook again for an hour on "low." Serve in soup bowls.

**NUTRITIONS:** Calories 172, Fats 4 g, Sodium 547 mg, Carbohydrates 24 mg, Fiber 4 g, Protein 11 g

# 369. BEAN SOUP

**COOKING: 5H**     **PREPARATION: 15'**     **SERVINGS: 4**

## INGREDIENTS

- » ½ cup Pinto Beans (dried)
- » ½ Bay Leaf
- » 1 clove Garlic
- » ½ onion (white)
- » 2 cups Water
- » 2 tbsp. Cilantro (chopped)
- » 1 cubed Avocado
- » 1/8 cup White Onion (chopped)
- » ¼ cup Roma Tomatoes (chopped)
- » 2 tbsp. Pepper Sauce (chipotle)
- » ¼ tsp. Kosher Salt
- » 2 tbsp. chopped Cilantro
- » 2 tbsp. Low Fat Monterrey Jack Cheese, shredded

## DIRECTIONS

1. Place water, salt, onion, pepper, garlic, bay leaf, and beans in the slow cooker. Cook on high for 5 6 hours. Discard the Bay leaf. Serve in heated bowls.

**NUTRITIONS:** Calories 258, Fats 19 g, Cholesterol 2 mg, Sodium 620 mg, Carbohydrates 25 mg, Fiber 11 g, Protein 8 g

# 370. BROWN RICE AND CHICKEN SOUP

**COOKING: 4H**     **PREPARATION: 15'**     **SERVINGS: 4**

## INGREDIENTS

- » 1/3 cups Brown Rice
- » 1 chopped Leek
- » 1 sliced Celery Rib
- » 1 ½ cups water
- » ½ tsp. Kosher Salt
- » ½ Bay Leaf
- » 1/8 tsp. Thyme (dried)
- » ¼ tsp. Black Pepper (ground)
- » 1 tbsp. chopped parsley
- » ½ quart Chicken Broth (low sodium)
- » 1 sliced Carrot
- » ¾ lb. of Chicken Thighs (skin and boneless)

## DIRECTIONS

1. Boil 1 cup of water with ½ tsp. of salt in a saucepan. Add the rice. Cook for 30 mins on medium flame. Brown chicken pieces in the oil. Transfer the chicken to a plate when done.

2. In the same pan, sauté the vegetables for 3 mins. Now, place the chicken pieces in the slow cooker. Add water and broth. Cook on "low" for 3 hrs. Put the rest of the fixing, the rice last. Cook again for 10 mins on "high." After discarding Bay leaf, serve in soup bowls

**NUTRITIONS:** Calories 208, Fats 6 g, Cholesterol 71 mg, Sodium 540 mg, Carbohydrates 18 mg, Fiber 2 g, Protein 20 g

# 371. BROCCOLI SOUP

**COOKING: 3H**     **PREPARATION: 15'**     **SERVINGS: 2**

## INGREDIENTS

- » 4 cups chopped broccoli
- » ½ cup chopped onion (white)
- » 1 ½ cup Chicken Broth (low sodium)
- » 1/8 tsp. Black Pepper (cracked)
- » 1 tbsp. Olive Oil
- » 1 Garlic Clove
- » 1/16 tsp. Pepper Flakes (chili)
- » ¼ cup Milk (low fat)

## DIRECTIONS

1. In the slow cooker, cover the broccoli with water and cook for an hour on "high." Set aside after draining. Sauté onion and garlic in oil and transfer them to slow cooker when done. Add the broth.

2. Cook on "low" for 2 hrs. Transfer the mixture to a blender and make a smooth puree. Add black pepper, milk, and pepper flakes to the puree. Boil briefly. Serve the soup in heated bowls.

**NUTRITIONS:** Calories 291, Fats 14 g, Cholesterol 24 mg, Sodium 227 mg, Carbohydrates 28 mg, Fiber 6 g, Protein 17 g

# 372. HEARTY GINGER SOUP

**COOKING: 5'**      **PREPARATION: 5'**      **SERVINGS: 4**

## INGREDIENTS

- » 3 cups coconut almond milk
- » 2 cups of water
- » ½ pound boneless chicken breast halves, cut into chunks
- » 3 tablespoons fresh ginger root, minced
- » 2 tablespoons fish sauce
- » ¼ cup fresh lime juice
- » 2 tablespoons green onions, sliced
- » 1 tablespoon fresh cilantro, chopped

## DIRECTIONS

1. Take a saucepan and add coconut almond milk and water. Bring the mixture to a boil and add the chicken strips. Adjust the heat to medium, then simmer for 3 minutes. Stir in the ginger, lime juice, and fish sauce. Sprinkle a few green onions and cilantro.

**NUTRITIONS:** Calories: 415, Fat: 39g, Carbohydrates: 8g, Protein: 14g, Sodium: 150 mg

# 373. TASTY TOFU AND MUSHROOM SOUP

**COOKING: 10'**      **PREPARATION: 15'**      **SERVINGS: 8**

## INGREDIENTS

- » 3 cups prepared dashi stock
- » ¼ cup shiitake mushrooms, sliced
- » 1 tablespoon miso paste
- » 1 tablespoon coconut aminos
- » 1/8 cup cubed soft tofu
- » 1 green onion, diced

## DIRECTIONS

1. Take a saucepan and add the stock; bring to a boil. Add mushrooms, cook for 4 minutes. Take a bowl and add coconut aminos, miso pastes, and mix well. Pour the mixture into stock and let it cook for 6 minutes on simmer. Add diced green onions and enjoy!

**NUTRITIONS:** Calories: 100, Fat: 4g, Carbohydrates: 5g, Protein: 11, Sodium: 87 mg

# 374. INGENIOUS EGGPLANT SOUP

**COOKING: 15'**     **PREPARATION: 15'**     **SERVINGS: 8**

## INGREDIENTS

- » 1 large eggplant, washed and cubed
- » 1 tomato, seeded and chopped
- » 1 small onion, diced
- » 2 tablespoons parsley, chopped
- » 2 tablespoons extra virgin olive oil
- » 2 tablespoons distilled white vinegar
- » ½ cup parmesan cheese, crumbled
- » Sunflower seeds as needed

## DIRECTIONS

1. Preheat your outdoor grill to medium-high. Pierce the eggplant a few times using a knife/fork. Cook the eggplants on your grill for about 15 minutes until they are charred. Put aside and allow them to cool.

2. Remove the eggplant's skin and dice the pulp. Put it in a mixing bowl and add parsley, onion, tomato, olive oil, feta cheese, and vinegar. Mix well and chill for 1 hour. Season with sunflower seeds and enjoy!

**NUTRITIONS:** Calories: 99, Fat: 7g, Carbohydrates: 7g, Protein:3.4g, Sodium: 90 mg

# 375. LOVING CAULIFLOWER SOUP

**COOKING: 10'**     **PREPARATION: 15'**     **SERVINGS: 6**

## INGREDIENTS

- » 4 cups vegetable stock
- » 1-pound cauliflower, trimmed and chopped
- » 7 ounces Kite ricotta/cashew cheese
- » 4 ounces almond butter
- » Sunflower seeds and pepper to taste

## DIRECTIONS

1. Put almond butter and melt in a skillet over medium heat. Add cauliflower and sauté for 2 minutes. Add stock and bring the mix to a boil.

2. Cook until cauliflower is al dente. Stir in cream cheese, sunflower seeds, and pepper. Puree the mix using an immersion blender. Serve and enjoy!

**NUTRITIONS:** Calories: 143, Fat: 16g, Carbohydrates: 6g, Protein: 3.4g, Sodium: 510 mg

# 376. GARLIC AND LEMON SOUP

**COOKING: 0'**     **PREPARATION: 15'**     **SERVINGS: 3**

## INGREDIENTS

- » 1 avocado, pitted and chopped
- » 1 cucumber, chopped
- » 2 bunches spinach
- » 1 ½ cups watermelon, chopped
- » 1 bunch cilantro, roughly chopped
- » Juice from 2 lemons
- » ½ cup coconut aminos
- » ½ cup lime juice

## DIRECTIONS

1. Add cucumber, avocado to your blender, and pulse well. Add cilantro, spinach, and watermelon and blend. Add lemon, lime juice, and coconut amino. Pulse a few more times. Transfer to a soup bowl and enjoy!

**NUTRITIONS:** Calories: 100, Fat: 7g, Carbohydrates: 6g, Protein: 3g, Sodium: 0 mg

# 377. CUCUMBER SOUP

**COOKING: 0'**     **PREPARATION: 15'**     **SERVINGS: 4**

## INGREDIENTS

- » 2 tablespoons garlic, minced
- » 4 cups English cucumbers, peeled and diced
- » ½ cup onions, diced
- » 1 tablespoon lemon juice
- » 1 ½ cups vegetable broth
- » ½ teaspoon sunflower seeds
- » ¼ teaspoon red pepper flakes
- » ¼ cup parsley, diced
- » ½ cup Greek yogurt, plain

## DIRECTIONS

1. Put the listed fixing in a blender and blend to emulsify (keep aside ½ cup of chopped cucumbers). Blend until smooth. Divide the soup amongst 4 servings and top with extra cucumbers. Enjoy chilled!

**NUTRITIONS:** Calories: 371, Fat: 36g, Carbohydrates: 8g, Protein: 4g, Sodium: 40 mg

# 378. ROASTED GARLIC SOUP

**COOKING: 60'**  **PREPARATION: 15'**  **SERVINGS: 10**

## INGREDIENTS

- » 1 tablespoon olive oil
- » 2 bulbs garlic, peeled
- » 3 shallots, chopped
- » 1 large head cauliflower, chopped
- » 6 cups vegetable broth
- » Sunflower seeds and pepper to taste

## DIRECTIONS

1. Warm your oven to 400 degrees F. Slice ¼ inch top of the garlic bulb and place it in aluminum foil. Oiled it using olive oil and roast in the oven for 35 minutes. Squeeze flesh out of the roasted garlic.

2. Heat-up oil in a saucepan and add shallots, sauté for 6 minutes. Add garlic and remaining ingredients. Adjust heat to low. Let it cook for 15-20 minutes.

3. Puree the mixture using an immersion blender. Season soup with sunflower seeds and pepper. Serve and enjoy!

**NUTRITIONS:** Calories: 142, Fat: 8g, Carbohydrates: 3.4g, Protein: 4g, Sodium: 548 mg

# 379. ROASTED CARROT SOUP

**COOKING: 50'**  **PREPARATION: 15'**  **SERVINGS: 4**

## INGREDIENTS

- » 8 large carrots, washed and peeled
- » 6 tablespoons olive oil
- » 1-quart broth
- » Cayenne pepper to taste
- » Sunflower seeds and pepper to taste

## DIRECTIONS

1. Warm your oven to 425 degrees F. Take a baking sheet, add carrots, drizzle olive oil, and roast for 30-45 minutes. Put roasted carrots into a blender and add broth, puree. Pour into saucepan and heat soup. Season with sunflower seeds, pepper and cayenne. Drizzle olive oil. Serve and enjoy!

**NUTRITIONS:** Calories: 222, Fat: 18g, Net Carbohydrates: 7g, Protein: 5g, Sodium: 266 mg

# 380. PUMPKIN SOUP

**COOKING: 6H**  **PREPARATION: 15'**  **SERVINGS: 4**

## INGREDIENTS

» 1 small pumpkin, halved, peeled, seeds removed, cubed
» 2 cups chicken broth
» 1 cup of coconut milk
» Pepper and thyme to taste

## DIRECTIONS

1. Add all the ingredients to a crockpot. Cook for 6-8 hours on low. Make a smooth puree by using a blender. Garnish with roasted seeds. Serve and enjoy!

**NUTRITIONS:** Calories: 60, Fat: 2g, Carbohydrates: 10g, Protein: 3g, Sodium: 10 mg

# 381. COCONUT AVOCADO SOUP

**COOKING: 15'**  **PREPARATION: 10'**  **SERVINGS: 4**

## INGREDIENTS

» 2 cups vegetable stock
» 2 teaspoons Thai green curry paste
» Pepper as needed
» 1 avocado, chopped
» 1 tablespoon cilantro, chopped
» Lime wedges
» 1 cup of coconut milk

## DIRECTIONS

1. Add milk, avocado, curry paste, pepper to a blender, and blend. Take a pan and place it over medium heat. Add mixture and heat, simmer for 5 minutes. Stir in seasoning, cilantro, and simmer for 1 minute. Serve and enjoy!

**NUTRITIONS:** Calories: 250, Fat: 30g, Carbohydrates: 2g, Protein: 4g, Sodium: 378 mg

# 382. COCONUT ARUGULA SOUP

**COOKING: 10'**   **PREPARATION: 15'**   **SERVINGS: 4**

## INGREDIENTS

- » 3 cups non-fat beef stock
- » 2 garlic cloves, minced
- » 1 tablespoon tomato paste
- » 2 cups cabbage, chopped
- » ½ yellow onion
- » ½ cup carrot, chopped
- » ½ cup green beans
- » ½ cup zucchini, chopped
- » ½ teaspoon basil
- » ½ teaspoon oregano
- » Sunflower seeds and pepper as needed

## DIRECTIONS

1. Grease a pot with non-stick cooking spray. Place it over medium heat and allow the oil to heat up. Add onions, carrots, and garlic, and sauté for 5 minutes. Add broth, tomato paste, green beans, cabbage, basil, oregano, sunflower seeds, and pepper.

2. Boil the whole mix and reduce the heat, simmer for 5-10 minutes until all veggies are tender. Add zucchini and simmer for 5 minutes more. Sever hot and enjoy!

**NUTRITIONS:** Calories: 22, Fat: 0g, Carbohydrates: 5g, Protein: 1g, Sodium: 200 mg

# 384. GINGER ZUCCHINI AVOCADO SOUP

**COOKING: 25'**   **PREPARATION: 15'**   **SERVINGS: 3**

## INGREDIENTS

- » 1 red bell pepper, chopped
- » 1 big avocado
- » 1 teaspoon ginger, grated
- » Pepper as needed
- » 2 tablespoons avocado oil
- » 4 scallions, chopped
- » 1 tablespoon lemon juice
- » 29 ounces vegetable stock
- » 1 garlic clove, minced
- » 2 zucchinis, chopped
- » 1 cup of water

## DIRECTIONS

1. Take a pan and place over medium heat, add onion and fry for 3 minutes. Stir in ginger, garlic and cook for 1 minute. Mix in seasoning, zucchini stock, water, and boil for 10 minutes.

2. Remove soup from fire and let it sit; blend in avocado and blend using an immersion blender. Heat over low heat for a while. Adjust your seasoning and add lemon juice, bell pepper. Serve and enjoy!

**NUTRITIONS:** Calories: 155, Fat: 11g, Carbohydrates: 10g, Protein: 7g, Sodium: 345 mg

# 385. GREEK LEMON AND CHICKEN SOUP

**COOKING: 30'**　　　**PREPARATION: 15'**　　　**SERVINGS: 4**

## INGREDIENTS

- » 2 cups cooked chicken, chopped
- » 2 medium carrots, chopped
- » ½ cup onion, chopped
- » ¼ cup lemon juice
- » 1 clove garlic, minced
- » 1 can cream of chicken soup, fat-free and low sodium
- » 2 cans of chicken broth, fat-free
- » ¼ teaspoon ground black pepper
- » 2/3 cup long-grain rice
- » 2 tablespoons parsley, snipped

## DIRECTIONS

1. Put all of the listed fixings in a pot (except rice and parsley). Season with sunflower seeds and pepper. Bring the mix to a boil over medium-high heat. Stir in rice and set heat to medium.

2. Simmer within 20 minutes until rice is tender. Garnish parsley, and enjoy!

**NUTRITIONS:** Calories: 582, Fat: 33g, Carbohydrates: 35g, Protein: 32g, Sodium: 210 mg

# 386. GARLIC AND PUMPKIN SOUP

**COOKING: 5H**　　　**PREPARATION: 15'**　　　**SERVINGS: 4**

## INGREDIENTS

- » 1 pound pumpkin chunks
- » 1 onion, diced
- » 2 cups vegetable stock
- » 1 2/3 cups coconut cream
- » ½ stick almond butter
- » 1 teaspoon garlic, crushed
- » 1 teaspoon ginger, crushed
- » Pepper to taste

## DIRECTIONS

1. Add all the fixing into your Slow Cooker. Cook for 4-6 hours on high. Puree the soup by using your immersion blender. Serve and enjoy!

**NUTRITIONS:** Calories: 235, Fat: 21g, Carbohydrates: 11g, Protein: 2g, Sodium: 395 mg

# 387. GOLDEN MUSHROOM SOUP

**COOKING: 8H**  **PREPARATION: 15'**  **SERVINGS: 6**

## INGREDIENTS

- » 1 onion, finely chopped
- » 1 carrot, peeled and finely chopped
- » 1 fennel bulb, finely chopped
- » 1-pound fresh mushrooms, quartered
- » 8 cups Vegetable Broth, Poultry Broth, or store-bought
- » ¼ cup dry sherry
- » 1 teaspoon dried thyme
- » 1 teaspoon garlic powder
- » ½ teaspoon of sea salt
- » 1/8 teaspoon freshly ground black pepper

## DIRECTIONS

1. In your slow cooker, combine all the ingredients, mixing to combine. Cover and set on low. Cook for 8 hours.

**NUTRITIONS:** Calories: 71, Fat: 0g, Carbohydrates: 15g, Fiber: 3g, Protein: 3g, Sodium: 650 mg

# 388. MINESTRONE

**COOKING: 9H**  **PREPARATION: 15'**  **SERVINGS: 6**

## INGREDIENTS

- » 2 carrots, peeled and sliced
- » 2 celery stalks, sliced
- » 1 onion, chopped
- » 2 cups green beans, chopped
- » 1 (16-ounce) can crushed tomatoes
- » 2 cups cooked kidney beans, rinsed
- » 6 cups Poultry Broth, Vegetable Broth, or store-bought
- » 1 teaspoon garlic powder
- » 1 teaspoon dried Italian seasoning
- » ¼ teaspoon of sea salt
- » ¼ teaspoon freshly ground black pepper
- » 1½ cups cooked whole-wheat elbow macaroni (or pasta shape of your choice)
- » 1 zucchini, chopped

## DIRECTIONS

1. In your slow cooker, combine the carrots, celery, onion, green beans, tomatoes, kidney beans, broth, garlic powder, Italian seasoning, salt, and pepper in the slow cooker. Cook on low within 8 hours. Stir in the macaroni and zucchini. Cook on low within 1 hour more.

**NUTRITIONS:** Calories: 193, Fat: 0g, Carbohydrates: 39g, Fiber: 10g, Protein: 10g, Sodium: 100 mg

# 389. BUTTERNUT SQUASH SOUP

**COOKING: 8H**     **PREPARATION: 15'**     **SERVINGS: 6**

## INGREDIENTS

- » 1 butternut squash, peeled, seeded, and diced
- » 1 onion, chopped
- » 1 sweet-tart apple (such as Braeburn), peeled, cored, and chopped
- » 3 cups Vegetable Broth or store-bought
- » 1 teaspoon garlic powder
- » ½ teaspoon ground sage
- » ¼ teaspoon of sea salt
- » ¼ teaspoon freshly ground black pepper
- » Pinch cayenne pepper
- » Pinch nutmeg
- » ½ cup fat-free half-and-half

## DIRECTIONS

1. In your slow cooker, combine the squash, onion, apple, broth, garlic powder, sage, salt, black pepper, cayenne, and nutmeg. Cook on low within 8 hours.

2. Using an immersion blender, counter-top blender, or food processor, purée the soup, adding the half-and-half as you do. Stir to combine, and serve.

**NUTRITIONS:** Calories: 106, Fat: 0g, Carbohydrates: 26g, Fiber: 4g, Protein: 3g, Sodium: 550 mg

# 390. BLACK BEAN SOUP

**COOKING: 8H**     **PREPARATION: 15'**     **SERVINGS: 6**

## INGREDIENTS

- » 1-pound dried black beans, soaked overnight and rinsed
- » 1 onion, chopped
- » 1 carrot, peeled and chopped
- » 2 jalapeño peppers, seeded and diced
- » 6 cups Vegetable Broth or store-bought
- » 1 teaspoon ground cumin
- » 1 teaspoon ground coriander
- » 1 teaspoon chili powder
- » ½ teaspoon ground chipotle pepper
- » ½ teaspoon of sea salt
- » ¼ teaspoon freshly ground black pepper
- » Pinch cayenne pepper
- » ¼ cup fat-free sour cream, for garnish (optional)
- » ¼ cup grated low-fat Cheddar cheese, for garnish (optional)

## DIRECTIONS

1. In your slow cooker, combine all the fixing listed, then cook on low for 8 hours. If you'd like, mash the beans with a potato masher, or purée using an immersion blender, blender, or food processor. Serve topped with the optional garnishes, if desired.

**NUTRITIONS:** Calories: 320, Fat: 3g, Carbohydrates: 57g, Fiber: 13g, Protein: 18g, Sodium: 430 mg

# 391. CHICKPEA & KALE SOUP

**COOKING: 9H**        **PREPARATION: 15'**        **SERVINGS: 6**

## INGREDIENTS

- » 1 summer squash, quartered lengthwise and sliced crosswise
- » 1 zucchini, quartered lengthwise and sliced crosswise
- » 2 cups cooked chickpeas, rinsed
- » 1 cup uncooked quinoa
- » 2 cans diced tomatoes, with their juice
- » 5 cups Vegetable Broth, Poultry Broth, or store-bought
- » 1 teaspoon garlic powder
- » 1 teaspoon onion powder
- » 1 teaspoon dried thyme
- » ½ teaspoon of sea salt
- » 2 cups chopped kale leaves

## DIRECTIONS

1. In your slow cooker, combine the summer squash, zucchini, chickpeas, quinoa, tomatoes (with their juice), broth, garlic powder, onion powder, thyme, and salt. Cover and cook on low within 8 hours. Stir in the kale. Cover and cook on low for 1 more hour.

**NUTRITIONS:** Calories: 221,Fat: 3g, Carbohydrates: 40g, Fiber: 7g, Protein: 10g, Sodium: 124 mg

# 392. CLAM CHOWDER

**COOKING: 8H**        **PREPARATION: 15'**        **SERVINGS: 6**

## INGREDIENTS

- » 1 red onion, chopped
- » 3 carrots, peeled and chopped
- » 1 fennel bulb and fronds, chopped
- » 1 (10-ounce) can chopped clams, with their juice
- » 1-pound baby red potatoes, quartered
- » 4 cups Poultry Broth or store-bought
- » ½ teaspoon of sea salt
- » 1/8 teaspoon freshly ground black pepper
- » 2 cups skim milk
- » ¼ pound turkey bacon, browned and crumbled, for garnish

## DIRECTIONS

1. In your slow cooker, combine the onion, carrots, fennel bulb and fronds, clams (with their juice), potatoes, broth, salt, and pepper. Cover and cook on low within 8 hours. Stir in the milk and serve garnished with the crumbled bacon.

**NUTRITIONS:** Calories: 172, Fat: 1g, Carbohydrates: 29g, Fiber: 4g, Protein: 10g, Sodium: 517 mg

# 393. CHICKEN & RICE SOUP

**COOKING: 8H**  **PREPARATION: 15'**  **SERVINGS: 6**

## INGREDIENTS

- » 1-pound boneless, skinless chicken thighs, cut into 1-inch pieces
- » 1 onion, chopped
- » 3 carrots, peeled and sliced
- » 2 celery stalks, sliced
- » 6 cups Poultry Broth or store-bought
- » 1 teaspoon garlic powder
- » 1 teaspoon dried rosemary
- » ¼ teaspoon of sea salt
- » ¼ teaspoon freshly ground black pepper
- » 3 cups cooked Brown Rice

## DIRECTIONS

1. In your slow cooker, combine the chicken, onion, carrots, celery, broth, garlic powder, rosemary, salt, and pepper. Cover and cook on low within 8 hours. Stir in the rice about 10 minutes before serving, and allow the broth to warm it.

**NUTRITIONS:** Calories: 354, Fat: 7g, Carbohydrates: 43g, Fiber: 3g, Protein: 28g, Sodium: 610 mg

# 394. TOM KHA GAI

**COOKING: 8H**  **PREPARATION: 15'**  **SERVINGS: 6**

## INGREDIENTS

- » 1-pound boneless, skinless chicken thighs, cut into 1-inch pieces
- » 1-pound fresh shiitake mushrooms halved
- » 2 tablespoons grated fresh ginger
- » 3 cups canned light coconut milk
- » 3 cups Poultry Broth or store-bought
- » 1 tablespoon Asian fish sauce
- » 1 teaspoon garlic powder
- » ¼ teaspoon freshly ground black pepper
- » Juice of 1 lime
- » 2 tablespoons chopped fresh cilantro

## DIRECTIONS

1. In your slow cooker, combine the chicken thighs, mushrooms, ginger, coconut milk, broth, fish sauce, garlic powder, and pepper. Cover and cook on low within 8 hours. Stir in the lime juice and cilantro just before serving.

**NUTRITIONS:** Calories: 481, Fat: 35g, Carbohydrates: 19g, Fiber: 5g, Protein: 28g, Sodium: 160 mg

# 395. CHICKEN CORN CHOWDER

**COOKING: 8H**      **PREPARATION: 15'**      **SERVINGS: 6**

## INGREDIENTS

» 1-pound boneless, skinless chicken thighs, cut into 1-inch pieces
» 2 onions, chopped
» 3 jalapeño peppers, seeded and minced
» 2 red bell peppers, seeded and chopped
» 1½ cups fresh or frozen corn
» 6 cups Poultry Broth or store-bought
» 1 teaspoon garlic powder
» ½ teaspoon of sea salt
» ¼ teaspoon freshly ground black pepper
» 1 cup skim milk

## DIRECTIONS

1. In your slow cooker, combine the chicken, onions, jalapeños, red bell peppers, corn, broth, garlic powder, salt, and pepper. Cover and cook on low within 8 hours. Stir in the skim milk just before serving.

**NUTRITIONS:** Calories: 236, Fat: 6g, Carbohydrates: 17g, Fiber: 3g, Protein: 27g, Sodium: 790 mg

# 396. TURKEY GINGER SOUP

**COOKING: 8H**      **PREPARATION: 15'**      **SERVINGS: 6**

## INGREDIENTS

» 1-pound boneless, skinless turkey thighs, cut into 1-inch pieces
» 1-pound fresh shiitake mushrooms halved
» 3 carrots, peeled and sliced
» 2 cups frozen peas
» 1 tablespoon grated fresh ginger
» 6 cups Poultry Broth or store-bought
» 1 tablespoon low-sodium soy sauce
» 1 teaspoon toasted sesame oil
» 2 teaspoons garlic powder
» 1½ cups cooked Brown Rice

## DIRECTIONS

1. In your slow cooker, combine the turkey, mushrooms, carrots, peas, ginger, broth, soy sauce, sesame oil, and garlic powder. Cover and cook on low within 8 hours. About 30 minutes before serving, stir in the rice to warm it through.

**NUTRITIONS:** Calories: 318, Fat: 7g, Carbohydrates: 42g, Fiber: 6g, Protein: 24g, Sodium: 690 mg

# 397. ITALIAN WEDDING SOUP

**COOKING: 7H**     **PREPARATION: 15'**     **SERVINGS: 6**

## INGREDIENTS

- » 1-pound ground turkey breast
- » 1½ cups cooked Brown Rice
- » 1 onion, grated
- » ¼ cup chopped fresh parsley
- » 1 egg, beaten
- » 1 teaspoon garlic powder
- » 1 teaspoon sea salt, divided
- » 6 cups Poultry Broth or store-bought
- » 1/8 teaspoon freshly ground black pepper
- » Pinch red pepper flakes
- » 1-pound kale, tough stems removed, leaves chopped

## DIRECTIONS

1. In a small bowl, combine the turkey breast, rice, onion, parsley, egg, garlic powder, and ½ teaspoon of sea salt. Roll the mixture into ½-inch meatballs and put them in the slow cooker.

2. Add the broth, black pepper, red pepper flakes, and the remaining ½ teaspoon of sea salt. Cover and cook on low for 7 to 8 hours. Before serving, stir in the kale. Cover and cook until the kale wilts.

**NUTRITIONS:** Calories: 302, Fat: 7g, Carbohydrates: 29g, Fiber: 3g, Protein: 29g, Sodium: 320 mg

# 398. TACO SOUP

**COOKING: 8H**     **PREPARATION: 15'**     **SERVINGS: 6**

## INGREDIENTS

- » 1-pound ground turkey breast
- » 1 onion, chopped
- » 1 can tomatoes and green chilis, with their juice
- » 6 cups Poultry Broth or store-bought
- » 1 teaspoon chili powder
- » 1 teaspoon ground cumin
- » ½ teaspoon of sea salt
- » ¼ cup chopped fresh cilantro
- » Juice of 1 lime
- » ½ cup grated low-fat Cheddar cheese

## DIRECTIONS

1. Crumble the turkey into the slow cooker. Add the onion, tomatoes, green chilis (with their juice), broth, chili powder, cumin, and salt. Cover and cook on low within 8 hours. Stir in the cilantro and lime juice. Serve garnished with the cheese.

**NUTRITIONS:** Calories: 281, Fat: 10g, Carbohydrates: 20g, Fiber: 5g, Protein: 30g, Sodium: 470 mg

# 399. ITALIAN SAUSAGE & FENNEL SOUP

**COOKING: 8H**     **PREPARATION: 15'**     **SERVINGS: 6**

## INGREDIENTS

- » 1-pound Italian chicken or turkey sausage, cut into ½-inch slices
- » 2 onions, chopped
- » 1 fennel bulb, chopped
- » 6 cups Poultry Broth or store-bought
- » ¼ cup dry sherry
- » 1½ teaspoons garlic powder
- » 1 teaspoon dried thyme
- » ½ teaspoon of sea salt
- » ¼ teaspoon freshly ground black pepper
- » Pinch red pepper flakes

## DIRECTIONS

1. In your slow cooker, combine all the ingredients. Cover and cook on low within 8 hours.

**NUTRITIONS:** Calories: 311, Fat: 22g, Carbohydrates: 8g, Fiber: 2g, Protein: 18g, Sodium: 660 mg

# 400. BEEF & BARLEY SOUP

**COOKING: 8H**     **PREPARATION: 15'**     **SERVINGS: 6**

## INGREDIENTS

- » 1-pound extra-lean ground beef
- » 2 onions, chopped
- » 3 carrots, peeled and sliced
- » 1-pound fresh mushrooms, quartered
- » 1½ cups dried barley
- » 6 cups Beef Broth or store-bought
- » 1 teaspoon ground mustard
- » 1 teaspoon dried thyme
- » 1 teaspoon garlic powder
- » ¼ teaspoon of sea salt
- » 1/8 teaspoon freshly ground black pepper

## DIRECTIONS

1. In your slow cooker, crumble the ground beef into small pieces. Add the remaining ingredients. Cover and cook on low within 8 hours.

**NUTRITIONS:** Calories: 319, Fat: 5g, Carbohydrates: 44g, Fiber: 11g, Protein: 28g, Sodium: 380 mg

# CHAPTER 12.
# SALADS

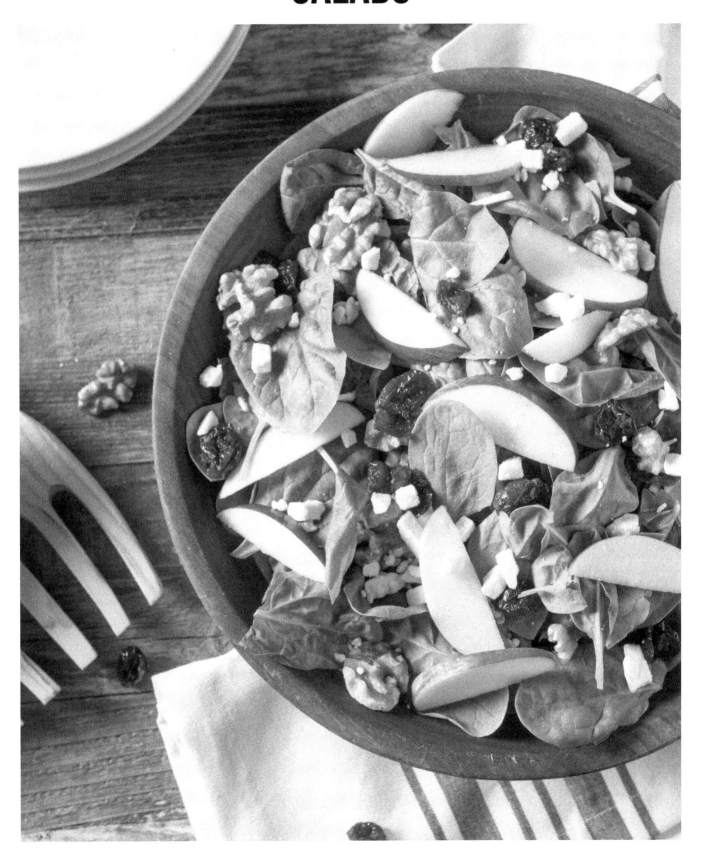

# 401. EDAMAME SALAD WITH CORN AND CRANBERRIES

**COOKING: 0'**             **PREPARATION: 15'**             **SERVINGS: 4**

## INGREDIENTS

- »   11/4 cups shelled edamame
- »   3/4 cup corn kernels
- »   1 red or orange bell pepper, chopped
- »   1/4 cup dried cranberries
- »   1 shallot, finely diced
- »   2 tablespoons red wine vinegar
- »   1 tablespoon olive oil
- »   1 teaspoon agave nectar
- »   1 teaspoon no-salt-added prepared mustard
- »   Freshly ground black pepper, to taste

## DIRECTIONS

1. Place the edamame, corn, bell pepper, cranberries, and shallot in a mixing bowl and stir to combine. Mix the vinegar, oil, agave nectar, and mustard into a small mixing bowl.

2. Pour the dressing over the salad. Flavor with freshly ground black pepper, to taste. Serve.

**NUTRITIONS:** Calories: 149, Fat: 5 g, Protein: 5 g, Sodium: 5 mg, Fiber: 3 g, Carbohydrates: 22 g, Sugar: 10 g

# 402. WARM ASIAN SLAW

**COOKING: 3H**             **PREPARATION: 15'**             **SERVINGS: 4**

## INGREDIENTS

- »   1 tablespoon sesame oil
- »   1 tablespoon peanut oil
- »   2 sliced scallions
- »   2 cloves garlic, minced
- »   1 tablespoon minced fresh ginger
- »   1 medium bok choy, chopped
- »   2 medium carrots, shredded
- »   1 tablespoon unflavored rice vinegar
- »   1/2 teaspoon sugar
- »   1/2 teaspoon ground white pepper
- »   1/2 tablespoon toasted sesame seeds (optional)

## DIRECTIONS

1. Heat both oils in a skillet over medium. Add scallions, garlic, and ginger and cook, stirring, for 1 minute. Add bok choy and carrots and sauté for 2 minutes. Remove from heat.

2. Place contents in a bowl. Stir in vinegar, sugar, and pepper. Garnish with sesame seeds, if desired. Serve immediately.

**NUTRITIONS:** Calories: 112, Fat: 7 g, Protein: 3 g, Sodium: 72 mg, Fiber: 3 g, Carbohydrates: 9 g, Sugar: 4 g

# 403. TANGY THREE-BEAN SALAD WITH BARLEY

**COOKING: 30'**         **PREPARATION: 15'**         **SERVINGS: 8**

## INGREDIENTS

- » 1 cup uncooked pearled barley
- » 21/4 cups water
- » 2 cups of green beans, slice into 2-inch pieces
- » 1 (15-ounce) can no-salt-added kidney beans
- » 1 (15-ounce) can no-salt-added garbanzo beans
- » 1 medium red bell pepper, diced
- » 1 small onion, finely chopped
- » 2 tablespoons chopped fresh cilantro or parsley
- » 1/3 cup canola oil
- » 1/3 cup apple cider vinegar
- » 1/3 cup pure maple syrup
- » Freshly ground black pepper, to taste

## DIRECTIONS

1. Measure the barley and water into a saucepan and boil over high heat. Once boiling, adjust heat to low, cover, and simmer until water is absorbed, 25–30 minutes. Remove pan from heat, then drain and rinse well.

2. Put the green beans in a bowl, then put the drained canned beans, bell pepper, onion, barley, and chopped cilantro or parsley. Stir well.

3. Mix the oil, vinegar, plus maple syrup in a small mixing bowl. Put on the salad and toss to coat. Flavor with ground black pepper, then serve.

**NUTRITIONS:** Calories: 367, Fat: 11 g, Protein: 11 g, Sodium: 10 mg, Fiber: 11 g, Carbohydrates: 57 g, Sugar: 11 g

# 404. BEAN SALAD WITH ORANGE VINAIGRETTE

**COOKING: 0'**         **PREPARATION: 15'**         **SERVINGS: 6**

## INGREDIENTS

- » 1 (15-ounce) can no-salt-added kidney beans
- » 1 (15-ounce) can no-salt-added garbanzo beans
- » 1 (15-ounce) can no-salt-added pinto beans
- » 2 shallots, chopped
- » 1 medium carrot, shredded
- » 1 small bell pepper, diced
- » 1 small stalk celery, diced
- » 1/4 cup pure maple syrup
- » 1/3 cup apple cider vinegar
- » 2 tablespoons freshly squeezed orange juice
- » 1 tablespoon olive oil
- » 1 teaspoon grated orange zest
- » 1/2 teaspoon freshly ground black pepper

## DIRECTIONS

1. Drain and rinse all the canned beans, then place them in a mixing bowl. Add the chopped shallot, shredded carrot, bell pepper, and celery and stir to combine.

2. Place the remaining fixing into a small mixing bowl and whisk well. Mix the dressing on the salad, then serve immediately.

**NUTRITIONS:** Calories: 393, Fat: 5 g, Protein: 19 g, Sodium: 70 mg, Fiber: 16 g, Carbohydrates: 69 g, Sugar: 13 g

# 405. FRESH CORN, PEPPER, AND AVOCADO SALAD

**COOKING: 0'**  **PREPARATION: 15'**  **SERVINGS: 6**

## INGREDIENTS

- » 3 ears freshly cooked corn
- » 1 medium red bell pepper
- » 1 ripe avocado
- » 1 jalapeño pepper, minced
- » 1 scallion, thinly sliced
- » 1 clove garlic, minced
- » Juice of 1 fresh lime
- » 2 tablespoons olive oil
- » Freshly ground black pepper, to taste

## DIRECTIONS

1. Slice the kernels using a very sharp knife. Place in a mixing bowl. Core and dice the red pepper and peel and dice the avocado. Add to the bowl, along with the jalapeño, sliced scallion (white and green parts), and minced garlic.

2. Mix the lime juice and oil in a small bowl. Drizzle over the salad and toss to coat. Flavor with freshly ground black pepper. Serve immediately.

**NUTRITIONS:** Calories: 135, Fat: 9 g, Protein: 2 g, Sodium: 5 mg, Fiber: 3 g, Carbohydrates: 13 g, Sugar: 2 g

# 406. GARLIC POTATO SALAD

**COOKING: 25'**  **PREPARATION: 15'**  **SERVINGS: 6**

## INGREDIENTS

- » 6 medium potatoes
- » 6 garlic scapes or 3 cloves garlic
- » 1 cup sliced scallions
- » 1/4 cup olive oil
- » 2 tablespoons unflavored rice vinegar
- » 2 teaspoons chopped fresh rosemary
- » Freshly ground black pepper, to taste

## DIRECTIONS

1. Boil the potatoes into a pot with water to cover by 1 inch over high heat. Boil until fork-tender but still solid, depending upon size, roughly 20–25 minutes.

2. Once cooked, remove from heat and place under cold running water. Drain and set potatoes aside to cool, then slice into cubes. Place cubed potato, garlic, and scallions into a mixing bowl and toss to combine.

3. Measure the olive oil, vinegar, and rosemary into a small mixing bowl. Put ground black pepper, and whisk well to combine. Pour the dressing over the salad and stir gently to coat. Cover and refrigerate within a few hours before serving.

**NUTRITIONS:** Calories: 204, Fat: 9 g, Protein: 2 g, Sodium: 6 mg, Fiber: 2 g, Carbohydrates: 28 g, Sugar: 1 g

# 407. CREAMY LOW-SODIUM COLESLAW

**COOKING: 0'**      **PREPARATION: 15'**      **SERVINGS: 6**

## INGREDIENTS

- 1/2 medium head green cabbage, shredded
- 1 medium carrot, shredded
- 1 small onion, grated
- 1/3 cup Salt-Free Mayonnaise
- 3 tablespoons sugar
- 3 tablespoons apple cider vinegar
- 1/2 teaspoon dry ground mustard
- 1/2 teaspoon freshly ground black pepper

## DIRECTIONS

1. Mix all the fixing in a large mixing bowl and stir well. Cover and refrigerate until ready to serve.

**NUTRITIONS:** Calories: 133, Fat: 8 g, Protein: 2 g, Sodium: 32 mg, Fiber: 3 g, Carbohydrates: 13 g, Sugar: 10 g

# 408. SOUTHWESTERN BEET SLAW

**COOKING: 0'**      **PREPARATION: 15'**      **SERVINGS: 6**

## INGREDIENTS

- 3 small medium beets
- 3 scallions, sliced
- 2 medium carrots, shredded
- 1/4 cup chopped fresh cilantro
- 2 cloves garlic
- Juice of 2 fresh limes
- 1 teaspoon olive oil
- 1/2 teaspoon salt-free chili seasoning
- 1/4 teaspoon freshly ground black pepper

## DIRECTIONS

1. Trim and peel the beets, then shred. Place into a mixing bowl. Add the scallions, carrots, cilantro, and garlic and stir well to combine.

2. Mix the lime juice, olive oil, chili seasoning, and black pepper in a small bowl. Pour dressing over the salad, then serve immediately.

**NUTRITIONS:** Calories: 38, Fat: 1 g, Protein: 1 g, Sodium: 46 mg, Fiber: 2 g, Carbohydrates: 7 g, Sugar: 4 g

# 409. WARM KALE SALAD

**COOKING: 12**      **PREPARATION: 15'**      **SERVINGS: 4**

## INGREDIENTS

- » 2 teaspoons olive oil
- » 1 small red onion, diced
- » 2 garlic cloves, minced
- » 1 small red bell pepper, diced
- » 8 cups chopped kale
- » Juice of 1 fresh orange
- » 1 medium carrot, shredded
- » 1/4 teaspoon ground cumin
- » 1/8 teaspoon dried red pepper flakes
- » 1 teaspoon grated orange zest
- » Freshly ground black pepper, to taste

## DIRECTIONS

1. Heat-up oil in a large skillet or sauté pan over medium. Add the onion and cook, stirring, for 2 minutes. Add the garlic, bell pepper, kale, and orange juice and stir well to combine. Adjust heat to medium-low, cover, and cook within 5 minutes.

2. Remove lid, add remaining ingredients, and stir well to combine. Cover and cook for another 5 minutes. Remove from heat and serve immediately.

**NUTRITIONS:** Calories: 137, Fat: 3 g, Protein: 5 g, Sodium: 76 mg, Fiber: 4 g, Carbohydrates: 25 g, Sugar: 7 g

# 410. TABOULEH SALAD

**COOKING: 0'**      **PREPARATION: 15'**      **SERVINGS: 4**

## INGREDIENTS

- » 2/3 cup dry couscous
- » 1 cup boiling water
- » 1 small ripe tomato, diced
- » 1 small green bell pepper, diced
- » 1 shallot, finely diced
- » 1/3 cup chopped fresh parsley
- » 1 clove garlic, minced
- » Juice of 1 fresh lemon
- » 1 tablespoon olive oil
- » 1/2 teaspoon freshly ground black pepper

## DIRECTIONS

1. Mix the dry couscous into a small bowl. Mix in the boiling water, cover, and set aside within 5 minutes. Place the tomato, green pepper, shallot, and parsley into a salad bowl.

2. Mix the garlic, lemon juice, oil, and pepper in a small mixing bowl. Put the cooked couscous in the salad bowl. Put the dressing over the top and stir well to combine. Serve immediately.

**NUTRITIONS:** Calories: 120, Fat: 3 g, Protein: 3 g, Sodium: 6 mg, Fiber: 1 g, Carbohydrates: 20 g, Sugar: 1 g

    

# 411. TART APPLE SALAD WITH FENNEL AND HONEY YOGURT DRESSING

**COOKING: 0'**     **PREPARATION: 15'**     **SERVINGS: 6**

## INGREDIENTS

» 2 tart green apples, diced
» 1 small bulb fennel, chopped
» 11/2 cups seedless red grapes, halved
» 2 tablespoons freshly squeezed lemon juice
» 1/4 cup low-fat vanilla yogurt
» 1 teaspoon honey

## DIRECTIONS

1. Mix all the fixing into a mixing bowl, then serve immediately.

**NUTRITIONS:** Calories: 70, Fat: 1 g, Protein: 1 g, Sodium: 26 mg, Fiber: 3 g, Carbohydrates: 16 g, Sugar: 11 g

# 412. ORCHID SALAD

**COOKING: 0'**     **PREPARATION: 15'**     **SERVINGS: 4**

## INGREDIENTS

» 2 cups shredded red cabbage
» 3 tablespoons freshly squeezed orange juice
» 1 teaspoon balsamic vinegar
» 1/8 teaspoon freshly ground black pepper
» 2 tart green apples, sliced thinly
» 1/2 teaspoon freshly squeezed lemon juice
» 1 medium ripe cantaloupe
» 1/4 cup chopped walnuts

## DIRECTIONS

1. Place the cabbage into a mixing bowl. Add the orange juice, vinegar, and pepper and toss well to coat. Set aside. Place the apple slices in another bowl, add the lemon juice, and toss gently to coat. Set aside.

2. Slice the cantaloupe in half and discard the seeds. Slice each half into 8 wedges and remove the rind. Slice each wedge in half across the middle, so you're left with 16 triangular parts.

3. Place 2 cantaloupe parts in the middle of a plate, cut-sides, so they look rejoined. Pull them slightly apart and then do the same with another two parts so that you have a sort of X with a space in the middle.

4. Arrange a trio of fanned apple slices in each of the 4 empty spots between the cantaloupe points. Then place 1/4 of the cabbage mixture in the space in the middle of the X. Top with 1/4 of the chopped walnuts. Serve immediately.

**NUTRITIONS:** Calories: 166, Fat: 5 g, Protein: 3 g, Sodium: 36 mg, Fiber: 4 g, Carbohydrates: 30 g, Sugar: 24 g

# 413. THAI PASTA SALAD

**COOKING: 14'**       **PREPARATION: 15'**       **SERVINGS: 4**

## INGREDIENTS

- » 1 (16-ounce) package dry spaghetti
- » 2 tablespoons peanut oil
- » 1 medium yellow squash, julienned
- » 1 medium zucchini, julienned
- » 1 medium green bell pepper, julienned
- » 1 red bell pepper, julienned
- » 1 orange bell pepper, julienned
- » 6 scallions, sliced
- » 3 cloves garlic, minced
- » 1 jalapeño pepper, minced
- » 3/4 cup chopped walnuts
- » 1/3 cup peanut oil
- » 1 tablespoon sesame oil
- » 1/4 cup unflavored rice vinegar
- » 2 tablespoons salt-free peanut butter
- » 1 tablespoon no-salt-added tomato paste
- » 1/4 cup chopped fresh cilantro
- » 1 tablespoon minced fresh ginger
- » 1 teaspoon sugar
- » 1/4 teaspoon salt-free chili seasoning

## DIRECTIONS

1. Cook the spaghetti in the pot with boiling water. Cook within 10 minutes, stirring once or twice. Remove from heat, drain, and set aside.

2. Warm 2 tablespoons peanut oil in a large sauté pan over medium heat. Add the julienned vegetables, scallions, garlic, jalapeño, and walnuts and cook, stirring, for 3–4 minutes.

3. Remove from heat and transfer to a huge bowl. Add cooked spaghetti. Whisk the remaining ingredients in a mixing bowl. Mix over the pasta salad. Serve immediately.

**NUTRITIONS:** Calories: 464, Fat: 24 g, Protein: 11 g, Sodium: 9 mg, Fiber: 5 g, Carbohydrates: 50 g, Sugar: 4 g

---

# 414. WHOLE-WHEAT COUSCOUS SALAD WITH CITRUS AND CILANTRO

**COOKING: 2'**       **PREPARATION: 15'**       **SERVINGS: 6**

## INGREDIENTS

- » 11/2 cups water
- » 1 cup whole-wheat couscous
- » 1 medium cucumber, slice in halve
- » 1-pint grape or cherry tomatoes halved
- » 1 jalapeño pepper, minced
- » 2 shallots, minced
- » 2 scallions, sliced
- » 2 cloves garlic, minced
- » 2 tablespoons freshly squeezed lemon juice
- » 2 tablespoons freshly squeezed lime juice
- » 1 teaspoon olive oil
- » 1/4 cup chopped fresh cilantro
- » Freshly ground black pepper, to taste

## DIRECTIONS

1. Mix water into a saucepan and boil over high heat. Once boiling, stir in the couscous, reduce heat to medium-low, cover, and simmer for 2 minutes.

2. Remove pot from heat, remove the lid, and fluff couscous with a fork. Set aside to cool for 5 minutes.

3. Scrape out the cucumber's seeds using a spoon, then dice and place into a mixing bowl. Put the rest of the fixing in the bowl along with the cooked couscous and toss well to coat. Flavor with freshly ground black pepper, then serve immediately.

**NUTRITIONS:** Calories: 126, Fat: 2 g, Protein: 4 g, Sodium: 5 mg, Fiber: 2 g, Carbohydrates: 24 g, Sugar: 3 g

# 415. SALAD NIÇOISE

**COOKING: 35'**          **PREPARATION: 5'**          **SERVINGS: 2**

## INGREDIENTS

» 1 small head butter lettuce
» 1 small cucumber
» 2 medium red potatoes
» 1 tablespoon white distilled vinegar
» 2 eggs
» 1 bunch fresh green beans, trimmed
» 2 tablespoons olive oil
» 2 tablespoons red wine vinegar
» 1 teaspoon salt-free prepared mustard
» 1 clove garlic, minced
» 1/2 teaspoon freshly ground black pepper
» 2 small tomatoes, quartered
» 1 (5-ounce) can no-salt-added tuna in water, drained

## DIRECTIONS

1. Rip-up the lettuce leaves into small pieces and set aside. Peel the cucumber, halve lengthwise, and remove seeds using a spoon. Slice and set aside.

2. Boil the potatoes into a pan with water over high heat, reduce heat slightly, and simmer until tender, about 20 minutes. Once cooked, dice, toss with white vinegar and set aside.

3. Boil the eggs into a saucepan, with enough water to cover over high heat within 12 minutes. Once cooked, carefully crack, peel, and slice into quarters. Set aside.

4. Boil a small pot of water, then once it's boiling, add the green beans and cook for 2 minutes. Remove beans from the pot and immediately place them in a bowl of ice water. Set aside.

5. In a small bowl, add the oil, vinegar, mustard, garlic, and pepper and whisk well to combine.

6. Assemble the salad on a platter, placing lettuce on the bottom and then grouping the cucumber, potatoes, eggs, green beans, tomatoes, and tuna on top. Drizzle the dressing evenly over the salad. Serve immediately.

**NUTRITIONS:** Calories: 471, Fat: 20 g, Protein: 30 g, Sodium: 111 mg, Fiber: 7 g, Carbohydrates: 41 g, Sugar: 5 g

# 416. SIMPLE GREEN SALAD

**COOKING: 5'**          **PREPARATION: 5'**          **SERVINGS: 4**

## INGREDIENTS

» ¼ cup extra-virgin olive oil
» 1 tablespoon fresh lemon juice
» ¼ teaspoon salt
» ¼ teaspoon freshly ground black pepper
» 6 cups loosely packed mixed greens
» ½ small red onion, thinly sliced
» 1 small cucumber, peeled and thinly sliced
» ¼ cup shredded Parmesan cheese

## DIRECTIONS

1. Mix the oil, lemon juice, salt, plus pepper in a small bowl. Store the dressing in 4 condiment cups. Mix the mixed greens, onion, and cucumber in a large bowl. Divide salad into 4 medium storage containers. Top each with 1 tablespoon of Parmesan cheese. To serve, toss the dressing and salad.

**NUTRITIONS:** Calories: 162g, Fat: 15g, Carbohydrates: 6g, Fiber: 2g, Protein: 3g, Sodium: 290mg

# 417. KALE-POPPY SEED SALAD

**COOKING: 5'**       **PREPARATION: 10'**       **SERVINGS: 6**

## INGREDIENTS

- » ½ cup nonfat plain Greek yogurt
- » 2 tablespoons apple cider vinegar
- » ½ tablespoon extra-virgin olive oil
- » 1 teaspoon poppy seeds
- » 1 teaspoon sugar
- » 4 cups firmly packed finely chopped kale
- » 2 cups broccoli slaw
- » 2 cups thinly sliced Brussels sprouts
- » 6 tablespoons dried cranberries
- » 6 tablespoons hulled pumpkin seeds

## DIRECTIONS

1. Mix the yogurt, vinegar, oil, poppy seeds, sugar in a small bowl. Store the dressing in 6 condiment cups.

2. In a large bowl, mix the kale, broccoli slaw, and Brussels sprout. Divide the greens into 6 large storage containers and top each salad with cranberries and pumpkin seeds. To serve, toss the greens with the poppy seed dressing to coat.

**NUTRITIONS:** Calories: 129g, Fat: 6g, Carbohydrates: 13g, Fiber: 3g, Protein: 8g, Sodium: 26mg

# 418. WEDGE SALAD WITH CREAMY BLUE CHEESE DRESSING

**COOKING: 0'**       **PREPARATION: 15'**       **SERVINGS: 4**

## INGREDIENTS

- » 1 cup nonfat plain Greek yogurt
- » Juice of ½ large lemon
- » ¼ teaspoon freshly ground black pepper
- » ¼ teaspoon salt
- » 1/3 cup crumbled blue cheese
- » 2 heads romaine lettuce, stem end trimmed, halved lengthwise
- » 1 cup grape tomatoes, halved
- » ½ cup slivered almonds

## DIRECTIONS

1. Mix the yogurt, lemon juice, pepper, salt, and cheese in a small bowl. Store the dressing in 4 condiment cups. Divide the lettuce halves and tomatoes among 4 large storage containers. Store the almonds separately.

2. To serve, arrange a half-head of romaine on a plate and top with the tomatoes. Sprinkle with 2 tablespoons of almonds and drizzle with the dressing.

**NUTRITIONS:** Calories: 216g, Fat: 11g, Carbohydrates: 20g, Fiber: 9g, Protein: 16g, Sodium: 329mg

# 419. SOUTHWESTERN BEAN SALAD WITH CREAMY AVOCADO DRESSING

**COOKING: 0**      **PREPARATION: 15'**      **SERVINGS: 4**

## INGREDIENTS

» 1 head romaine lettuce, chopped
» 1 can no-salt-added black beans, drained
» 2 cups fresh corn kernels
» 2 cups grape tomatoes, halved
» 2 small avocados, halved and pitted 1 cup chopped fresh cilantro
» 1 cup nonfat plain Greek yogurt 8 scallions, chopped
» 3 garlic cloves, quartered zest, and juice of 1 large lime
» ½ teaspoon sugar

## DIRECTIONS

1. Mix the lettuce, beans, corn, and tomatoes in a large bowl. Toss you well combined. Divide the salad into 4 large storage containers. Put the avocado flesh into your blender or food processor.

2. Add the yogurt, scallions, garlic, lime zest and juice, and sugar. Blend until well combined. Divide the dressing into 4 condiment cups. To serve, toss the salad and the dressing.

**NUTRITIONS:** Calories: 349g, Fat: 11g, Carbohydrates: 53g, Fiber: 16g, Protein: 19g, Sodium: 77mg

# 420. COBB PASTA SALAD

**COOKING: 10'**      **PREPARATION: 15'**      **SERVINGS: 6**

## INGREDIENTS

» 1-pound whole wheat rotini pasta
» 2 cups cooked chicken breast, chopped
» 8 low-sodium turkey bacon slices, cooked and chopped 4 scallions, sliced
» 1½ cups cherry tomatoes halved
» ¼ teaspoon freshly ground black pepper
» 4 hard-boiled eggs, peeled and coarsely chopped
» 1/3 cup crumbled blue cheese
» 1 cup frozen avocado cubes
» ¾ cup Greek Yogurt Dill Dressing

## DIRECTIONS

1. Cook the pasta until al dente as stated to package directions. Rinse under cold water, then drain. Mix the pasta, chicken, bacon, scallions, tomatoes, pepper in a large bowl. Toss until well combined.

2. Add the eggs and blue cheese and fold until mixed well. Divide the salad into 6 storage containers. Divide the avocado into 6 small storage containers. Make the dressing as directed and store in 6 condiment cups.

3. The night before you're planning on having a salad, add the portion off the avocado to the salad so they will be soft by mealtime the next day. Serve drizzled with the dressing.

**NUTRITIONS:** Calories: 550g, Fat: 18g, Carbohydrates: 62g, Fiber: 9.5g, Protein: 40g, Sodium: 619mg

# CHAPTER 13.
# SNACKS

# 421. GARLIC COTTAGE CHEESE CRISPY

**COOKING: 2'**          **PREPARATION: 5'**          **SERVINGS: 4**

## INGREDIENTS

» 1 cup cottage cheese
» ½ teaspoon Garlic powder
» Pinch of pepper
» Pinch of onion powder

## DIRECTIONS

1. Take a bowl and mix in cheese and spices. Scoop half a teaspoon of the cheese mix and place it in the pan. Cook in a skillet over medium heat within 1 minute per side. Repeat until done.

**NUTRITIONS:** Calories: 70, Fat: 6g, Carbohydrates: 1g, Protein: 6g, Sodium: 195 mg

# 422. LEMON FAT BOMBS

**COOKING: 0'**          **PREPARATION: 10'**          **SERVINGS: 3**

## INGREDIENTS

» 1 whole lemon
» 4 ounces cream cheese
» 2 ounces butter
» 2 teaspoons natural sweetener

## DIRECTIONS

1. Take a fine grater and zest your lemon. Squeeze lemon juice into a bowl alongside the zest. Add butter, cream cheese to a bowl, and add zest, salt, sweetener, and juice.

2. Stir well using a hand mixer until smooth. Spoon mix into molds and freeze for 2 hours. Serve and enjoy!

**NUTRITIONS:** Calories: 404, Carbs: 4g, Fiber: 1g, Protein: 4g, Fat: 43g, Sodium: 19 mg

# 423. CHOCOLATE COCONUT BOMBS

**COOKING: 0'**  **PREPARATION: 20'**  **SERVINGS: 12**

## INGREDIENTS

- » ½ cup dark cocoa powder
- » ½ tablespoon vanilla extract
- » 5 drops stevia
- » 1 cup coconut oil, solid
- » 1 tablespoon peppermint extract

## DIRECTIONS

1. Take a high-speed food processor and add all the ingredients. Blend until combined. Take a teaspoon and drop a spoonful onto parchment paper. Refrigerate until solidified and keep refrigerated.

**NUTRITIONS:** Calories: 126, Carbs: 0g, Fiber: 0g, Protein: 0g, Fat: 14g, Sodium: 30 mg

# 424. ESPRESSO FAT BOMBS

**COOKING: 0'**  **PREPARATION: 20'**  **SERVINGS: 24**

## INGREDIENTS

- » 5 tablespoons butter, tender
- » 3 ounces cream cheese, soft
- » 2 ounces espresso
- » 4 tablespoons coconut oil
- » 2 tablespoons coconut whipping cream
- » 2 tablespoons stevia

## DIRECTIONS

1. Prepare your double boiler and melt all ingredients (except stevia) for 3-4 minutes and mix. Add sweetener and mix using a hand mixer.

2. Spoon mixture into silicone muffin molds and freeze for 4 hours. Remove fat bombs and serve!

**NUTRITIONS:** Carbs: 1.3g, Fiber: 0.2g, Protein: 0.3g, Fat: 7g, Sodium: 50 mg

# 425. CRISPY COCONUT BOMBS

**COOKING: 0'**  **PREPARATION: 10'**  **SERVINGS: 6**

## INGREDIENTS

- » 14 ½ ounces coconut milk
- » ¾ cup of coconut oil
- » 1 cup unsweetened coconut flakes
- » 20 drops stevia

## DIRECTIONS

1. Microwave your coconut oil for 20 seconds in the microwave. Mix in coconut milk and stevia in the hot oil. Stir in coconut flakes and pour the mixture into molds. Let it chill for 60 minutes in the fridge. Serve and enjoy!

**NUTRITIONS:** Carbs: 2g, Fiber: 0.5g, Protein: 1g, Fat: 13g, Calories: 123, Carbs: 1g, Sodium: 0mg

# 426. PUMPKIN PIE FAT BOMBS

**COOKING: 5'**  **PREPARATION: 35'**  **SERVINGS: 12**

## INGREDIENTS

- » 2 tablespoons coconut oil
- » 1/3 cup pumpkin puree
- » 1/3 cup almond oil
- » ¼ cup almond oil
- » 3 ounces sugar-free dark chocolate
- » 1 ½ teaspoon of pumpkin pie spice mix
- » Stevia to taste

## DIRECTIONS

1. Melt almond oil and dark chocolate over a double boiler. Take this mixture and layer the bottom of 12 muffin cups. Freeze until the crust has set. Meanwhile, take a saucepan and combine the rest of the ingredients.

2. Put the saucepan on low heat. Heat until softened and mix well. Pour this over the initial chocolate mixture. Let it chill within 1 hour, then serve.

**NUTRITIONS:** Calories: 124, Carbs: 3g, Fiber: 1g, Protein: 3g, Fat: 13g, Sodium: 0mg

# 427. SWEET ALMOND AND COCONUT FAT BOMBS

**COOKING: 0'**    **PREPARATION: 10'**    **SERVINGS: 6**

## INGREDIENTS

» ¼ cup melted coconut oil
» 9 ½ tablespoons almond butter
» 90 drops liquid stevia
» 3 tablespoons cocoa
» 9 tablespoons melted butter, salted

## DIRECTIONS

1. Take a bowl and add all of the listed ingredients. Mix them well. Pour scant 2 tablespoons of the mixture into as many muffin molds as you like. Chill for 20 minutes and pop them out. Serve and enjoy!

**NUTRITIONS:** Calories: 72, Carbs: 2g, Fiber: 0g, Protein: 2.53g, Fat: 14g, Sodium: 0mg

# 428. ALMOND AND TOMATO BALLS

**COOKING: 0'**    **PREPARATION: 10'**    **SERVINGS: 6**

## INGREDIENTS

» 1/3 cup pistachios, de-shelled
» 10 ounces cream cheese
» 1/3 cup sun-dried tomatoes, diced

## DIRECTIONS

1. Chop pistachios into small pieces. Add cream cheese, tomatoes in a bowl and mix well. Chill for 15-20 minutes and turn into balls. Roll into pistachios. Serve and enjoy!

**NUTRITIONS:** Calories: 183, Fat: 18g, Carb: 5g, Protein: 5g, Sodium: 10 mg

# 429. AVOCADO TUNA BITES

**COOKING: 0'**   **PREPARATION: 10'**   **SERVINGS: 4**

## INGREDIENTS

- » 1/3 cup coconut oil
- » 1 avocado, cut into cubes
- » 10 ounces of canned tuna, drained
- » ¼ cup parmesan cheese, grated
- » ¼ teaspoon garlic powder
- » 1/4 teaspoon onion powder
- » 1/3 cup almond flour
- » ¼ teaspoon pepper
- » ¼ cup low-fat mayonnaise
- » Pepper as needed

## DIRECTIONS

1. Take a bowl and add tuna, mayo, flour, parmesan, spices, and mix well. Fold in avocado and make 12 balls out of the mixture. Dissolve coconut oil in a pan and cook over medium heat until all sides are golden. Serve and enjoy!

**NUTRITIONS:** Calories: 185, Fat: 18g, Carbohydrates: 1g, Protein: 5g, Sodium: 0mg

# 430. MEDITERRANEAN POP CORN BITES

**COOKING: 2-3'**   **PREPARATION: 5' + 20' TO CHIL**   **SERVINGS: 4**

## INGREDIENTS

- » 3 cups Medjool dates, chopped
- » 12 ounces brewed coffee
- » 1 cup pecan, chopped
- » ½ cup coconut, shredded
- » ½ cup of cocoa powder

## DIRECTIONS

1. Soak dates in warm coffee for 5 minutes. Remove dates from coffee and mash them, making a fine smooth mixture. Stir in remaining ingredients (except cocoa powder) and form small balls out of the mixture. Coat with cocoa powder, serve and enjoy!

**NUTRITIONS:** Calories: 265, Fat: 12g, Carbohydrates: 43g, Protein 3g, Sodium: 75 mg

# 431. HEARTY BUTTERY WALNUTS

**COOKING: 0'**      **PREPARATION: 10'**      **SERVINGS: 4**

## INGREDIENTS

» 4 walnut halves
» ½ tablespoon almond butter

## DIRECTIONS

1. Spread butter over two walnut halves. Top with other halves. Serve and enjoy!

**NUTRITIONS:** Calories: 90, Fat: 10g, Carbohydrates: 0g, Protein: 1g, Sodium: 1 mg

# 432. REFRESHING WATERMELON SORBET

**COOKING: 0'**      **PREPARATION: 20' + 20' TO CHIL**      **SERVINGS: 4**

## INGREDIENTS

» 4 cups watermelon, seedless and chunked
» ¼ cup of coconut sugar
» 2 tablespoons lime juice

## DIRECTIONS

1. Add the listed fixing to a blender and puree. Freeze the mix for about 4-6 hours until you have gelatin-like consistency.

2. Puree the mix once again in batches and return to the container. Chill overnight. Allow the sorbet to stand for 5 minutes before serving and enjoy!

**NUTRITIONS:** Calories: 91, Fat: 0g, Carbohydrates: 25g, Protein: 1g, Sodium: 0mg

# 433. FAUX MAC AND CHEESE

**COOKING: 45'**      **PREPARATION: 15'**      **SERVINGS: 4**

## INGREDIENTS

- » 5 cups cauliflower florets
- » Salt and pepper to taste
- » 1 cup of coconut milk
- » ½ cup vegetable broth
- » 2 tablespoons coconut flour, sifted
- » 1 organic egg, beaten
- » 2 cups cheddar cheese

## DIRECTIONS

1. Warm your oven to 350 degrees F. Season florets with salt and steam until firm. Place florets in a greased ovenproof dish. Heat-up coconut milk over medium heat in a skillet; make sure to season the oil with salt and pepper.

2. Stir in broth and add coconut flour to the mix, stir. Cook until the sauce begins to bubble. Remove heat and add beaten egg. Pour the thick sauce over cauliflower and mix in cheese. Bake for 30-45 minutes. Serve and enjoy!

**NUTRITIONS:** Calories: 229, Fat: 14g, Carbohydrates: 9g, Protein: 15g, Sodium: 125 mg

# 434. BANANA CUSTARD

**COOKING: 25'**      **PREPARATION: 10'**      **SERVINGS: 3**

## INGREDIENTS

- » 2 ripe bananas, peeled and mashed finely
- » ½ teaspoon of vanilla extract
- » 14-ounce unsweetened almond milk
- » 3 eggs

## DIRECTIONS

1. Warm your oven to 350 degrees F. Grease 8 custard glasses lightly. Arrange the glasses in a large baking dish. Take a large bowl and mix all of the ingredients and mix them well until combined nicely.

2. Divide the mixture evenly between the glasses. Pour water into the baking dish. Bake for 25 minutes. Take out and serve.

**NUTRITIONS:** Calories: 59, Fat: 2.4g, Carbohydrates: 7g, Protein: 3g, Sodium: 92 mg

# 435. HEALTHY TAHINI BUNS

**COOKING: 15-20'**  **PREPARATION: 10'**  **SERVINGS: 3**

## INGREDIENTS

- » 1 whole egg
- » 5 tablespoons Tahini paste
- » ½ teaspoon baking soda
- » 1 teaspoon lemon juice
- » 1 pinch salt

## DIRECTIONS

1. Warm your oven to 350 degrees F. Line a baking sheet with parchment paper and keep it on the side. Put the listed fixing in a blender and blend until you have a smooth batter.

2. Scoop batter onto prepared sheet forming buns. Bake for 15-20 minutes. Remove, then let them cool. Serve and enjoy!

**NUTRITIONS:** Calories: 172, Carbs: 7g, Fiber: 2g, Protein: 6g, Fat: 14g, Sodium: 112 mg

# CHAPTER 14.
# DESSERTS

# 436. POACHED PEARS

**COOKING: 30'**　　　　**PREPARATION: 15'**　　　　**SERVINGS: 4**

## INGREDIENTS

- » ¼ cup apple juice extract
- » ½ cup fresh raspberries
- » 1 cup of orange juice extract
- » 1 teaspoon cinnamon, ground
- » 1 teaspoon ground nutmeg
- » 2 tablespoons orange zest
- » 4 whole pears, peeled, destemmed, core removed

## DIRECTIONS

1. In a bowl, combine the fruit juices, nutmeg, and cinnamon, and then stir evenly. In a shallow pan, pour the fruit juice mixture, and set to medium fire.

2. Adjust the heat to simmer within 30 minutes; turn pears frequently to maintain poaching, do not boil. Transfer poached pears to a serving bowl; garnish with orange zest and raspberries.

**NUTRITIONS:** Calories 140, Fats 0.5 g, Proteins 1 g, Carbohydrates 34 g, Fibers 2 g, Sodium 9 mg

# 437. PUMPKIN WITH CHIA SEEDS PUDDING

**COOKING: 0'**　　　　**PREPARATION: 60'**　　　　**SERVINGS: 4**

## INGREDIENTS

**For the Pudding:**
- » ½ cup organic chia seeds
- » ¼ cup raw maple syrup
- » 1 ¼ cup low-fat milk
- » 1 cup pumpkin puree extract

**For the Toppings:**
- » ¼ cup organic sunflower seeds
- » ¼ cup coarsely chopped almonds
- » ¼ cup blueberries

## DIRECTIONS

1. Add all the ingredients for the pudding in a bowl and mix until blended. Cover and store in a chiller for 1-hour. Remove from the chiller, transfer contents to a jar and add the ingredients for the toppings. Serve immediately.

**NUTRITIONS:** Calories 189, Sodium 42 mg, Fats 7 g, Potassium 311 mg, Carbohydrates 27 g, Fibers 4 g, Proteins 5 g, Sugar 18 g

# 438. CHOCOLATE TRUFFLES

**COOKING: 0'**   **PREPARATION: 15'**   **SERVINGS: 24**

## INGREDIENTS

**For the truffles:**
- » ½ cup cacao powder
- » ¼ cup chia seeds
- » ¼ cup flaxseed meal
- » ¼ cup maple syrup
- » 1 cup flour
- » 2 tablespoons almond milk

**For the Coatings:**
- » Cacao powder
- » Chia seeds
- » Flour
- » Shredded coconut, unsweetened

## DIRECTIONS

1. Place all the fixing for the truffle in a blender; pulse until it is thoroughly blended; transfer contents to a bowl. Form into chocolate balls, then cover with the coating ingredients. Serve immediately.

**NUTRITIONS:** Calories 70, Sodium 2 mg, Fats 1 g, Carbohydrates 14 g, Fibers 2 g, Sugar 11 g, Proteins 1 g

# 439. GRILLED PINEAPPLE STRIPS

**COOKING: 5'**   **PREPARATION: 15'**   **SERVINGS: 6**

## INGREDIENTS

- » Vegetable oil
- » Dash of iodized salt
- » 1 pineapple
- » 1 tablespoon lime juice extract
- » 1 tablespoon olive oil
- » 1 tablespoon raw honey
- » 3 tablespoons brown sugar

## DIRECTIONS

1. Peel the pineapple, remove the eyes of the fruit, and discard the core. Slice lengthwise, forming six wedges. Mix the rest of the fixing in a bowl until blended.

2. Brush the coating mixture on the pineapple (reserve some for basting). Grease an oven or outdoor grill rack with vegetable oil.

3. Place the pineapple wedges on the grill rack and heat for a few minutes per side until golden brownish, basting it frequently with a reserved glaze. Serve on a platter.

**NUTRITIONS:** Calories 97, Fats 2 g, Carbohydrates 20 g, Sodium 2 mg, Sugar 17 g, Fibers 1 g, Proteins 1 g

# 440. RASPBERRY PEACH PANCAKE

**COOKING: 30'**          **PREPARATION: 15'**          **SERVINGS: 4**

## INGREDIENTS

- » ½ teaspoon sugar
- » ½ cup raspberries
- » ½ cup fat-free milk
- » ½ cup all-purpose flour
- » ¼ cup vanilla yogurt
- » 1/8 teaspoon iodized salt
- » 1 tablespoon butter
- » 2 medium peeled, thinly sliced peaches
- » 3 lightly beaten organic eggs

## DIRECTIONS

1. Preheat oven to 400 °F. Toss peaches and raspberries with sugar in a bowl. Melt butter in a 9-inch round baking plate. Mix eggs, milk, plus salt in a small bowl until blended; whisk in the flour.

2. Remove the round baking plate from the oven, tilt to coat the bottom and sides with the melted butter; pour in the flour mixture.

3. Put it in the oven until it becomes brownish and puffed. Remove the pancake from the oven. Serve immediately with more raspberries and vanilla yogurt.

**NUTRITIONS:** Calories 199, Sodium 173 mg, Fats 7 g, Cholesterol 149 g, Carbohydrates 25 g, Sugar 11 g, Fibers 3 g, Proteins 9 g

# 441. MANGO RICE PUDDING

**COOKING: 35'**          **PREPARATION: 15'**          **SERVINGS: 4**

## INGREDIENTS

- » ½ teaspoon ground cinnamon
- » ¼ teaspoon iodized salt
- » 1 teaspoon vanilla extract
- » 1 cup long-grain uncooked brown rice
- » 2 mediums ripe, peeled, cored mango
- » 1 cup vanilla soymilk
- » 2 tablespoons sugar
- » 2 cups of water

## DIRECTIONS

1. Bring saltwater to a boil in a saucepan to cook rice; after a few minutes, simmer covered within 30-35 minutes until the rice absorbs the water. Mash the mango with a mortar and pestle or stainless-steel fork.

2. Pour milk, sugar, cinnamon, and the mashed mango into the rice; cook uncovered on low heat, stirring frequently. Remove the mango rice pudding from the heat, then stir in the vanilla soymilk. Serve immediately.

**NUTRITIONS:** Calories 275, Sodium 176 mg, Fats 3 g, Carbohydrates 58 mg, Sugar 20 g, Fibers 3 g

# 442. CHOCO BANANA CAKE

**COOKING: 30'**   **PREPARATION: 15'**   **SERVINGS: 18**

## INGREDIENTS

- » ½ cup semisweet dark chocolate
- » ½ cup brown sugar
- » ½ teaspoon baking soda
- » ¼ cup unsweetened cocoa powder
- » ¼ cup canola oil
- » ¾ cup soymilk
- » 1 large egg
- » 1 egg white
- » 1 large, ripe, mashed banana
- » 1 tablespoon lemon juice extract
- » 1 teaspoon vanilla extract
- » 2 cups all-purpose flour

## DIRECTIONS

1. Preheat the oven to 350 °F. Coat a baking pan with a non-stick spray. Whisk brown sugar, flour, baking soda, and cocoa powder in a bowl.

2. In another bowl, whisk bananas, lemon juice extract, vanilla extract, oil, soymilk, egg, and egg whites. Create a hole in the flour mixture's core or center, then pour in the banana mixture and mix in the dark chocolate.

3. Stir all the fixing with a spoon until thoroughly blended; spoon the batter onto the baking pan. Place in the oven and bake within 25-30 minutes until the center springs back when pressed lightly using your fingertips.

**NUTRITIONS:** Calories 150, Sodium 52 mg, Cholesterol 12 mg, Fats 3 g, Carbohydrates 27 g, Proteins 3 g

# 443. ZESTY ZUCCHINI MUFFINS

**COOKING: 30'**   **PREPARATION: 15'**   **SERVINGS: 12**

## INGREDIENTS

- » Vegetable oil cooking spray
- » ½ cup of sugar
- » ¼ teaspoon iodized salt
- » ¼ teaspoon ground nutmeg
- » ¾ cup skim milk
- » 1 cup shredded zucchini
- » 1 tablespoon baking powder
- » 1 large egg
- » 2 teaspoons grated lemon rind
- » 2 cups of all-purpose flour
- » 3 tablespoons vegetable oil

## DIRECTIONS

1. Mix the flour, baking powder, sugar, salt, plus lemon rinds in a bowl. Create a well in the center of the flour batter. In another bowl, mix zucchini, milk, vegetable oil, and egg. Coat muffin cups with vegetable oil cooking spray.

2. Divide the batter equally into 12 muffin cups. Transfer the muffin cups to the baking pan, put it in a microwave oven, and bake at 400 °F within 30 minutes until light golden brown. Remove, then allow to cool on a wire rack before serving.

**NUTRITIONS:** Calories 169, Sodium 211.5 mg, Fats 4.8 g, Potassium 80.2 g, Carbohydrates 29.1 g, Fibers 2.5 g, Sugar 12.8 g, Proteins 0 g

# 444. BLUEBERRY OAT MUFFINS

**COOKING: 30'**   **PREPARATION: 15'**   **SERVINGS: 12**

## INGREDIENTS

- » ½ cup raw oatmeal
- » ½ teaspoon baking powder
- » ½ teaspoon iodized salt
- » ½ cup dry milk
- » ¼ cup of vegetable oil
- » ¼ teaspoon baking soda
- » 1/3 cup sugar
- » 1 ½ cup flour
- » 1 cup milk
- » 1 cup blueberries

## DIRECTIONS

1. Preheat oven to 350 °F. Coat the muffin tins with vegetable oil. Mix or combine the flour, baking soda, baking powder, oats, sugar, and salt in a bowl. Mix milk, dry milk, egg, and vegetable oil in another bowl.

2. Pour the bowl of wet fixing into the bowl of dry fixing and mix partially. Add the blueberries and mix until the consistency turns lumpy. Scoop blueberry batter into the muffin tins.

3. Bake within 30 minutes until the muffins turn golden brown on the edges. Serve warm immediately or put it in an airtight container and store it in the refrigerator to chill.

**NUTRITIONS:** Calories 150, Sodium 180 mg, Fats 5 g, Carbohydrates 22 g, Proteins 4 g, Fibers 1 g

# 445. BANANA BREAD

**COOKING: 60'**   **PREPARATION: 15'**   **SERVINGS: 14**

## INGREDIENTS

- » Vegetable oil cooking spray
- » ½ cup brown rice flour
- » ½ cup amaranth flour
- » ½ cup tapioca flour
- » ½ cup millet flour
- » ½ cup quinoa flour
- » ½ cup of raw sugar
- » ¾ cup egg whites
- » 1/8 teaspoon iodized salt
- » 1 teaspoon baking soda
- » 2 tablespoons grapeseed oil
- » 2 pieces of mashed banana

## DIRECTIONS

1. Preheat oven to 350 °F. Coat a loaf pan with a vegetable oil cooking spray, dust evenly with a bit of flour, and set aside. In a bowl, mix the brown rice flour, amaranth flour, tapioca flour, millet flour, quinoa flour, and baking soda.

2. Coat a separate bowl with vegetable oil, then mix eggs, sugar, and mashed bananas. Pour the bowl of wet fixing into the bowl of dry fixing and mix thoroughly. Scoop the mixture into the loaf pan. Bake within an hour.

3. To check the doneness, insert a toothpick in the center of the loaf pan; if you remove the toothpick and it has no batter sticking to it, remove the bread from the oven. Slice and serve immediately and store the remaining banana bread in a refrigerator to prolong shelf life.

**NUTRITIONS:** Calories 150, Sodium 150 mg, Fats 3 g, Fibers 2 g, Proteins 4 g, Sugar 7 g

# 446. MILK CHOCOLATE PUDDING

**COOKING: 15'**     **PREPARATION: 15'**     **SERVINGS: 4**

## INGREDIENTS

- » ½ teaspoon vanilla extract
- » 1/3 cup chocolate chips
- » 1/8 teaspoon salt
- » 2 cups nonfat milk
- » 2 tablespoons cocoa powder
- » 2 tablespoons sugar
- » 3 tablespoons cornstarch

## DIRECTIONS

1. Mix cocoa powder, cornstarch, sugar, and salt in a saucepan and whisk in milk; frequently stir over medium heat.

2. Remove, put the chocolate chips and vanilla extract, stir until the chocolate chips and vanilla melt into the pudding. Pour contents into serving bowls and store in a chiller. Serve chilled.

**NUTRITIONS:** Calories 197, Sodium 5 mg, Fats 5 g, Carbohydrates 9 g, Proteins 0.5 g

# 447. MINTY LIME AND GRAPEFRUIT YOGURT PARFAIT

**COOKING: 0'**     **PREPARATION: 15'**     **SERVINGS: 6**

## INGREDIENTS

- » A handful of torn mint leaves
- » 2 teaspoons grated lime zest
- » 2 tablespoons lime juice extract
- » 3 tablespoons raw honey
- » 4 large red grapefruits
- » 4 cups reduced-fat plain yogurt

## DIRECTIONS

1. Cut the top and lower part of the red grapefruits and stand the fruit upright on a cutting board. Discard the peel with a knife and slice along the membrane of each segment to remove the skin.

2. Mix yogurt, lime juice extract, and lime zest in a bowl. Layer half of the grapefruit and yogurt mixture into 6 parfait glasses; add another layer until the glass is filled and then drizzle with honey and top with mint leaves. Serve immediately.

**NUTRITIONS:** Calories 207, Sodium 115 mg, Fats 3 g, Cholesterol 10 mg, Carbohydrates 39 mg, Sugar 36 g, Fibers 3 g

# 448. PEACH TARTS

**COOKING: 55'**     **PREPARATION: 15'**     **SERVINGS: 8**

## INGREDIENTS

**Tart Ingredients:**
» ¼ cup softened butter
» ¼ teaspoon ground nutmeg
» 1 cup all-purpose flour
» 3 tablespoons sugar

**Filling Ingredients:**
» ¼ teaspoon ground cinnamon
» ¼ cup coarsely chopped almonds
» 1/8 teaspoon almond extract
» 1/3 cup sugar
» 2 pounds peaches medium, peeled, thinly sliced

## DIRECTIONS

1. Preheat oven to 375 °F. Mix butter, nutmeg, and sugar in a bowl until light and fluffy. Add and beat in flour until well-blended. Place the batter on an ungreased fluted tart baking pan and press firmly on the bottom and topsides.

2. Put it in the medium rack of the preheated oven and bake for about 10 minutes until it turns to a crust. In a bowl, coat peaches with sugar, flour, cinnamon, almond extract, and almonds.

3. Open the oven, put the tart crust on the lower rack of the oven, and pour in the peach filling; bake for about 40-45 minutes. Remove, cool, and serve; or cover with a cling wrap and refrigerate to serve chilled.

**NUTRITIONS:** Calories 222, Sodium 46 milligrams, Fats 8 g, Cholesterol 15 mg, Carbohydrates 36 g, Sugar 21 g, Fibers 3 g, Proteins 4 g

# 449. RASPBERRY NUTS PARFAIT

**COOKING: 10'**     **PREPARATION: 15'**     **SERVINGS: 1**

## INGREDIENTS

» ¼ cup frozen raspberries
» ¼ cup frozen blueberries
» ¼ cup toasted, thinly sliced almonds
» 1 cup nonfat, plain Greek yogurt
» 2 teaspoons raw honey

## DIRECTIONS

1. First, layer Greek yogurt in a parfait glass; add berries; layer yogurt again, top with almonds and more berries; drizzle with honey. Serve chilled.

**NUTRITIONS:** Calories 378, Sodium 83 mg, Fats 15 g, Fibers 6 g, Carbohydrates 35 g, Proteins 30 g, Sugar 25 g

# 450. STRAWBERRY BRUSCHETTA

**COOKING: 0'**          **PREPARATION: 15'**          **SERVINGS: 12**

## INGREDIENTS

» 1 loaf sliced Ciabatta bread
» 8 ounces goat cheese
» 1 cup basil leaves
» 2 containers of strawberries, sliced
» 5 tablespoons balsamic glaze

## DIRECTIONS

1. Wash and slice strawberries; set aside. Wash and chop the basil leaves; set aside. Slice the ciabatta bread and spread some goat cheese evenly on each slice; add strawberries, balsamic glaze, and top with basil leaves. Serve on a platter.

**NUTRITIONS:** Calories 80, Sodium 59 mg, Fats 2 g, Carbohydrates 12 g, Proteins 3 g

# 451. VANILLA CUPCAKES WITH CINNAMON-FUDGE FROSTING

**COOKING: 18'**          **PREPARATION: 10'**          **SERVINGS: 12**

## INGREDIENTS

» 11/2 cups white whole-wheat flour
» 3/4 cup sugar
» 3/4 teaspoon sodium-free baking powder
» 1/2 teaspoon sodium-free baking soda
» 1 cup nondairy milk
» 6 tablespoons canola oil
» 1 tablespoon apple cider vinegar
» 1 tablespoon pure vanilla extract

**Frosting:**
» 2 cups powdered sugar
» 1/3 cup unsweetened cocoa powder
» 4 tablespoons non-hydrogenated vegetable shortening
» 4 tablespoons nondairy milk
» 1 teaspoon ground cinnamon
» 1 teaspoon pure vanilla extract

## DIRECTIONS

1. Warm oven to 350 F. Line a 12-muffin tin with paper liners and put aside. Mix or combine the flour, sugar, baking powder, and baking soda into a mixing bowl. Add the remaining batter fixing and stir just until combined.

2. Split the batter evenly between the muffin cups, then bake within 18 minutes. Remove, then put on a wire rack to cool. Beat until fluffy the frosting fixings into a mixing bowl. Frost cupcakes. Serve immediately.

**NUTRITIONS:** Calories: 347, Fat: 7 g, Protein: 13 g, Sodium: 46 mg, Fiber: 4 g, Carbohydrates: 60 g, Sugar: 3 g

# 452. CHOCOLATE CUPCAKES WITH VANILLA FROSTING

**COOKING: 20'**  **PREPARATION: 15'**  **SERVINGS: 12**

## INGREDIENTS

- » 11/2 cups white whole-wheat flour
- » 1 cup of sugar
- » 2 teaspoons sodium-free baking soda
- » 1/4 cup unsweetened cocoa powder
- » 1 cup of water
- » 4 tablespoons canola oil
- » 4 tablespoons unsweetened applesauce
- » 1 tablespoon pure vanilla extract
- » 1 teaspoon distilled white vinegar

**Frosting:**
- » 11/2 cups powdered sugar
- » 4 tablespoons non-hydrogenated vegetable shortening
- » 21/2 tablespoons nondairy milk
- » 1 tablespoon pure vanilla extract

## DIRECTIONS

1. Warm oven to 350°F. Prepare a 12-muffin tin with paper liners and set aside. Measure the flour, sugar, and baking soda into a mixing bowl and whisk well to combine. Put the rest of the batter ingredients and stir just until combined.

2. Divide the batter evenly into the muffin cups. Bake within 20 minutes or until a toothpick inserted in the center of cupcakes comes out clean.

3. Remove, then put on a wire rack to cool. Mix the frosting fixing into a clean mixing bowl, then frost cupcakes. Serve immediately.

**NUTRITIONS:** Calories: 272, Fat: 9 g, Protein: 2 g, Sodium: 2 mg, Fiber: 1 g, Carbohydrates: 45 g, Sugar: 32 g

# 453. CHOCOLATE CHIP BANANA MUFFIN TOP COOKIES

**COOKING: 15'**  **PREPARATION: 15'**  **SERVINGS: 16**

## INGREDIENTS

- » 1 cup quick oats
- » 1 cup white whole-wheat flour
- » 1/4 cup sugar
- » 1 tablespoon sodium-free baking powder
- » 1 teaspoon ground cinnamon
- » 3 ripe medium bananas, mashed
- » 4 tablespoons canola oil
- » 1 tablespoon pure vanilla extract
- » 3/4 cup chocolate chips

## DIRECTIONS

1. Preheat oven to 350°F. Put aside a baking sheet with parchment paper. Measure the oats, flour, sugar, baking powder, and cinnamon into a mixing bowl and whisk. Put the rest of the fixing and stir just until combined.

2. Using a medium-sized ice cream scoop, scoop the batter onto the prepared baking sheet, leaving an inch or two between cookies. Bake within 15 minutes. Remove, then put on a wire rack to cool. Serve immediately.

**NUTRITIONS:** Calories: 150, Fat: 6 g, Protein: 2 g, Sodium: 0 mg, Fiber: 1 g, Carbohydrates: 23 g, Sugar: 10 g

# 454. LEMON COOKIES

**COOKING: 10'**      **PREPARATION: 15'**      **SERVINGS: 36**

## INGREDIENTS

- » 21/2 cups white whole-wheat flour
- » 11/2 cups sugar
- » 1 tablespoon sodium-free baking powder
- » 3/4 cup canola oil
- » 2 large lemons, juice, and grated zest
- » 1 tablespoon pure vanilla extract

## DIRECTIONS

1. Preheat oven to 350°F. Mix the flour, sugar, plus baking powder into a mixing bowl. Put the rest of the fixing and stir to form a stiff dough.

2. Drop by rounded tablespoons onto an ungreased baking sheet. Bake within 10 minutes. Remove, then let cool on sheet for a few minutes before transferring to a wire rack to cool fully. Serve immediately.

**NUTRITIONS:** Calories: 106, Fat: 5 g, Protein: 1 g, Sodium: 0 mg, Fiber: 0 g, Carbohydrates: 15 g, Sugar: 8 g

# 455. PEANUT BUTTER CHOCOLATE CHIP BLONDIES

**COOKING: 20'**      **PREPARATION: 15'**      **SERVINGS: 24**

## INGREDIENTS

- » 1/4 cup salt-free peanut butter
- » 3/4 cup light brown sugar
- » 1/2 cup unsweetened applesauce
- » 1/4 cup canola oil
- » 2 egg whites
- » 1 tablespoon pure vanilla extract
- » 2 teaspoons sodium-free baking powder
- » 1 cup unbleached all-purpose flour
- » 1/2 cup white whole-wheat flour
- » 1/2 cup semisweet chocolate chips

## DIRECTIONS

1. Preheat oven to 400°F. Oiled and flour a 9" × 13" baking pan and set aside. Measure the peanut butter, sugar, applesauce, oil, egg whites, and vanilla into a mixing bowl and stir well to combine.

2. Add the baking powder and mix. Gradually add in the flours, stirring well. Fold in the chocolate chips. Spread batter in prepared pan and smooth to even.

3. Bake within 20 minutes. Remove, then let it cool. Cool before cutting into bars and serving.

**NUTRITIONS:** Calories: 18, Fat: 5 g, Protein: 2 g, Sodium: 7 mg, Fiber: 1 g, Carbohydrates: 17 g, Sugar: 10 g

# 456. GINGER SNAPS

**COOKING: 10'**     **PREPARATION: 15'**     **SERVINGS: 18**

## INGREDIENTS

- » 4 tablespoons unsalted butter
- » 1/2 cup light brown sugar
- » 2 tablespoons molasses
- » 1 egg white
- » 21/2 teaspoons ground ginger
- » 1/4 teaspoon ground allspice
- » 1 teaspoon sodium-free baking soda
- » 1/2 cup unbleached all-purpose flour
- » 12 cup white whole-wheat flour
- » 1 tablespoon sugar

## DIRECTIONS

1. Warm oven to 375°F. Put aside a baking sheet with parchment paper. Put the butter, sugar, plus molasses into a mixing bowl and beat well.

2. Mix the egg white, ginger, and allspice. Mix in the baking soda, then put the flours, then beat.

3. Roll the dough into small balls. Put the balls on a prepared baking sheet and press down using a glass dipped in the tablespoon sugar.

4. Once the glass presses on the dough, it will moisten sufficiently to coat with sugar. Bake within 10 minutes. Let it cool, then serve.

**NUTRITIONS:** Calories: 81, Fat: 2 g, Protein: 1 g, Sodium: 6 mg, Fiber: 0 g, Carbohydrates: 14 g, Sugar: 8 g

# 457. CARROT CAKE COOKIES

**COOKING: 12'**     **PREPARATION: 15'**     **SERVINGS: 36**

## INGREDIENTS

- » 3 medium carrots, shredded
- » 11/2 cups white whole-wheat flour
- » 3/4 cup oat flour
- » 3/4 cup light brown sugar
- » 1 egg white
- » 1/3 cup canola oil
- » 1 tablespoon pure vanilla extract
- » 1 teaspoon sodium-free baking powder
- » 11/2 teaspoons ground cinnamon
- » 1/2 teaspoon ground nutmeg
- » 1/4 teaspoon ground ginger
- » 1/8 teaspoon ground cloves

## DIRECTIONS

1. Preheat oven to 375°F. Prepare and line a baking sheet with parchment paper and set aside. Place all the ingredients into a mixing bowl and stir well to combine. The dough will be quite sticky.

2. Put onto a lined baking sheet. Bake within 12 minutes. Remove, then transfer cookies to a wire rack to cool. Store in an airtight container.

**NUTRITIONS:** Calories: 67, Fat: 2 g, Protein: 1 g, Sodium: 7 mg, Fiber: 0 g, Carbohydrates: 10 g, Sugar: 4 g

# 458. CHEWY PUMPKIN OATMEAL RAISIN COOKIES

**COOKING: 16'**     **PREPARATION: 15'**     **SERVINGS: 48**

## INGREDIENTS

- » 1 cup pumpkin purée
- » 12/3 cups sugar
- » 2 tablespoons molasses
- » 11/2 teaspoons pure vanilla extract
- » 2/3 cup canola oil
- » 1 tablespoon ground flaxseed
- » 2 teaspoons Ener-G Baking Soda Substitute
- » 1 teaspoon ground cinnamon
- » 1/2 teaspoon ground nutmeg
- » 1 cup unbleached all-purpose flour
- » 1 cup white whole-wheat flour
- » 11/3 cups rolled or quick oats
- » 1 cup seedless raisins

## DIRECTIONS

1. Preheat oven to 350°F. Spray 2 baking sheets lightly with oil and set aside. Measure the ingredients into a large mixing bowl and stir using a rubber spatula.

2. Scoop batter out by tablespoons—a small retractable ice cream scoop works wonderfully here—and place on the prepared baking sheets.

3. Put sheets on the middle rack in the oven and bake 16 minutes. Remove, then transfer cookies to a wire rack to cool. Repeat process with remaining batter. Cool, and serve.

**NUTRITIONS:** Calories: 97, Fat: 3 g, Protein: 1 g, Sodium: 1 mg, Fiber: 0.6 g, Carbohydrates: 16 g, Sugar: 9 g

# 459. EASY APPLE CRISP

**COOKING: 25'**     **PREPARATION: 15'**     **SERVINGS: 8**

## INGREDIENTS

- » 6 medium apples
- » 1 tablespoon lemon juice
- » 1/3 cup sugar
- » 1/2 cup rolled or quick oats
- » 1/2 cup white whole-wheat flour
- » 1/2 cup light brown sugar
- » 1 tablespoon pure vanilla extract
- » 1 teaspoon ground cinnamon
- » 1/2 teaspoon ground ginger
- » 3 tablespoons unsalted butter

## DIRECTIONS

1. Preheat oven to 425°F. Take out a 2-quart baking pan and set aside. Slice each apple into 16 wedges. Put into a mixing bowl, place the lemon juice and sugar, and toss well to coat.

2. Turn batter out into the baking pan, then set aside. Place the oats, flour, sugar, vanilla, and spices into a mixing bowl and stir to combine.

3. Slice the butter into the mixture using your hands and process until a wet crumb has formed. Sprinkle mixture over the fruit. Bake within 25 minutes. Remove, then let it cool and serve.

**NUTRITIONS:** Calories: 232, Fat: 5 g, Protein: 2 g, Sodium: 5 mg, Fiber: 2 g, Carbohydrates: 46 g, Sugar: 34 g

# 460. MANGO CRUMBLE

**COOKING: 25'**     **PREPARATION: 15'**     **SERVINGS: 8**

## INGREDIENTS

- » 2 barely ripe mangoes
- » 2 tablespoons light brown sugar
- » 1 tablespoon cornstarch
- » 11/2 teaspoons minced fresh ginger
- » 1/2 cup unbleached all-purpose flour
- » 1/2 cup white whole-wheat flour
- » 1/2 cup sugar
- » 1 teaspoon ground cinnamon
- » 1/4 teaspoon ground ginger
- » 3 tablespoons unsalted butter

## DIRECTIONS

1. Preheat oven to 375°F. Take out an 8-inch square baking pan and set aside. Peel mangoes and cut into 1-inch chunks. Place in a mixing bowl.

2. Add the brown sugar, cornstarch, and minced ginger and toss to coat. Put the batter out into the baking pan and spread to even. In another bowl, whisk the flours, sugar, cinnamon, and ginger.

3. Slice the butter into pieces, and put it in the bowl. Work the butter into the mixture using your hands until it resembles damp sand and sticks when squeezed. Sprinkle mixture evenly over the fruit.

4. Bake within 25 minutes, until fruit is tender. Remove, and put on a wire rack to cool. Serve warm or cool.

**NUTRITIONS:** Calories: 190, Fat: 5 g, Protein: 3 g, Sodium: 3 mg, Fiber: 2 g, Carbohydrates: 37 g, Sugar: 23 g

# 461. HOMEMADE BANANA ICE CREAM

**COOKING: 0'**     **PREPARATION: 5'**     **SERVINGS: 4**

## INGREDIENTS

- » 4 ripe bananas

## DIRECTIONS

1. Place bananas in the freezer and freeze until solid. Remove bananas from the freezer, peel, and slice into chunks. Pulse chunks into a blender or food processor. Scoop mixture out and serve immediately.

**NUTRITIONS:** Calories: 105, Fat: 0 g, Protein: 1 g, Sodium: 1 mg, Fiber: 3 g, Carbohydrates: 26 g, Sugar: 14 g

# 462. KAREN'S APPLE KUGEL

**COOKING: 25'**      **PREPARATION: 15'**      **SERVINGS: 8**

## INGREDIENTS

» 3 sheets unsalted matzo
» 2 cups of water
» 4 tart green apples
» 1 tablespoon freshly squeezed lemon juice
» 3 tablespoons unsalted butter, melted
» 1/4 cup brown sugar
» 1/2 cup seedless raisins
» 3 egg whites
» 11/2 teaspoons ground cinnamon

## DIRECTIONS

1. Preheat oven to 400°F. Take out an 8" × 11" baking dish and set aside. Place the matzo in an 8-inch square baking pan. Pour the water into the pan and set aside to rehydrate.

2. Peel apples, core, and cut into quarters. Cut each quarter crosswise into thirds and then lengthwise into slices no more than 1/4 inch thick. Transfer apples to a mixing bowl.

3. Check on the matzo. When soft, drain the matzo and squeeze out excess water. Place matzo into the mixing bowl. Put the rest of the fixing and stir well to combine.

4. Pour mixture into the 8" × 11" baking dish. Bake within 25 minutes. Remove from the oven. Set on a wire rack to cool. Cut into portions and serve warm or cool.

**NUTRITIONS:** Calories: 181, Fat: 4 g, Protein: 3 g, Sodium: 24 mg, Fiber: 2 g, Carbohydrates: 34 g, Sugar: 21 g

# 463. PEACH COBBLER

**COOKING: 25'**      **PREPARATION: 15'**      **SERVINGS: 8**

## INGREDIENTS

» 6 ripe peaches, peeled and sliced
» 3 tablespoons sugar
» Juice of 1 fresh lemon
» 11/4 cups unbleached all-purpose flour
» 1/2 cup white whole-wheat flour
» 2/3 cup sugar
» 1 teaspoon sodium-free baking powder
» 4 tablespoons unsalted butter, melted and cooled
» 1 egg white
» 1/2 cup low-fat milk
» 1 tablespoon pure vanilla extract

## DIRECTIONS

1. Preheat oven to 425°F. Take out a 9" × 13" baking dish and set aside. Put the sliced peaches into a mixing bowl, put sugar plus lemon juice, and toss well to coat. Transfer to the baking dish. Set aside.

2. Mix the flours, sugar, plus baking powder into a mixing bowl. Add the melted butter, egg white, milk, and vanilla and stir well to combine. Scoop batter over sliced peaches.

3. Put baking dish on middle rack in the oven, then bake for 25 minutes. Remove dish from oven and place on a wire rack to cool. Serve warm or cool.

**NUTRITIONS:** Calories: 273, Fat: 6 g, Protein: 5 g, Sodium: 15 mg, Fiber: 3 g, Carbohydrates: 50 g, Sugar: 28 g

# 464. BLUEBERRY PUDDING CAKE

**COOKING: 25'**            **PREPARATION: 15'**            **SERVINGS: 6**

## INGREDIENTS

- » 3 cups blueberries
- » 3/4 cup sugar, divided
- » 1 tablespoon freshly squeezed lemon juice
- » 6 tablespoons unsalted butter, softened
- » 2 teaspoons pure vanilla extract
- » 1 teaspoon freshly grated lemon zest
- » 1 egg white
- » 11/2 teaspoons sodium-free baking powder
- » 2 tablespoons low-fat milk
- » 2/3 cup white whole-wheat flour

## DIRECTIONS

1. Preheat oven to 400°F. Oiled an 8-inch square baking pan lightly with oil and set aside. Place blueberries into a mixing bowl. Add 1/4 cup sugar and the lemon juice and toss well to coat.

2. Pour berries into the prepared baking pan, place on the middle rack in the oven, and bake for 5 minutes. Remove from the oven and set aside. Place the butter and remaining 1/2 cup sugar into a mixing bowl and beat to combine.

3. Add the vanilla, lemon zest, and egg white and mix well. Add the baking powder and milk and stir. Gradually add in the flour, mixing until combined.

4. Pour batter over the cooked blueberries. Bake within 20 minutes, until golden brown. Serve warm or cool.

**NUTRITIONS:** Calories: 300, Fat: 12 g, Protein: 2 g, Sodium: 14 mg, Fiber: 2 g, Carbohydrates: 46 g, Sugar: 32 g

# 465. VEGAN RICE PUDDING

**COOKING: 20'**            **PREPARATION: 15'**            **SERVINGS: 8**

## INGREDIENTS

- » 1-quart vanilla nondairy milk
- » 1 cup basmati or jasmine rice, rinsed
- » 1/4 cup sugar
- » 1 teaspoon pure vanilla extract
- » 1/8 teaspoon pure almond extract
- » 1/2 teaspoon ground cinnamon
- » 1/8 teaspoon ground cardamom

## DIRECTIONS

1. Mix all of the fixings into a saucepan and stir well to combine. Bring to a boil over medium-high heat. Adjust heat to low and simmer, stirring very frequently, about 15–20 minutes. Remove from heat and cool. Serve sprinkled with additional ground cinnamon if desired.

**NUTRITIONS:** Calories: 148, Fat: 2 g, Protein: 4 g, Sodium: 48 mg, Fiber: 1 g, Carbohydrates: 26 g, Sugar: 10 g

# 466. BEETROOT AND BERRY SMOOTHIE

**COOKING: 0'**          **PREPARATION: 5'**          **SERVINGS: 1**

## INGREDIENTS

» 1/2 cup pineapple juice
» 1/2 cup low-fat vanilla yogurt
» 1/2 cup frozen strawberries
» 1/4 cup frozen blueberries
» 1/4 cup beetroot (peeled, washed, and sliced)

## DIRECTIONS

1. Combine all the ingredients in a blender and blend until you obtain a smooth puree. Serve cold.

**NUTRITIONS:** Calories 218 g, Fat 1.9 g, Carbohydrates 40.7 g, Protein 8.4 g, Sodium- 121 mg

# 467. BERRY BLAST

**COOKING: 40'**          **PREPARATION: 15'**          **SERVINGS: 1**

## INGREDIENTS

» 4 cups blueberries (2 cups fresh and 2 cups frozen)
» 1 cup rolled oats
» 1 tsp cinnamon
» 2 tbsp all-purpose flour
» 2 tsp unsalted butter
» 1 tbsp maple syrup

## DIRECTIONS

1. Coat a pie pan with cooking spray and set it aside. Put the blueberries on the pie plate. Preheat the oven to 250 degrees Fahrenheit.

2. Combine the flour, butter, oats, maple syrup, and cinnamon in a large mixing bowl and whisk until you obtain a grainy mixture.

3. Transfer the oats mixture to the pie pan and bake for forty minutes until the mixture is golden brown. Serve warm.

**NUTRITIONS:** Calories 824 g, Fat 15.2 g, Carbohydrates 166.6 g, Protein 16.9 g, Sodium 65 mg

# 468. OATS AND FRUIT BAR CRACKER

**COOKING: 0'**          **PREPARATION: 15'**          **SERVINGS: 3**

## INGREDIENTS

- » 1 cup quinoa
- » 1 cup oats
- » 1/2 cup figs (dried)
- » 1/2 cup honey
- » 1/2 cup almonds (chopped)
- » 1/2 cup apricots (dried)
- » 1/2 cup wheat germ
- » 1/2 cup pineapple (dried and chopped)
- » 1 tbsp cornstarch

## DIRECTIONS

1. Mix the fixing in a mixing bowl until you obtain a well-balanced mixture. Put the batter on a baking tray or plate and flatten it. Ensure that the mixture is at least one inch thick. Let it cool before you cut it into pieces and serve.

**NUTRITIONS:** Calories 766 g, Fat 15.7 g, Carbohydrates 144.2 g, Protein 22.2 g, Sodium 12 mg

# 469. COLORFUL POPS

**COOKING: 0'**          **PREPARATION: 15'**          **SERVINGS: 6**

## INGREDIENTS

- » 2 cups of watermelon, strawberries, and cantaloupe (diced)
- » 2 cups pure apple juice
- » 2 cups fresh blueberries
- » 6 craft sticks
- » 6 paper cups

## DIRECTIONS

1. Mix all the fruit in a mixing bowl. Divide the fruit salad into the paper cups and pour the apple juice. Ensure that the apple juice only covers half the paper cup. Deep-freeze the cups for an hour or until they are partially frozen.

2. Remove the cups and add the sticks to the cups, and deep freeze for one more hour. Serve them as colorful pops!

**NUTRITIONS:** Calories 83 g, Fat 0.2 g, Carbohydrates 20.8 g, Protein 0.7 g, Sodium 8 mg

# 470. PUMPKIN PIE RECIPE

**COOKING: 50'**     **PREPARATION: 15'**     **SERVINGS: 2**

## INGREDIENTS

- » 1 cup ginger snaps
- » 8 ounces canned pumpkin
- » 1/4 cup egg whites
- » 1/4 cup erythritol
- » 1 tsp pumpkin pie spice
- » 6 ounces evaporated skim milk
- » Cooking spray

## DIRECTIONS

1. Preheat the oven to 300 degrees Fahrenheit. Oiled a glass pie pan with cooking spray. Crumble the ginger snaps and pat them into the glass pan. Mix the rest of the fixing in a mixing bowl and pour it into the prepared glass pie pan.

2. Bake the dish for fifty minutes or until a knife inserted in the center comes out clean. Transfer the pie pan into the refrigerator and allow it to cool. Serve cold.

**NUTRITIONS:** Calories 792 g, Fat 16.6 g, Carbohydrates 172.7 g, Protein 20 g, Sodium 1181 mg

# 471. WALNUT AND OATMEAL CHOCOLATE CHIP COOKIES

**COOKING: 20'**     **PREPARATION: 15'**     **SERVINGS: 4**

## INGREDIENTS

- » 1 cup rolled oats
- » 1/4 cup all-purpose flour
- » 1/4 cup whole-wheat pastry flour
- » 1/2 tsp ground cinnamon
- » 1/4 tsp baking soda
- » 1/4 tsp salt
- » 1/4 tsp tahini
- » 2 tbsp unsalted butter (cubed)
- » 1/2 cup erythritol
- » 1/2 cup maple syrup
- » 2 eggs (one whole and one egg white)
- » 1/2 tbsp vanilla extract
- » 1/2 cup bittersweet chocolate chips
- » 1/4 cup chopped walnuts

## DIRECTIONS

1. Place racks in the oven's upper and lower parts and preheat the oven to 300 degrees Fahrenheit. Prepare or arrange two lined baking sheets with parchment paper. Combine the oats, whole-wheat flour, all-purpose flour, baking soda, cinnamon, and salt in a bowl and whisk.

2. Beat butter and tahini in a large mixing bowl and blend until you obtain a paste. Add maple syrup and granulated sugar to the bowl and continue to beat until you get a well-combined mixture. Note that the mixture will still be slightly grainy.

3. Now, add the vanilla extract, egg white, and whole egg to the bowl and continue to whisk until you obtain a well-combined mixture.

4. Stir in the oat's mixture, chocolate chips, and walnuts into the bowl. Wet your hands slightly, roll one tablespoon of the batter into a small ball, and place it on the baking sheet. Flatten the ball out but ensure that the sides do not crack. Continue with the remaining batter and leave at least a two-inch space between each cookie.

5. Bake the cookies for twenty minutes or until golden brown. Cool the cookies for two minutes before you transfer them onto the wire rack to cool completely.

**NUTRITIONS:** Calories 530 g, Fat 14.8 g, Carbohydrates 98.6 g, Protein 10.6 g, Sodium 280 mg

# 472. APPLE DUMPLINGS

**COOKING: 30'**     **PREPARATION: 10'**     **SERVINGS: 6**

## INGREDIENTS

**Dough:**
- » 1 tablespoon butter
- » 1 teaspoon honey
- » 1 cup whole-wheat flour
- » 2 tablespoons buckwheat flour
- » 2 tablespoons rolled oats
- » 2 tablespoons brandy or apple liquor

**Apple filling:**
- » 6 large tart apples, thinly sliced
- » 1 teaspoon nutmeg
- » 2 tablespoons honey
- » Zest of one lemon

## DIRECTIONS

1. Warm oven to heat at 350 degrees F. Combine flours with oats, honey, and butter in a food processor. Pulse this mixture for few times, then stirs in apple liquor or brandy. Mix until it forms a ball. Wrap it in a plastic sheet.

2. Refrigerate for 2 hours. Mix apples with honey, nutmeg, and lemon zest, then set it aside. Spread the dough into ¼ inch thick sheet. Cut it into 8-inch circles and layer the greased muffin cups with the dough circles.

3. Divide the apple mixture into the muffin cups and seal the dough from the top. Bake for 30 minutes at 350 degrees F until golden brown. Enjoy.

**NUTRITIONS:** Calories 178, Fat 5.7 g, Cholesterol 15 mg, Sodium 114 mg, Carbs 12.4 g, Fiber 0.2g, Sugar 15 g, Protein 9.1 g

# 473. BERRIES MARINATED IN BALSAMIC VINEGAR

**COOKING: 0'**     **PREPARATION: 10'**     **SERVINGS: 2**

## INGREDIENTS

- » 1/4 cup balsamic vinegar
- » 2 tablespoons brown sugar
- » 1 teaspoon vanilla extract
- » 1/2 cup sliced strawberries
- » 1/2 cup blueberries
- » 1/2 cup raspberries
- » 2 shortbread biscuits

## DIRECTIONS

1. Combine balsamic vinegar, vanilla, and brown sugar in a small bowl. Toss strawberries with raspberries and blueberries in a bowl. Pour the vinegar mixture on top and marinate them for 15 minutes. Serve immediately.

**NUTRITIONS:** Calories 176, Fat 11.9 g, Cholesterol 78 mg, Sodium 79 mg, Carbs 33 g, Fiber 1.1 g, Sugar 10.3 g, Protein 13 g

# 474. LEMON PUDDING CAKES

**COOKING: 40'**　　　**PREPARATION: 10'**　　　**SERVINGS: 4**

## INGREDIENTS

» 2 eggs
» 1/4 teaspoon salt
» 3/4 cup sugar
» 1 cup skim milk
» 1/3 cup freshly squeezed lemon juice
» 3 tablespoons all-purpose flour
» 1 tablespoon finely grated lemon peel
» 1 tablespoon melted butter

## DIRECTIONS

1. Warm oven at 350 degrees F. Grease the custard cups with cooking oil. Whisk egg whites with salt and ¼ cup sugar in a mixer until it forms stiff peaks. Beat egg yolks with ½ cup sugar until mixed.

2. Stir in lemon juice, milk, butter, flour, and lemon peel. Mix it until smooth. Fold in the egg white mixture. Divide the batter into the custard cups. Bake them for 40 minutes until golden from the top. Serve.

**NUTRITIONS:** Calories 174, Fat 10.2 g, Cholesterol 120 mg, Sodium 176 mg, Carbs 19 g, Fiber 1.9 g, Sugar 11.4 g, Protein 12.8 g

# 475. MIXED BERRY WHOLE-GRAIN COFFEE CAKE

**COOKING: 30'**　　　**PREPARATION: 10'**　　　**SERVINGS: 6**

## INGREDIENTS

» 1/2 cup of skim milk
» 1 tbsp vinegar
» 2 tbsp canola oil
» 1 tsp vanilla
» 1 egg
» 1/3 cup of packed brown sugar
» 1 cup of whole-wheat pastry flour
» 1/2 tsp baking soda
» 1/2 tsp ground cinnamon
» 1/8 tsp salt
» 1 cup of frozen mixed berries
» 1/4 cup of low-fat granola, slightly crushed

## DIRECTIONS

1. Warm oven to heat at 350 degrees F. Grease an 8-inch baking pan with cooking spray and dust it with flour. Combine milk with vanilla, oil, vinegar, brown sugar, and egg until smooth.

2. Add baking soda, cinnamon, salt, and flour. Mix well. Fold in half of the berries and transfer the batter to the pan. Top it with the berries and granola. Bake for 30 minutes until golden brown. Serve.

**NUTRITIONS:** Calories 135, Fat 24g, Cholesterol 61 mg, Sodium 562 mg, Carbs 23 g, Fiber 1.7 g, Sugar 39 g, Protein 11g

# 476. STRAWBERRIES AND CREAM CHEESE CREPES

**COOKING: 10'**      **PREPARATION: 10'**      **SERVINGS: 2**

## INGREDIENTS

- » 4 tbsp cream cheese, softened
- » 2 tbsp powdered sugar, sifted
- » 2 tsp vanilla extract
- » 2 pre-packaged crepes, each about 8 inches in diameter
- » 8 strawberries, hulled and sliced

## DIRECTIONS

1. Set the oven to heat at 325 degrees F. Grease a baking dish with cooking spray. Mix cream cheese with vanilla plus powdered sugar in a mixer. Spread the cream cheese mixture on each crepe and top it with 2 tablespoons strawberries.

2. Roll the crepes and place them in the baking dish. Bake them within 10 minutes until golden brown. Garnish as desired. Serve.

**NUTRITIONS:** Calories 144, Fat 4.9 g, Cholesterol 11 mg, Sodium 13 mg, Carbs 19.3 g, Fiber 1.9 g, Sugar 9.7 g , Protein 3.4 g

# 477. HEALTHY BLUEBERRY & BANANA MUFFINS

**COOKING: 25'**      **PREPARATION: 30'**      **SERVINGS: 12**

## INGREDIENTS

- » 3/4 cup mashed ripe banana
- » 3/4 cup + 2 tbsp almond milk, unsweetened
- » 1 teaspoon apple cider vinegar
- » 1/4 cup pure maple syrup
- » 1 teaspoon pure vanilla extract
- » 1/4 cup coconut oil, melted
- » 1/2 teaspoon baking soda
- » 2 teaspoons baking powder
- » 4 tablespoons coconut sugar
- » 1 1/2 teaspoons cinnamon
- » 2 cups white spelt flour
- » 1 1/4 cups of blueberries
- » 1/2 cup walnut halves, chopped

## DIRECTIONS

1. Prepare lined 12-muffin tin with muffin liners and preheat oven to 3500F. In a large mixing bowl, whisk well-mashed bananas, almond milk, vinegar, maple syrup, vanilla, melted coconut oil, baking soda, baking powder, coconut sugar, and cinnamon.

2. Whisk well until thoroughly incorporated. Fold in spelt flour. Add blueberries and walnut halves. Evenly divide batter into prepared muffin tins. Bake within 25 minutes. Cool completely. Serve.

**NUTRITIONS:** Calories: 226.5, Protein: 5g, Carbs: 33.4g, Fat: 8.1g, Sodium: 67mg

# 478. TART RASPBERRY CRUMBLE BAR

**COOKING: 45'**     **PREPARATION: 50'**     **SERVINGS: 9**

## INGREDIENTS

- » 1/2 cup whole toasted almonds
- » 1 3/4 cups whole wheat flour
- » 1/4 tsp salt
- » 3/4 cup cold butter, unsalted, cut into cubes
- » 3 tbsp cold water, or more if needed
- » 1/2 cup granulated sugar
- » 18-ounce fresh raspberries

## DIRECTIONS

1. Pulse almonds using a food processor until chopped coarsely. Transfer to a bowl. Add flour and salt into the food processor and pulse until a bit combined. Put butter, then pulse until you have a coarse batter. Evenly divide batter into two bowls.

2. In the first bowl of batter, knead well until it forms a ball. Wrap in cling wrap, flatten a bit, and chill for an hour for easy handling. In the second bowl of batter, add sugar. In a pinching motion, pinch batter to form clusters of streusels. Set aside.

3. When ready to bake, warm oven to 375oF and lightly grease an 8x8-inch baking pan with cooking spray. Discard cling wrap and evenly press dough on the bottom of the pan, up to 1-inch up the pan's sides, making sure that everything is covered in dough.

4. Evenly spread raspberries. Top with streusel. Bake within 45 minutes. Remove from oven and cool within 20 minutes before slicing into 9 equal bars. Serve and enjoy or store in a lidded container for 10-days in the fridge.

**NUTRITIONS:** Calories: 235.7, Protein: 4.4g, Carbs: 29.1g, Fat: 11.3g, Sodium: 73mg

# 479. EASY STRAWBERRY SHEET CAKE

**COOKING: 60'**     **PREPARATION: 1H**     **SERVINGS: 16**

## INGREDIENTS

- » 9 tablespoons unsalted butter
- » 3/4 teaspoon salt
- » 1 1/2 cups granulated sugar, divided
- » 1 large egg
- » 1 large egg yolk
- » 1 1/2 teaspoons vanilla extract
- » 3/4 cup low-fat milk
- » 2 1/4 teaspoons baking powder
- » 2 1/4 cups whole wheat flour
- » 1 1/2 pounds fresh and a bit overripe strawberry, hulled and halved

## DIRECTIONS

1. Oiled a 9x13-inch baking pan with cooking spray and preheat oven to 350oF. Remove 3 tbsp of sugar and set aside. In a blender, blend well butter, salt, sugar, egg, egg yolk, vanilla extract, milk, and baking powder until smooth and creamy.

2. Add flour and blend until thoroughly incorporated. Scrape down sides of the blender and blend once more. Pour batter evenly into prepared pan. Evenly spread halved strawberries on top of batter. Sprinkle the set aside 3 tbsp sugar on top of strawberries.

3. Pop in the oven and bake within 45 minutes or until golden brown. Remove from oven and cool within 20 minutes before slicing into 16 equal pieces. Serve.

**NUTRITIONS:** Calories: 182.4, Protein: 5g, Carbs: 25.3g, Fat: 6.8g, Sodium: 163mg

# 480. EASY COCONUT-CARROT CAKE BALLS

**COOKING: 0'**     **PREPARATION: 10'**     **SERVINGS: 16**

## INGREDIENTS

- » 3/4 cup carrot, peeled and finely shredded
- » 1 cup packed Medjool date, pitted
- » 1 ¾ cups raw walnuts
- » 3/4 tsp ground cinnamon
- » 1/2 tsp ground ginger
- » 1 pinch ground nutmeg
- » 2 tsp vanilla extract
- » 5 tbsp almond flour
- » 1/4 cup raisins
- » ¼ cup desiccated coconut flakes

## DIRECTIONS

1. In a food processor, process dates until it clumps. Transfer to a bowl. In the same food processor, process walnuts, cinnamon, ginger, and nutmeg. Process until it resembles a fine meal.

2. Add the processed dates, extract, almond flour, and shredded carrots. Pulse until you form a loose dough but not mushy. Do not over-pulse. Transfer to a bowl.

3. Pulse desiccated coconut into tinier flakes and transfer to a small plate. Divide the carrot batter into 4 and then divide each part into 4 to make a total of 16 equal-sized balls. Roll it in the coconut flakes, place in a lidded container, and refrigerate for 2 hours before enjoying.

**NUTRITIONS:** Calories: 77.9, Protein: 1.5g, Carbs: 3.8g, Fat: 6.3g, Sodium: 8mg

# 481. BANANA DELIGHT

**COOKING: 12'**     **PREPARATION: 15'**     **SERVINGS: 4**

## INGREDIENTS

- » 1 tbsp sodium-free baking powder
- » 1 tbsp sugar
- » 1 cup flour
- » 1 tbsp oil
- » ¼ cup egg substitute
- » ½ tsp nutmeg
- » 1 cup banana (chopped)
- » 1 tbsp oil
- » ½ cup skim milk

## DIRECTIONS

1. In a bowl, mix and stir baking powder, sugar, and flour. Mix oil, egg, and milk, then add nutmeg and banana in a separate bowl. Add the mixture into the bowl of dry ingredients.

2. In a hot frying pan, drop just by tablespoonfuls and fry for about 2 to 3 minutes. Wait until it is golden brown, then drain and serve.

**NUTRITIONS:** Calories: 210.1, Protein: 5.7g, Carbs: 37.6g, Fat: 4.1g, Sodium: 141mg

# 482. HEALTHY BANANA-CHOCO ICE CREAM

**COOKING: 0'**          **PREPARATION: 10'**          **SERVINGS: 4**

## INGREDIENTS

- » 3 medium bananas, peeled and frozen
- » 3 tbsp Unsweetened Cocoa Powder
- » 1/2 tsp peppermint extract

## DIRECTIONS

1. Place all the fixing in a blender and puree until it resembles soft-serve ice cream. Evenly divide into 4 bowls. Serve and enjoy

**NUTRITIONS:** Calories: 88, Protein: 1.7g, Carbs: 22.6g, Fat: 0.8g, Sodium: 2.0 mg

# 483. HEALTHY CHOCOLATE MOUSSE

**COOKING: 0'**          **PREPARATION: 10'**          **SERVINGS: 4**

## INGREDIENTS

- » 1 large, ripe avocado
- » 1/4 cup sweetened almond milk
- » 1 tbsp coconut oil
- » 1/4 cup cocoa or cacao powder
- » 1 tsp vanilla extract

## DIRECTIONS

1. Process all the fixing using a food processor until smooth and creamy. Chill within 4 hours. Serve and enjoy.

**NUTRITIONS:** Calories: 125, Protein: 1.2g, Carbs: 6.9g, Fat: 11.0g, Sodium: 22.0 mg

# 484. ALMOND RICE PUDDING

**COOKING: 20'**     **PREPARATION: 25'**     **SERVINGS: 6**

## INGREDIENTS

- » 3 cups 1% milk
- » 1 cup white rice
- » 1/4 cup sugar
- » 1 teaspoon vanilla
- » 1/4 teaspoon almond extract
- » Cinnamon
- » 1/4 cup toasted almonds

## DIRECTIONS

1. Mix milk plus rice in a medium saucepan. Bring them to a boil. Reduce heat and simmer for 20 minutes with the lid on until the rice is soft.

2. Remove, then put the sugar, vanilla, almond extract, and cinnamon. Put toasted almonds on top, then serve warm.

**NUTRITIONS:** Calories 180, Fat 1.5 g, Carbohydrates 36 g, Protein 7 g, Fiber 1 g, Sodium 65 mg, Potassium 1 mg

# 485. APPLES AND CREAM SHAKE

**COOKING: 0'**     **PREPARATION: 10'**     **SERVINGS: 4**

## INGREDIENTS

- » 2 cups vanilla low-fat ice cream
- » 1 cup apple sauce
- » 1/4 teaspoon ground cinnamon
- » 1 cup fat-free skim milk

## DIRECTIONS

1. In a blender container, combine the low-fat ice cream, applesauce, and cinnamon. Cover and blend until smooth. Add fat-free skim milk. Cover and blend until mixed. Pour into glasses. Serve immediately.

**NUTRITIONS:** Calories 160, Fat 3 g, Carbohydrates 27 g, Protein 6 g, Fiber 1 g, Sodium 80 mg, Potassium 46 mg

# 486. BAKED STUFFED APPLES

**COOKING: 8'**　　　　　**PREPARATION: 10'**　　　　　**SERVINGS: 4**

## INGREDIENTS

- » 4 Jonagold apples
- » 1/4 cup flaked coconut
- » 1/4 cup chopped dried apricots
- » 2 teaspoons grated orange zest
- » 1/2 cup orange juice
- » 2 tablespoons brown sugar

## DIRECTIONS

1. Peel the apples 1/3, then hollow out the center with a knife. Arrange, peeled end up, in microwave-safe baking dish. Combine coconut, apricots, and orange zest. Divide to fill centers of apples evenly.

2. Mix orange juice plus brown sugar, then put over apples. Microwave on high within 8 minutes or until apples are tender. Cool before serving.

**NUTRITIONS:** Calories 192, Fat 2 g, Carbohydrates 46 g, Protein 1 g, Fiber 6 g, Sodium 19 mg

# 487. CARROT-CAKE SMOOTHIE

**COOKING: 0'**　　　　　**PREPARATION: 5'**　　　　　**SERVINGS: 2**

## INGREDIENTS

- » 1 frozen banana, peeled and diced
- » 1 cup carrots, diced (peeled if preferred)
- » 1 cup nonfat or low-fat milk
- » ½ cup ice
- » ¼ cup diced pineapple, frozen
- » ½ teaspoon ground cinnamon
- » Pinch nutmeg
- » ½ cup nonfat or low-fat vanilla Greek yogurt
- » Optional toppings: chopped walnuts, grated carrots

## DIRECTIONS

1. Add all of the fixing listed to a blender and process until smooth and creamy. Serve immediately with optional toppings as desired.

**NUTRITIONS:** Calories: 180, Fat: 1 g, Cholesterol: 5 mg, Sodium: 114 mg, Carbs: 36 g, Fiber: 4 g, Sugar: 25 g, Protein: 10 g

# 488. EASY CINNAMON BAKED APPLES

**COOKING: 45'**　　　**PREPARATION: 5'**　　　**SERVINGS: 4**

## INGREDIENTS

» 4 apples, cored, peeled, and sliced thin
» ½ tablespoon ground cinnamon
» ¼ cup brown sugar
» ¼ teaspoon ground nutmeg
» Optional: 2 teaspoons freshly squeezed lemon juice

## DIRECTIONS

1. Preheat the oven to 375°F. Place apples in a mixing bowl and gently mix all the other ingredients. Put apples in a nonstick pan.

2. Bake within 45 minutes, stirring at least once every 15 minutes. Once they are soft, cook for another few minutes to thicken the cinnamon sauce. Serve.

**NUTRITIONS:** Calories: 117, Fat: 1 g, Sodium: 4 mg, Carbs: 34 g, Fiber: 5 g, Sugar: 28 g, Protein: 0 g

# 489. CHOCOLATE CAKE IN A MUG

**COOKING: 1'**　　　**PREPARATION: 5'**　　　**SERVINGS: 1**

## INGREDIENTS

» 3 tablespoons white whole-wheat flour
» 2 tablespoons unsweetened cocoa powder
» 2 teaspoons sugar
» 1/8 teaspoon baking powder
» 1 egg white
» ½ teaspoon olive oil
» 3 tablespoons nonfat or low-fat milk
» ½ teaspoon vanilla extract
» Cooking spray

## DIRECTIONS

1. Place the flour, cocoa, sugar, and baking powder in a small bowl and whisk until combined. Then add in the egg white, olive oil, milk, and vanilla extract, and mix to combine.

2. Oiled a mug with cooking spray and pour batter into mug. Microwave on high for 60 seconds or until set. Serve.

**NUTRITIONS:** Calories: 217, Fat: 4 g, Cholesterol: 1 mg, Sodium: 139 mg, Carbs: 35 g, Fiber: 7 g, Sugar: 12 g, Protein: 11 g

# 490. PEANUT BUTTER BANANA "ICE CREAM"

**COOKING: 0'**     **PREPARATION: 10'**     **SERVINGS: 4**

## INGREDIENTS

» 2 tablespoons peanut butter
» 4 bananas, very ripe, peeled and sliced into ½-inch rings

## DIRECTIONS

1. On a large baking sheet or plate, spread the banana slices in an even layer. Freeze for 1 to 2 hours. Puree the frozen banana until it forms a smooth and creamy mixture in a food processor or blender, scraping down the bowl as needed.

2. Add the peanut butter, pureeing until just combined. For a soft-serve ice cream consistency, serve immediately. For a harder consistency, place the ice cream in the freezer for a few hours before serving.

**NUTRITIONS:** Calories: 153, Fat: 4 g, Sodium: 4 mg, Carbs: 29 g, Fiber: 4 g, Sugar: 15 g, Protein: 3 g

# 491. BANANA-CASHEW CREAM MOUSSE

**COOKING: 0'**     **PREPARATION: 55'**     **SERVINGS: 2**

## INGREDIENTS

» ½ cup cashews, presoaked
» 1 tablespoon honey
» 1 teaspoon vanilla extract
» 1 cup plain nonfat Greek yogurt
» 1 large banana, sliced (reserve 4 slices for garnish)

## DIRECTIONS

1. Put the cashews in your small bowl, then cover with 1 cup of water. Dip at room temperature within 2 to 3 hours. Drain, rinse and set aside. Place honey, vanilla extract, cashews, and bananas in a blender or food processor.

2. Blend until smooth. Place mixture in a medium bowl. Fold in yogurt, mix well. Cover, then chill within 45 minutes. Portion mousse into 2 serving bowls. Garnish each with 2 banana slices.

**NUTRITIONS:** Calories: 329, Fat: 14 g, Sodium: 64 mg, Carbs: 37 g, Fiber: 3 g, Sugar: 24 g, Protein: 17 g

# 492. GRILLED PLUMS WITH VANILLA BEAN FROZEN YOGURT

**COOKING: 15'**　　　**PREPARATION: 10'**　　　**SERVINGS: 4**

## INGREDIENTS

- » 4 large plums, sliced in half and pitted
- » 1 tablespoon olive oil
- » 1 tablespoon honey
- » 1 teaspoon ground cinnamon
- » 2 cups vanilla bean frozen yogurt

## DIRECTIONS

1. Preheat the grill to medium heat. Brush the plum halves with olive oil. Grill, flesh-side down, for 4 to 5 minutes, then flip and cook for another 4 to 5 minutes, until just tender.

2. Mix the honey plus cinnamon in a small bowl. Scoop the frozen yogurt into 4 bowls. Place 2 plum halves in each bowl and drizzle each with the cinnamon-honey mixture.

**NUTRITIONS:** Calories: 192, Fat: 8 g, Sodium: 63 mg, Carbs: 30 g, Fiber: 1 g, Sugar: 28 g, Protein: 3 g

# 493. KEY LIME CHERRY "NICE" CREAM

**COOKING: 15'**　　　**PREPARATION: 10'**　　　**SERVINGS: 4**

## INGREDIENTS

- » 4 frozen bananas, peeled
- » 1 cup frozen dark sweet cherries
- » Zest and juice of 1 lime, divided
- » ½ teaspoon vanilla extract
- » ¼ teaspoon kosher or sea salt

## DIRECTIONS

1. Blend the fixing in a food processor and enjoy a frozen treat. Place the bananas, cherries, lime juice, vanilla extract, and salt in a food processor and purée until smooth, scraping the sides as needed.

2. Transfer the "nice" cream to bowls and top with the lime zest. For leftovers, place the "nice" cream in airtight containers and store them in the freezer for up to 1 month. Let thaw for 30 minutes, until it reaches a soft-serve ice cream texture.

**NUTRITIONS:** Calories: 150, Fat: 0 g, Sodium: 147 mg, Carbs: 37 g, Fiber: 4 g, Sugar: 21 g, Protein: 2 g

# 494. OATMEAL DARK CHOCOLATE CHIP PEANUT BUTTER COOKIES

**COOKING: 10'**     **PREPARATION: 15'**     **SERVINGS: 4**

## INGREDIENTS

- » 1½ cups natural creamy peanut butter
- » ½ cup dark brown sugar
- » 2 large eggs
- » 1 cup old-fashioned rolled oats
- » 1 teaspoon baking soda
- » ½ teaspoon kosher or sea salt
- » ½ cup dark chocolate chips

## DIRECTIONS

1. Preheat the oven to 350°F. Line a baking sheet with parchment paper. Whip the peanut butter in the bowl of a stand mixer until very smooth. Continue beating and add the brown sugar, then one egg at a time, until fluffy.

2. Beat in the oats, baking soda, and salt until combined. Fold in the dark chocolate chips. Put the cookie dough on the baking sheet, about 2 inches apart. Bake within 8 to 10 minutes, depending on your preferred level of doneness.

**NUTRITIONS:** Calories: 152, Fat: 10 g, Sodium: 131 mg, Carbs: 12 g, Fiber: 2 g, Sugar: 8 g, Protein: 4 g

# 495. PEACH CRUMBLE MUFFINS

**COOKING: 25'**     **PREPARATION: 25'**     **SERVINGS: 15**

## INGREDIENTS

**For the crumble:**
- » 2 tablespoons dark brown sugar
- » 1 tablespoon honey
- » 1 teaspoon ground cinnamon
- » 2 tablespoons canola oil
- » ½ cup old-fashioned rolled oats

**For the peach muffins:**
- » 1 teaspoon baking powder
- » 1 teaspoon baking soda
- » 1 teaspoon ground cinnamon
- » ½ teaspoon ground ginger
- » ½ teaspoon kosher or sea salt
- » ¼ cup canola oil
- » ¼ cup dark brown sugar
- » 2 large eggs
- » 1½ teaspoons vanilla extract
- » ¼ cup plain nonfat Greek yogurt
- » 3 peaches, diced (about 1½ cups)
- » 1¾ cups whole-wheat flour or whole-wheat pastry flour

## DIRECTIONS

1. In a small bowl, mix the brown sugar, honey, cinnamon, canola oil, and oats until combined for the crumble. For your muffins, mix the flour, baking powder, baking soda, cinnamon, ginger, and salt in a large bowl.

2. Beat the canola oil, brown sugar, and one egg at a time in a separate bowl, using a hand mixer until fluffy. Beat in the vanilla extract and yogurt. Put the flour mixture in the bowl and whisk until the ingredients are just combined.

3. Fold in the diced peaches with a spatula. Preheat the oven to 425°F. Oiled a 12-cup muffin tin with muffin liners. Fill each muffin well with batter about three-quarters of the way full. Scoop the crumble batter on top of each.

4. Bake for 5 to 6 minutes, then reduce the oven temperature to 350°F and bake for 15 to 18 additional minutes. Cool before removing from the muffin tin. Once completely cooled, serve.

**NUTRITIONS:** Calories: 187, Fat: 8 g, Sodium: 216 mg, Carbs: 26 g, Fiber: 3 g, Sugar: 10 g, Protein: 4 g

# 496. PEANUT BUTTER BANANA BREAD BITES

**COOKING: 20'**  **PREPARATION: 10'**  **SERVINGS: 4**

## INGREDIENTS

- » 1½ cups whole-wheat pastry flour
- » 2 tablespoons ground flaxseed
- » 1 teaspoon baking powder
- » ½ teaspoon kosher or sea salt
- » ½ teaspoon ground cinnamon
- » 3 ripe bananas, peeled
- » 2 large eggs
- » 2 tablespoons canola oil
- » ½ cup dark brown sugar
- » 2 tablespoons honey
- » ½ cup natural creamy peanut butter
- » ¼ cup nonfat Greek yogurt
- » 1 teaspoon vanilla extract
- » ¼ cup unsalted roasted peanuts, crushed

## DIRECTIONS

1. Preheat the oven to 350°F. Oiled a 24-cup mini muffin tin with cooking spray. In a bowl, whisk the flour, flaxseed, baking powder, salt, and cinnamon. Beat the bananas in a separate bowl with a hand mixer set on low.

2. Add the eggs, one at a time, then add the canola oil, brown sugar, and honey. Adjust the speed to medium and beat until fluffy. Add the peanut butter, Greek yogurt, and vanilla extract and mix until combined. Lower the speed to low, then beat in the dry ingredient mixture until just combined.

3. Put the mixture into each of the muffin wells about three-quarters of the way full. Tap it on the counter until the batter is evenly spread out.

4. Top with the crushed peanuts. Bake within 20 minutes, until a toothpick inserted into the center of a bite, comes out clean. Let rest on the counter until cooled. Remove the bites from the muffin tin. Serve.

**NUTRITIONS:** Calories: 123, Fat: 5 g, Sodium: 81 mg, Carbs: 17 g, Fiber: 2 g, Sugar: 8 g, Protein: 3 g

# 497. TOASTED ALMOND AMBROSIA

**COOKING: 20'**  **PREPARATION: 10'**  **SERVINGS: 2**

## INGREDIENTS

- » ½ Cup Almonds, Slivered
- » ½ Cup Coconut, Shredded & Unsweetened
- » 3 Cups Pineapple, Cubed
- » 5 Oranges, Segment
- » 2 Red Apples, Cored & Diced
- » 2 Tablespoons Cream Sherry
- » Mint Leaves, Fresh to Garnish
- » 1 Banana, Halved Lengthwise, Peeled & Sliced

## DIRECTIONS

1. Start by heating your oven to 325, and then get out a baking sheet. Roast your almonds for ten minutes, making sure they're spread out evenly. Transfer them to a plate and then toast your coconut on the same baking sheet.

2. Toast for ten minutes. Mix your banana, sherry, oranges, apples, and pineapple in a bowl. Divide the mixture, not serving bowls and top with coconut and almonds. Garnish with mint before serving.

**NUTRITIONS:** Calories: 177, Fat: 4.9 g, Sodium: 13 mg, Carbs: 36 g, Fiber: 0 g, Sugar: 0 g, Protein: 3.4 g

# 498. APRICOT BISCOTTI

**COOKING: 50'**  **PREPARATION: 10'**  **SERVINGS: 4**

## INGREDIENTS

- » 2 Tablespoons Honey, Dark
- » 2 Tablespoons Olive Oil
- » ½ Teaspoon Almond Extract
- » ¼ Cup Almonds, Chopped Roughly
- » 2/3 Cup Apricots, Dried
- » 2 Tablespoons Milk, 1% & Low Fat
- » 2 Eggs, Beaten Lightly
- » ¾ Cup Whole Wheat Flour
- » ¾ Cup All-Purpose Flour
- » ¼ Cup Brown Sugar, Packed Firm
- » 1 Teaspoon Baking Powder

## DIRECTIONS

1. Start by heating the oven to 350, then mix your baking powder, brown sugar, and flours in a bowl. Whisk your canola oil, eggs, almond extract, honey, and milk. Mix until it forms a smooth dough. Fold in the apricots and almonds.

2. Put your dough on plastic wrap, and then roll it out to a twelve-inch-long and three-inch wide rectangle. Place this dough on a baking sheet, and bake for twenty-five minutes. It should turn golden brown. Allow it to cool, slice it into ½ inch thick slices, and then bake for another fifteen minutes. It should be crispy.

**NUTRITIONS:** Calories: 291, Fat: 2 g, Sodium: 123 mg, Carbs: 12 g, Fiber: 0 g, Sugar: 0 g, Protein: 2 g

# 499. APPLE & BERRY COBBLER

**COOKING: 40'**  **PREPARATION: 10'**  **SERVINGS: 4**

## INGREDIENTS

- » Filling:
- » 1 Cup Blueberries, Fresh
- » 2 Cups Apples, Chopped
- » 1 Cup Raspberries, Fresh
- » 2 Tablespoons Brown Sugar
- » 1 Teaspoon Lemon Zest
- » 2 Teaspoon Lemon Juice, Fresh
- » ½ Teaspoon Ground Cinnamon
- » 1 ½ Tablespoons Corn Starch
- » Topping:
- » ¾ Cup Whole Wheat Pastry Flour
- » 1 ½ Tablespoon Brown Sugar
- » ½ Teaspoon Vanilla Extract, Pure
- » ¼ Cup Soy Milk
- » ¼ Teaspoon Sea Salt, Fine
- » 1 Egg White

## DIRECTIONS

1. Turn your oven to 350, and get out six small ramekins. Grease them with cooking spray. Mix your lemon juice, lemon zest, blueberries, sugar, cinnamon, raspberries, and apples in a bowl. Stir in your cornstarch, mixing until it dissolves.

2. Beat your egg white in a different bowl, whisking it with sugar, vanilla, soy milk, and pastry flour. Divide your berry mixture between the ramekins and top with the vanilla topping. Put your ramekins on a baking sheet, baking for thirty minutes. The top should be golden brown before serving.

**NUTRITIONS:** Calories: 131, Fat: 0 g, Sodium: 14 mg, Carbs: 13.8 g, Fiber: 0 g, Sugar: 0 g, Protein: 7.2 g

# 500. MIXED FRUIT COMPOTE CUPS

**COOKING: 15'**       **PREPARATION: 5'**       **SERVINGS: 2**

## INGREDIENTS

- » 1 ¼ Cup Water
- » ½ Cup Orange juice
- » 12 Ounces Mixed Dried Fruit
- » 1 Teaspoon Ground Cinnamon
- » ¼ Teaspoon Ground Ginger
- » ¼ Teaspoon Ground Nutmeg
- » 4 Cups Vanilla Frozen Yogurt, Fat-Free

## DIRECTIONS

1. Mix your dried fruit, nutmeg, cinnamon, water, orange juice, and ginger in a saucepan. Cover, and allow it to cook over medium heat for ten minutes. Remove the cover and then cook for another ten minutes. Add your frozen yogurt to serving cups, and top with the fruit mixture.

**NUTRITIONS:** Calories: 228, Fat: 5.7 g, Cholesterol: 15 mg, Sodium: 114 mg, Carbs: 12.4 g, Fiber: 0 g, Sugar: 0 g, Protein: 9.1 g

# 7-DAY MEAL PLAN

| Day | Breakfast | Lunch | Snack | Dinner | Dessert |
|-----|-----------|-------|-------|--------|---------|
| 1 | Blueberry Waffles | Creamy Chicken Breast | Garlic Cottage Cheese Crispy | Shrimp Cocktail | Beetroot and Berry Smoothie |
| 2 | Apple Pancakes | Indian Chicken Stew | Lemon Fat Bombs | Quinoa and Scallops Salad | Berry Blast |
| 3 | Super-Simple Granola | Chicken, Bamboo and Chestnuts Mix | Avocado Tuna Bites | Squid and Shrimp Salad | Oats and Fruit Bar Cracker |
| 4 | Savory Yogurt Bowls | Tomato Soup | Faux Mac and Cheese | Parsley Seafood Cocktail | Colorful Pops |
| 5 | Energy Sunrise Muffins | Cod Soup | Mediterranean Pop Corn Bites | Fruit Shrimp Soup | Pumpkin Pie Recipe |
| 6 | Spinach, Egg, and Cheese Breakfast Quesadillas | Easy Lunch Salmon Steak | Almond and Tomato Balls | Fish Stew | Apple Dumplings |
| 7 | Simple Cheese and Broccoli Omelets | Light Balsamic Salad | Hearty Buttery Walnuts | Parsley Cod Mix | Lemon Pudding Cake |

# CONCLUSION

Congrats! Making this far on your DASH-journey and embracing the Dash diet as its best! Dash Diet has gained popularity in the past few years as it is beneficial in strengthening metabolism and controlling hypertension. Contrary to the popular belief that while following the dash diet, one gets to eat vegetarian foods while getting a balanced diet that includes fresh fruits, vegetables, nuts, low-fat dairy products, and whole grains. You do not have to cut down on meat; instead, you have to reduce sodium and fat content from your everyday diet.

The diet also has many health benefits as it helps reduce hypertension and obesity, lower osteoporosis, and prevent cancer. This well-balanced diet strengthens metabolism, which further helps in decomposing the fat deposits stored in the body. As a result, it improves and enhance the overall health of a person.

This cookbook has provided you different Dash meals from breakfast, lunch, dinner, mains, side dishes, fish and seafood, poultry, vegetables, soups, salads, snacks, and desserts. However, you can consult experts if you suffer from current health conditions or follow certain exercise routines, as this will help you customize the diet as per your requirement.

This diet is easy to follow as you get to everything but in a healthier fashion and limited quantity. Talking about the DASH diet outside the theory and more in practice reveals its efficiency as a diet. Besides excess research and experiments, the real reasons for people looking into this diet are its specific features. It gives the feeling of ease and convenience, making the users more comfortable with its rules and regulations.

Here are the following reasons why the DASH Diet works

amazingly:

Easy to Adopt: The broad range of options available under the DASH diet label makes it more flexible for all. It is the reason that people find it easier to switch to and harness its real health benefits. It makes adaptability easier for its users.

Promotes Exercise: It is most effective than all the other factors because not only does it focus on the food and its intake, but it also duly stresses daily exercises and routine physical activities. It is the reason that it produces quick, visible results.

All-Inclusive: With a few limitations, this diet has taken every food item into its fold with certain modifications. It rightly guides about the Dos and Don'ts of all the ingredients and prevents us from consuming those harmful to the body and its health.

A Well-Balanced Approach: One of its most significant advantages is that it maintains balance in our diet, in our routine, our caloric intake, and our nutrition.

Satisfactory Caloric Check: Every meal we plan on the DASH diet is pre-calculated in terms of calories. We can easily keep track of the daily caloric intake and consequently restrict them easily by cutting off certain food items.

Prohibits Bad Food: The DASH diet suggests using more organic and fresh food and discourages the use of processed food and junk items available in stores. So, it creates better eating habits in the users.

Focused on Prevention: Though it is proven to be a cure for many diseases, it is described as more of a preventive strategy.

Slow Yet Progressive Changes: The diet is not highly restrictive and accommodates gradual changes towards achieving the ultimate health goal. You can set up your daily, weekly, or even monthly targets at your convenience.

Long Term Effects: The DASH diet results are not just incredible, but they are also long-lasting. It is considered slow in progress, but the effects last longer.

Accelerates Metabolism: With its healthy approach to life, the DASH diet can activate our metabolism and boost it for better functioning of the body.

Does this all flatter your hearts out? Of course, it does! So, start cooking now, and let us all be healthier and happier.

CPSIA information can be obtained
at www.ICGtesting.com
Printed in the USA
LVHW061400040621
689379LV00013B/721